Glaucoma Imaging

Antonio Ferreras
Editor

Glaucoma Imaging

Springer

Editor
Antonio Ferreras
Ophthalmology
Miguel Servet University Hospital
Zaragona
Spain

ISBN 978-3-319-18958-1 ISBN 978-3-319-18959-8 (eBook)
DOI 10.1007/978-3-319-18959-8

Library of Congress Control Number: 2015950942

Springer Cham Heidelberg New York Dordrecht London

Printed on acid-free paper

Springer International Publishing AG Switzerland is part of Springer Science+Business Media (www.springer.com)

Contents

Chapter 1
Standard Automated Perimetry

Francisco Javier Goñi and Krapez Maja

1.1 Introduction

Human beings interact with their environment through mechanisms designed to *perceive* or in other words to detect, process, and interpret some of its physical characteristics. Among them, we have evolved to detect a specific range of the electromagnetic wave spectrum that the earth's atmosphere freely permits to pass through: the light [1].

The human eye is able to discriminate some light properties including luminosity, contrast, and color perception, as well as dynamic characteristics like spatial and temporal changes. Thus, the human visual system has been arranged anatomically to accomplish different visual functions working together to provide vision.

The visual system detects a wide extension of our environment at the same time, the so-called visual field (VF). Within the VF, the central area gathers most of the neuronal resources to perceive contrast and color, while the peripheral area is more sensitive to movement. The posterior pole – the retinal area within temporal vascular arcades – covers approximately the 15 central degrees of the VF (Fig. 1.1).

F.J. Goñi
Centro de Tratamiento Integral del Glaucoma (CTIG), Hospital Quiron Teknon, Barcelona, Spain
e-mail: francisgoni@yahoo.com

K. Maja
Zdravstveni dom, Department of Ophthalmology, Nova Gorica, Slovenia
e-mail: mkrapez@yahoo.com

A. Ferreras (ed.), *Glaucoma Imaging*, DOI 10.1007/978-3-319-18959-8_1

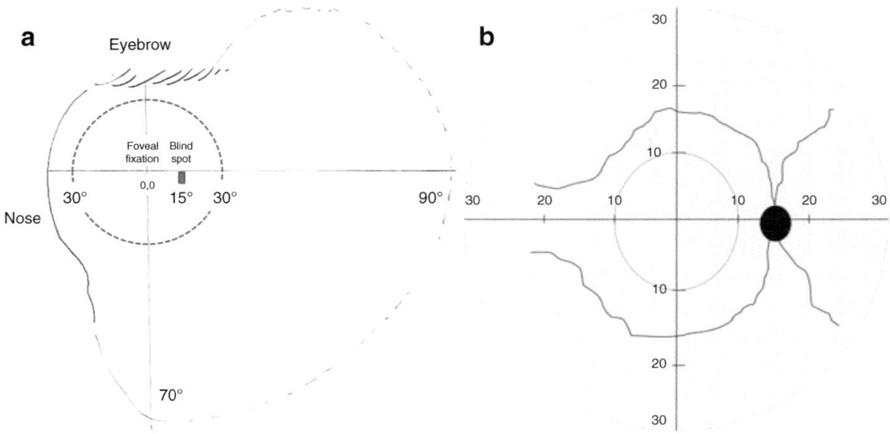

Fig. 1.1 (*Left*) Visual field representation of a right eye. The horizontal and vertical meridians separate superior and inferior, and nasal and temporal hemifields, respectively. The fovea represents the fixation (coordinates 0,0) and the blind spot is located 15° temporally and 1° inferiorly (15,-1). The visual field extension examined in glaucoma disease is usually restricted to the central 30° (blue dotted circumference). (*Right*) The limits of the retinal posterior pole of a right eye, superimposed on a 30° central visual field (inverted image has been turned for better understanding)

1.2 How Can the Visual Field Be Measured and Displayed?

The VF can be examined using several methods to test the different visual functions. The most widely and accepted technique is Standard Automated Perimetry (SAP). SAP measures both achromatic light and contrast perception and is used in clinical practice to diagnose and monitor visual diseases more characteristically affecting the visual field, like glaucoma. Among the different strategies to examine the VF with SAP, standard conditions (size III Goldmann stimulus) within the 30° central VF are most frequently used.

VF results can be displayed by several formats[1]. The single field printout is generally represented as a seven-in-one format (Fig. 1.2). The source of true, observed data is shown at the thresholds map. Every location shows a number representing the patient's differential light sensitivity threshold, expressed in decibels (dB). The other maps are obtained from statistical corrections according to age (from a database of normality), sensitivity cutoff at percentile 85 (to remove diffuse sensitivity loss), and corresponding, interpolated gray or color scale representations.

VF data are summarized in global summary indices [2, 3]. Mean Defect (MD) expresses the difference between observed and expected mean sensitivity. Pattern Standard Deviation (PSD) represents the standard deviation of thresholds' distribution. Visual Field Index (VFI) reflects the amount of VF capacity, in terms of percentage, ascribing a stronger weight to the macular area than periphery [4]. A normal subject will show MD, PSD, and VFI values around cero. When a cataract is present, only MD is generally affected. In the case of any pathology eliciting the appearance of a scotoma, as seen in glaucoma, the three indices will likely be altered.

Glaucoma is a progressive condition, and VF deterioration continues over the course of the disease. VF series must be obtained over time to detect and measure progression. They can also be displayed by different formats. Guided Progression Analysis (GPA, HFA) software yields the GPA summary report, a single page, user-friendly printout showing the most relevant results of a VF series, including the first two reliable VF (baseline), the last VF and a graph displaying VFI evolution over time against the patient's age. MD and PSD values are also displayed for baseline and last fields. A regression analysis helps to interpret the statistical significance of VFI trends (Fig. 1.3) [5].

It is important to note that the relation between MD and PSD is not linear across the entire SAP dynamic range. Glaucoma progression manifests as a linear-like, parallel change of both MD and PSD till approximately half of the VF capacity is damaged. From this point, VF deterioration will continue increasing MD[2] but decreasing PSD (Fig. 1.4).

[1] In this chapter, all the examples of VF printouts come from Carl Zeiss-Meditec Humprey Field Analyzer (HFA) system.

[2] In the HFA system, MD values are represented as negative values, but terms like "increased" or "elevated" are frequently used in clinical practice, as MD is intuitively considered an absolute number. In the written text, we will preserve the negative sign for MD and VFI, and "increased" or "elevated" will actually refer to more negative values.

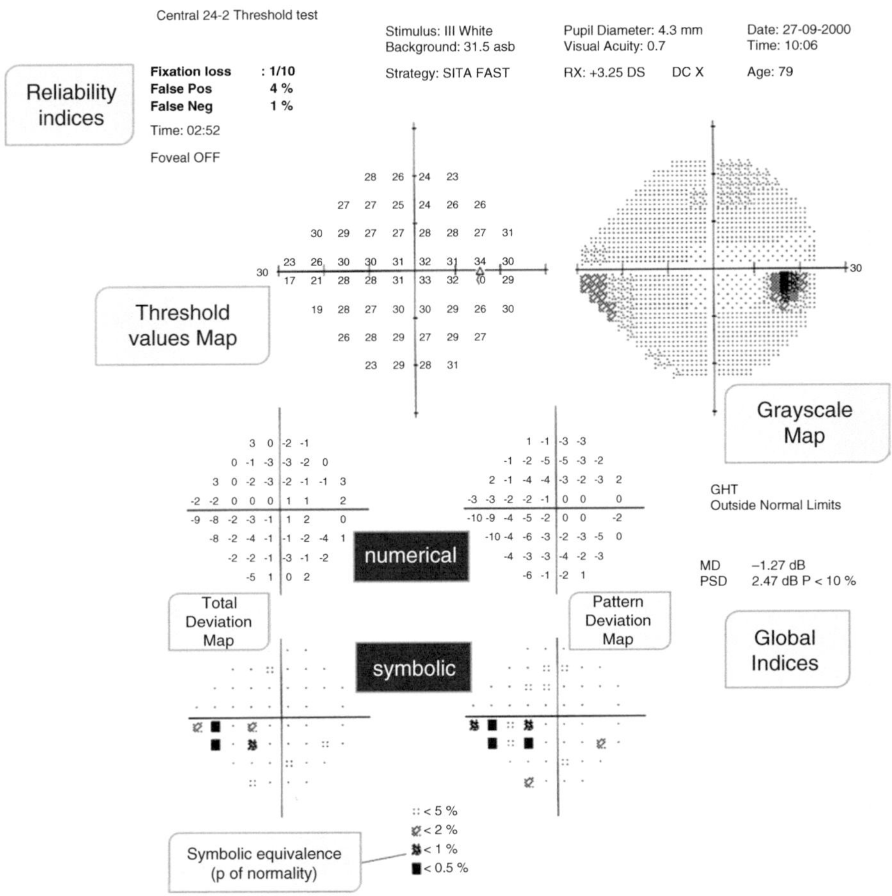

Fig. 1.2 Single visual field printout, central visual field of a right eye. First, reliability indices must be checked to evaluate the quality of results. At the threshold values map, the number displayed at each location of the grid represents the individual light sensitivity. Note that at the level of the blind spot, sensitivity is <0 dB, meaning no response after projecting the strongest, totally unfiltered light stimulus. Total and pattern maps identify significant deviations from age and highest sensitivity of data distribution, respectively. Deviations are highlighted as dots or boxes on the map of symbols. The lower the probability of normality, the darker the box. Both maps show a clustering of dots and boxes at the nasal inferior aspect of the field, also depicted at the gray-scale map, a typical appearance of early glaucoma focal damage

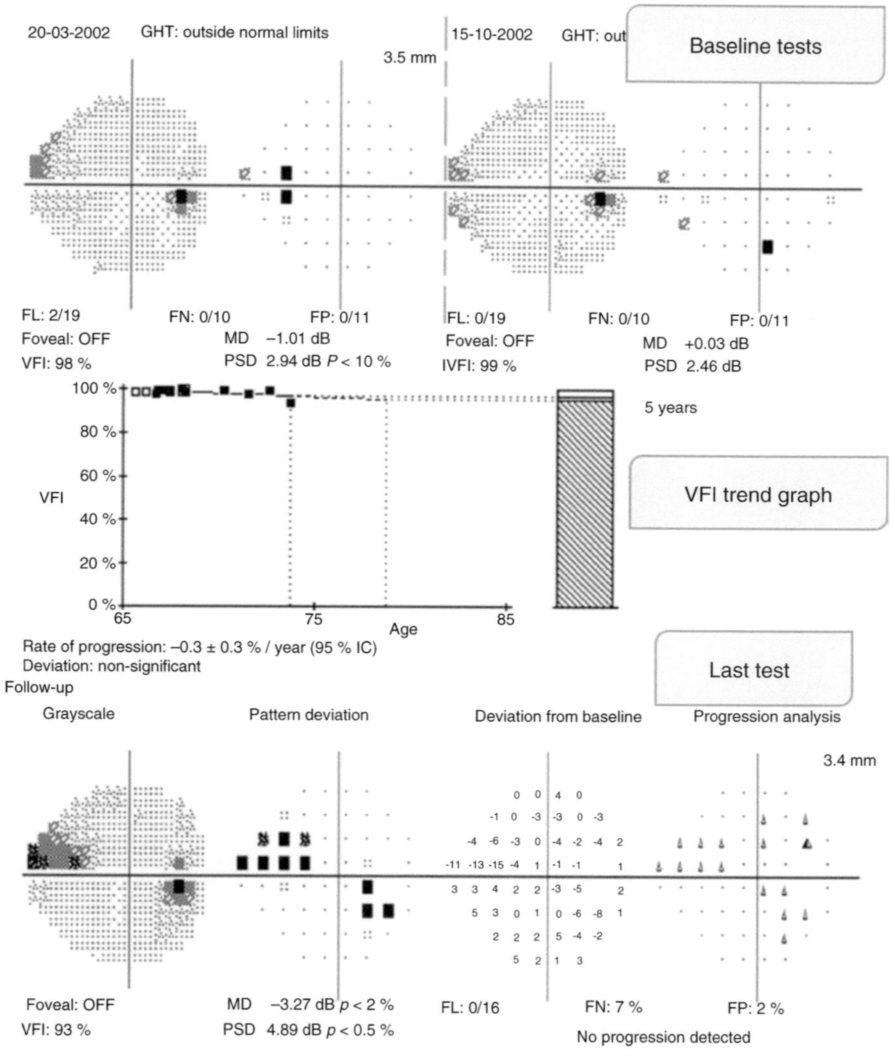

Fig. 1.3 Guided Progression Analysis (GPA) printout, central visual field series of a right eye. Baseline tests (*top*) must be reliable and similar. Last test (*bottom*) shows the last available visual field of the series. Events' Progression Analysis (*bottom, right*) depicts change from baseline mainly as open triangles, and no progression is detected yet. The VFI trend graph (*middle*) displays VFI evolution over time against the patient's age. After 8 years follow-up, VFI regression analysis has classified the trend as nonsignificant. Although some indicators suggest progression (global indices have increased absolute numbers and the nasal superior aspect of the field apparently shows a deepening of the scotoma), confirmation is required according to the statistical analysis approach

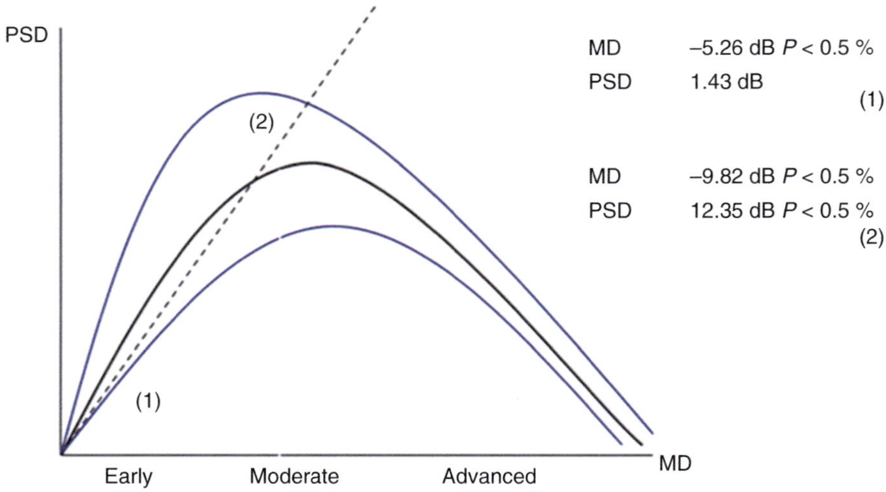

Fig. 1.4 Schematic representation of the nonlinear relationship between PSD and MD in glaucoma. The black and blue lines represent the central tendency and 95 % interval of confidence, respectively. Note that at the ascendant part of the curve the relationship between PSD and MD is linear-like, as represented by the dotted line. Case (*1*) shows a typical situation of VF loss due to cataract. MD is significantly affected (p of normality <0.5 %), but PSD remains within the normal limits. Case (*2*) shows an example of moderate glaucoma, where both PSD and MD will usually show abnormal values. When an early/moderate glaucoma progresses, both indices generally increase at the same time. From the top of the curve to the right, any worsening of MD due to glaucoma progression will be associated by a PSD decrease. Differently than MD or VFI, PSD is not useful to follow glaucoma across the entire dynamic range of SAP.

1.3 Quality of Results

SAP results must have sufficient quality to provide useful information in clinical practice. There are two different aspects of VF examination that can be considered separately when evaluating quality: (i) the single test and (ii) a series of tests.

1.3.1 Single Field Examination

When judging a single field examination, it must be both reliable and consistent with the clinical picture. Reliability is estimated using catch trials to calculate the so-called reliability indices (Fig. 1.2). Most frequently, the original manufacturer's standard for a reliable field using HFA (false positive [FP] and false negative [FN] responses less than 33 % and less than 20 % for fixation losses [FL]) had been used. For the *Swedish Interactive Thresholding Algorithm* (SITA), the limits of the FP response rate have been reduced to 15 %. SITA examinations showing higher FP rates are considered unreliable and excluded for analysis within a VF series. SITA has been reported to underestimate the rate of FP, in comparison to classic catch trials used in full threshold algorithms [6, 7] and quality control during VF testing by the technician has also been stressed [8]. Low-quality results may influence the ability of SAP to correctly diagnose glaucoma [9] but frequencies of unreliable examinations appear to be low in clinical trials. The *Ocular Hypertension Treatment Study* (OHTS) reported a rate of 2.4 % unreliable VF results [10]. The first SAP examination has a limited specificity, depending on the different criteria used to classify the VF. This is related to both the algorithm selected and subject inexperience. Next examination usually reduces the number of false positives and improves overall test performance, the so-called *learning effect*. Even this phenomenon is mainly seen between the first and second examination [11]. It may continue after several examinations [12]. In fact, a study has reported frequencies of prolonged learning effect in 31 % of glaucoma patients [13]. Thus a learning effect must be considered when selecting baseline examinations and evaluating a VF series. Baseline is composed of two fields which must be reliable, similar and consistent with the clinical picture. In general it can be recommended to exclude only clearly unreliable tests, in order to preserve as much information as possible.

A single field examination must be consistent with the clinical picture. The presence of a visual field defect should correlate with clinical findings. *Artifacts* are frequently seen in perimetry, including those produced by physical barriers (nose, superior lid, eyebrow, trial frames), blur (media opacity, uncorrected refractive errors) and poor collaboration or malingering (Fig. 1.5). In other cases, VF defects are due to anatomical or pathological reasons occurring at the retina. Here, an evaluation of spatial correlations between retinal and functional changes will help to identify causality (Fig. 1.1). Optic nerve diseases must also be considered, as they can mimic glaucomatous VF loss. Chiasmal and retrochiasmal diseases may elicit specific visual field defects that require careful evaluation and comparison of both right and left VF at the same time.

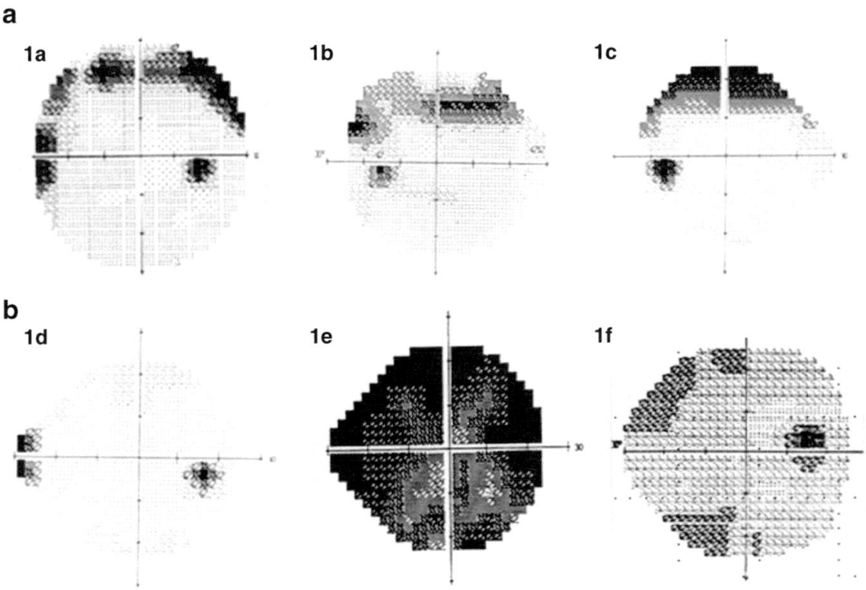

Fig. 1.5 Examples of typical perimetric artifacts. 1a and 1b Trial (a) and glasses frame (b). 1c Ptosis. 1d Nose interference. 1e Fatigue, cloverleaf pattern (only for HFA). 1f diffuse loss, first exam in naïve subject

1.3.2 Visual Field Series

A VF series including a sufficient group of examinations to generate a regression analysis, will depict a trend over time. The main factor influencing the quality of a trend is *variability*. When a test is repeated over time, results are not exactly reproduced. This is more evident for subjective exams like perimetry, where cognitive mechanisms are involved. Variability is related to intrinsic and extrinsic reasons. Intrinsic reasons are due to physiological characteristics of human perception. For example, response variability increases with decreasing sensitivity, in perimetry [14] and Visual Acuity measurement [15]. VF testing at the macular area of a normal subject will provide a better performance and lower variability than testing at the periphery. In case of disease, functional damage will increase intra-test [16] and inter-test [17] intrinsic variability. Extrinsic reasons are related to external factors, including methodology, instrumentation, and subject's collaboration.

A trend must have a sufficient number of tests, *goodness of fit*, and elapsed time. Goodness of fit relates to both intrinsic and extrinsic variability, and helps to predict a functional outcome with enough confidence (Fig. 1.6).

The variability of any VF series can be estimated evaluating the amount of dispersion associated to the trend. This is shown as the 95 % Interval of Confidence (95 % IC) of the values distribution of VFI at GPA of the HFA instrument (Fig. 1.3). When the 95 % IC is ≥5, no outcome can be predicted with sufficient power (Fig. 1.7).

A follow-up time of at least 5 years will increase the ratio between global change and variability, thus improving trend robustness [18]. The longer the elapsed time, the higher will be the confidence to predict an outcome, beyond variability and/or number of examinations. In the very long term, trend estimations can be in fact replaced by the measurement of true, total amount of change (Fig. 1.8).

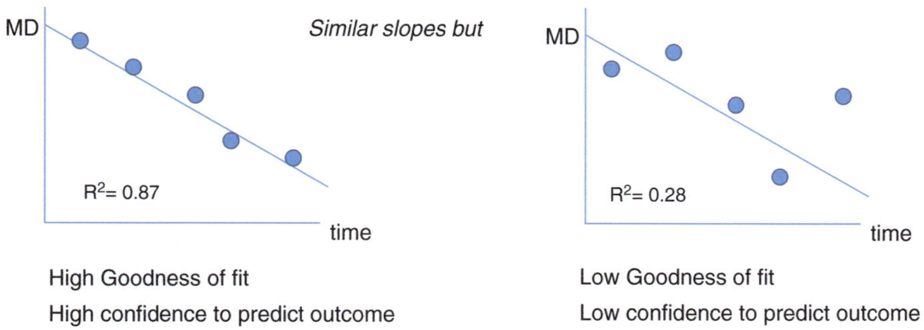

Fig. 1.6 Example of a VF series where the global index MD represents each examination, plotted against time. (*Left*) The distribution of MD values around the regression line shows a high goodness of fit, due to low inter-test variability. The confidence to predict an outcome, according to the measured change is high. (*Right*) MD dispersion is wide and goodness of fit is low, due to high inter-test variability. The low quality of the regression analysis does not allow the outcome to be predicted with confidence. Note that both trends show similar slopes but this information can be misleading if variability is not considered

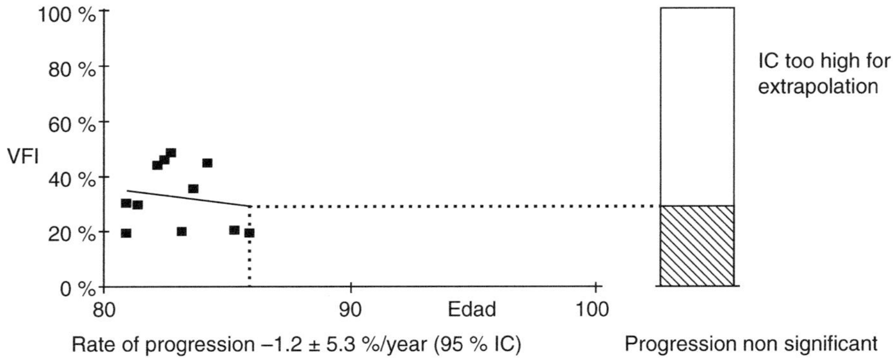

Fig. 1.7 Example of a VF series with a very high VFI variability. Note that 95 % IC is 5.3 %, too high to permit any prediction. The estimated value of the Rate must be disregarded

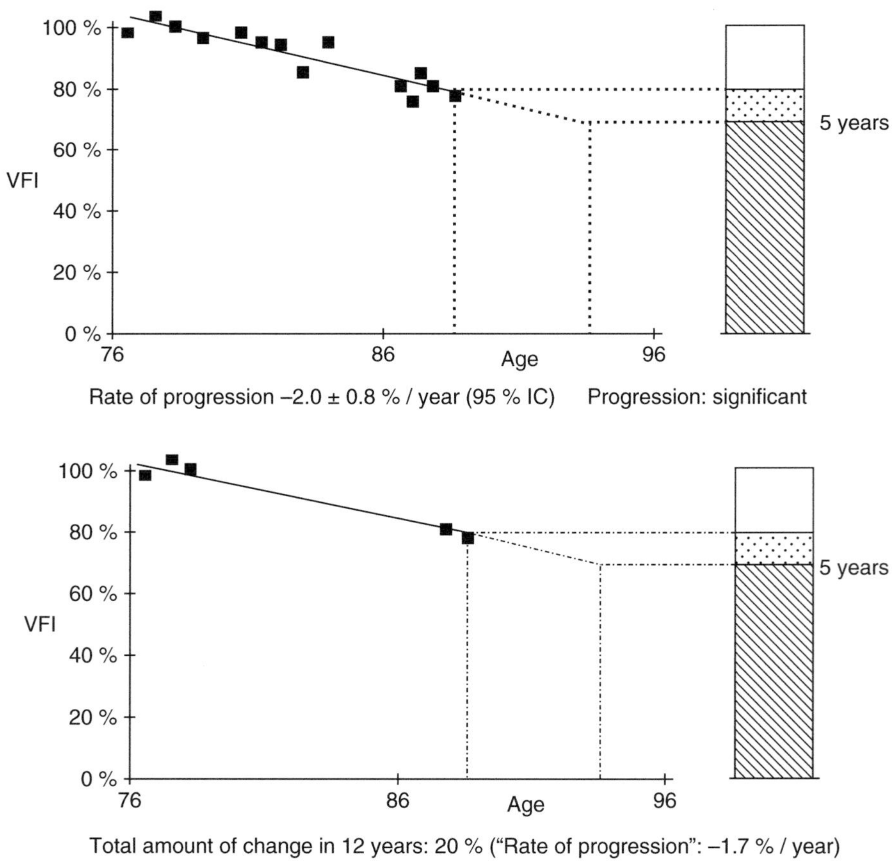

Fig. 1.8 Example of a long-term VF series including all examinations during 12 years (*upper graph*). Note that VFI trend slope and outcome prediction do not change significantly after excluding intermediate tests (*lower graph*). The total amount of change is about 20 % in 12 years

1.4 Where Do Glaucoma Visual Field Defects Appear Initially?

In glaucoma, the optic nerve head is most frequently damaged following specific topographical patterns. As a rule, temporal-inferior and temporal-superior aspects of the neuro-retinal rim (NRR) show morphological changes first. NRR loss and retinal nerve fiber layer (RNFL) degradation are responsible for the corresponding functional changes observed in the VF.

The earliest manifestations of glaucomatous functional damage appear more frequently at the Bjerrum area of the central VF of the superior hemifield [19] as partial arcuate and nasal scotomas in approximately 70 % of the cases (Fig. 1.9) [20]. Glaucoma is usually an intra- and inter-eye asymmetric disease. On the same eye, one hemifield will usually be affected earlier than the opposite, and one eye will show damage sooner than the contralateral one. This represents useful information in glaucoma diagnosis.

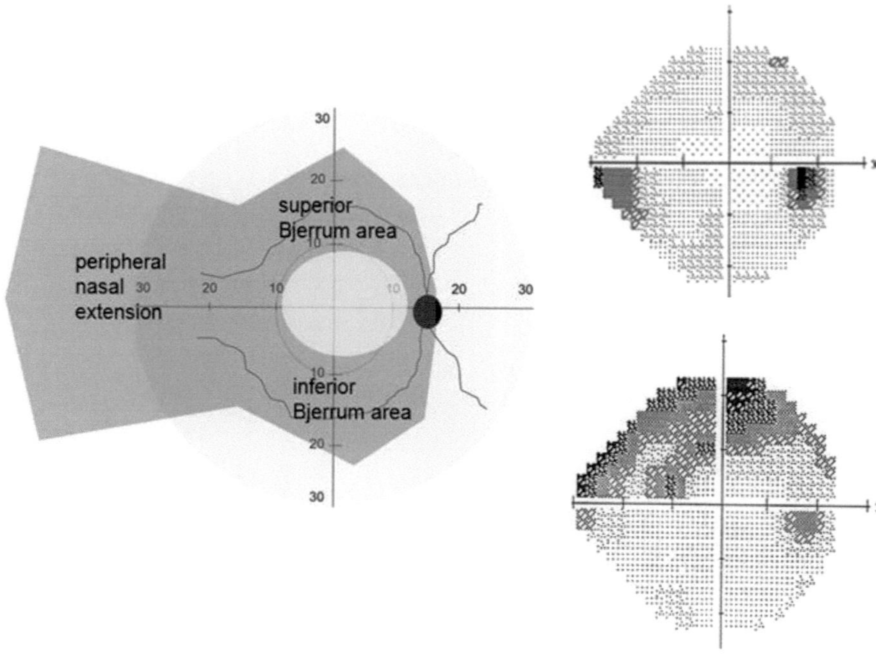

Fig. 1.9 (*Left*) Visual field representation of a right eye. The region within 10–20 central degrees corresponds to the Bjerrum area, superior and inferior. The nasal region extends beyond the 30 central degrees but it is not generally examined in clinical practice. (*Right*) Two examples of a mild, nasal inferior defect (*upper graph*) and a double, partial arcuate defect (*lower graph*) (only the gray-scale map is displayed for illustration)

1.5 Perimetric Criteria of Glaucoma

Criteria to define *perimetric glaucoma* vary according to the different technologies and algorithms most frequently used in clinical practice. Classic criteria are summarized in Table 1.1 and shown in Fig. 1.10 [21, 22]. They have been employed as binary classifiers (disease or nondisease). Their usefulness is limited to confirm or reject glaucoma, with a level of certainty that depends on the trade-off between sensitivity and specificity. Alternatively, as glaucoma is a progressive disease, longitudinal information can be used for this purpose. This method can be especially useful in ocular hypertensives converting to glaucoma, as it provides quantitative information (Figs. 1.11 and 1.12), either through event and or trend analysis, as described later in the text.

Table 1.1 HFA criteria suggested to define perimetric glaucoma in clinical practice

HFA criteria
In ≥2 consecutive VF or in 3 nonconsecutive of a 5 VF series, one or more of the following indicators:
1. Glaucoma Hemifield Test (GHT) outside the normal limits
2. A group of ≥3 contiguous locations at the pattern deviation map (same hemifield) with p values <5 %, one of them showing a p of normality <1 %, excluding peri-cecal and peripheral row of points (when 24–2 grid, peripheral row is not excluded)
3. PSD with a p of normality <5 %. Pattern Standard Deviation (PSD) with a p of normality <5 %.

Partially modified by the authors

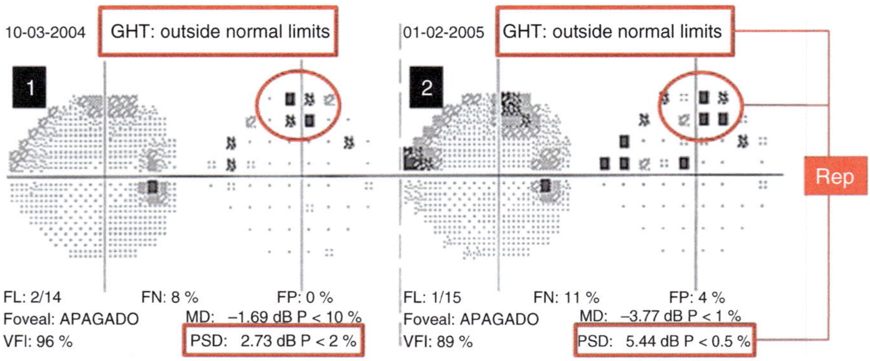

Fig. 1.10 Two visual fields of a right eye, determined approximately 1 year apart. According to classic criteria listed in Table 1.1, the three of them (GHT outside normal limits, number of abnormal locations ≥3 and PSD <5 %) are reproducible (*Rep*) in this case, and perimetric glaucoma criteria are fully met

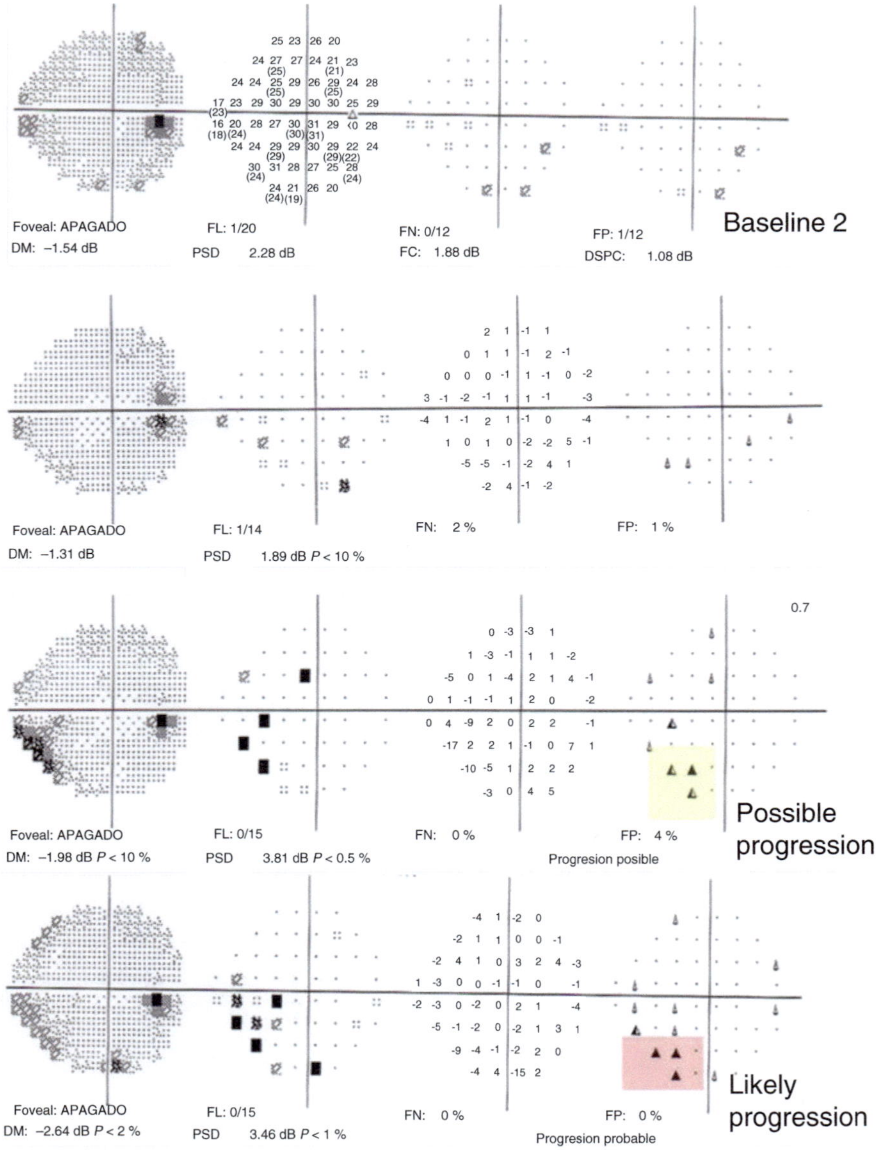

Fig. 1.11 Example of part of a VF series on a right eye showing perimetric glaucoma, defined as VF conversion by event analysis (5 years follow-up). At baseline, fields were classified as normal. The GPA program shows a reproducible change at the nasal inferior quadrant where three locations are flagged first as possible progression (*two half-black* and *one black triangles*, *yellow patch*) and then as likely progression (*three black triangles*, *red patch*) on the change map. This method can also be used as an alternative criterion to define perimetric glaucoma. Note that classic criteria were also met (only PSD is displayed)

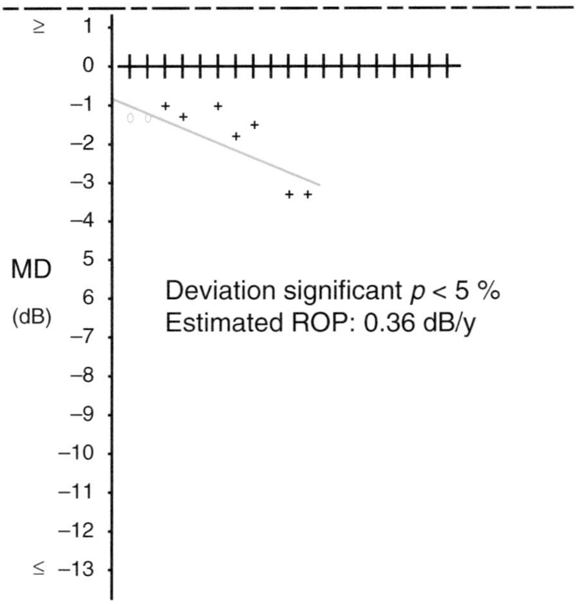

Fig. 1.12 Example of the same VF series as Fig. 1.10, including all tests. MD values of each examination are plotted against time. A statistically significant, negative-slope trend is depicted after regression analysis. This method can also be used as an alternative criterion to define perimetric glaucoma as early as a significant trend is detected. ROP: Rate of Progression (see below)

1.6 Glaucoma Progression

VF progression is the rule in glaucoma disease. There are two main methods to detect a functional change: event analysis and trend analysis [23]. When judging progression, the authors recommend considering the results from both methods, as they play a complementary role at different stages of the disease. Event analysis detects changes earlier than trend analysis [24], mainly in early to moderate glaucoma damage, but trend analysis provide more specific results and useful information across the entire functional range.

1.6.1 Event Analysis

As described above, a VF series starts with two reliable and similar examinations. They can be considered as a baseline functional situation that will be used as the reference for comparison every time a new examination is obtained. Every field location at baseline will show a threshold value and its expected variability range. Each individual threshold value obtained at the same location in the following examinations will be compared with its baseline reference. When a value deviates beyond the range of its baseline reference, it is considered as a significant change flagged at the change map. GPA will show an open triangle when this change is detected at one location for the first time, a half-black triangle if this change is detected again on a next examination, and a black triangle if confirmed again on a third test (Fig. 1.11). The appearance of ≥3 black triangles is considered an event of likely progression, according to criteria of the Early Manifest Glaucoma Trial [25]. Event analysis provides spatial information about where on the visual field the change occurs.

1.6.2 Trend Analysis

To find a trend, a time series regression model of a global index value, like MD or VFI, must be used. Trends can show a positive, neutral, or negative slope. Positive trends are frequently seen in clinical practice, and they probably represent a continuous improvement of patient's performance after serial VF examination (Fig. 1.13). Negative trends represent continuous functional decay over time. They may be flagged as statistically significant (see Fig. 1.11), but the clinical value of any amount of functional loss is related to the time for this change to take place: the speed or *Rate of Progression* (ROP).

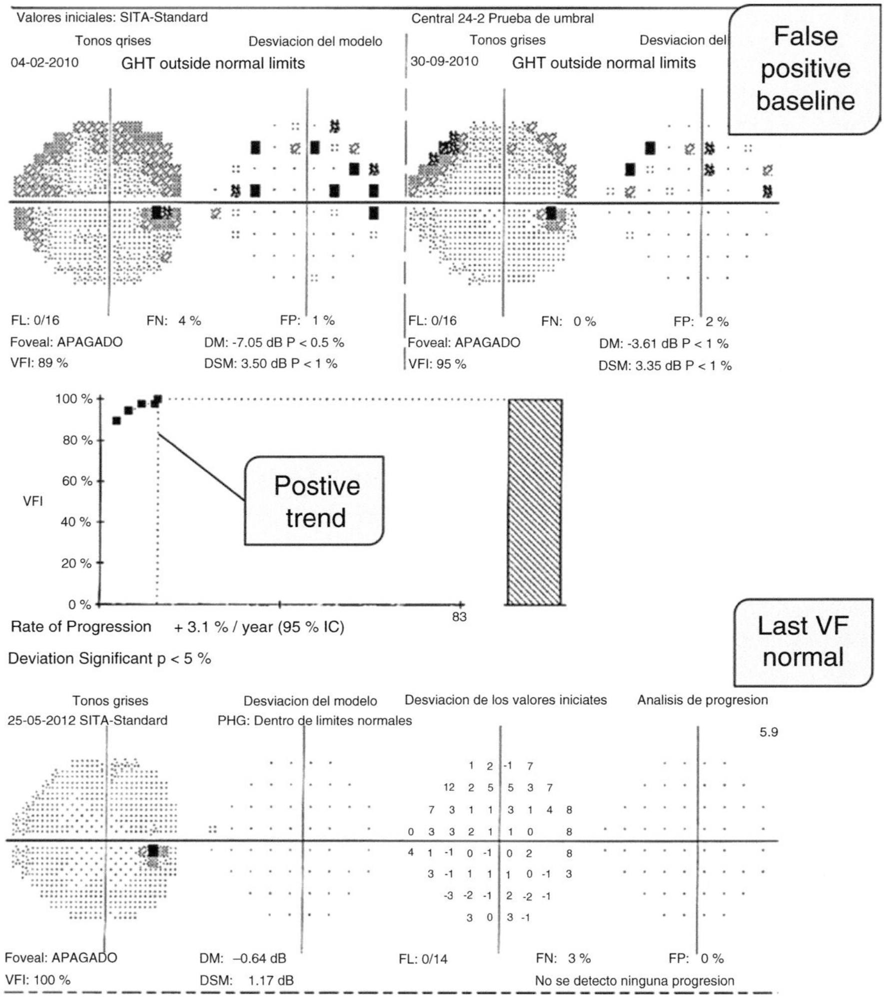

Fig. 1.13 Example of a persistent VF learning effect, right eye. At baseline, both fields show all classic criteria consistent with perimetric glaucoma, apparently due to mild, superior hemifield damage. Over time, VF indicators show a continuous improvement, and VFI increases up to 100 % at the last examination. Regression analysis is not available due to insufficient time follow-up, but a tentative positive trend is depicted. VF is consistent with normality 2 years later

1.6.3 Rate of Progression

ROP is expressed in terms of dB or percentage of loss per year, for MD and VFI, respectively. Linearity, variability, and the number or tests are all important factors that must be considered when calculating a ROP. It has been shown that ROPs can be estimated with sufficient power according to a minimum number of examinations undertaken during a period of time. As an example, to detect a ROP of –2 dB loss per year with sufficient statistical power, at least six examinations must be obtained in 2 years [26]. More examinations and time will be required to detect slower ROPs. The longer the follow-up, the more likely will be the probability to estimate ROPs with confidence [18].

ROPs can be classified as slow, average or fast, but no numerical definition has been proposed for each level. According to studies on glaucoma progression in treated patients, MD rates varies from –0.05 to –0.8 dB per year [27–33]. Thus for practical purposes it can be said that fast and slow rates are those at the top (more negative) and bottom (less negative) of this range, respectively. In clinical practice, a rate of –1 dB per year represents a useful round number referring to a fast progression (Fig. 1.14).

VFI and MD rates are not strictly comparable but show an acceptable correlation [34]. For practical purposes, a VFI/MD ratio of 3:1 can be accepted, mainly in those fields where damage progression is focal and not affecting the macular region. As an example, a MD rate of –1 dB per year corresponds approximately to a VFI rate of –3 % per year. This correlation is weaker in cases showing purely diffuse progression, where MD worsens faster than VFI, and in cases where macular progression is seen, where VFI decays faster. This is due to characteristics defining each specific VF index.

Whenever a significant intervention to treat glaucoma is made during the course of the disease (ie: a strong intraocular pressure reduction after filtering surgery), or any concurring nonglaucomatous reason impacts the VF, it may be considered to reset the VF baseline and establish a new trend. In such situations the authors recommend to obtain both the original trend (including all tests) and a partial trend, after resetting a new baseline. The reason for that is to maintain an unbiased, global perspective of the eye's functional evolution and not only a part of it (Fig. 1.15).

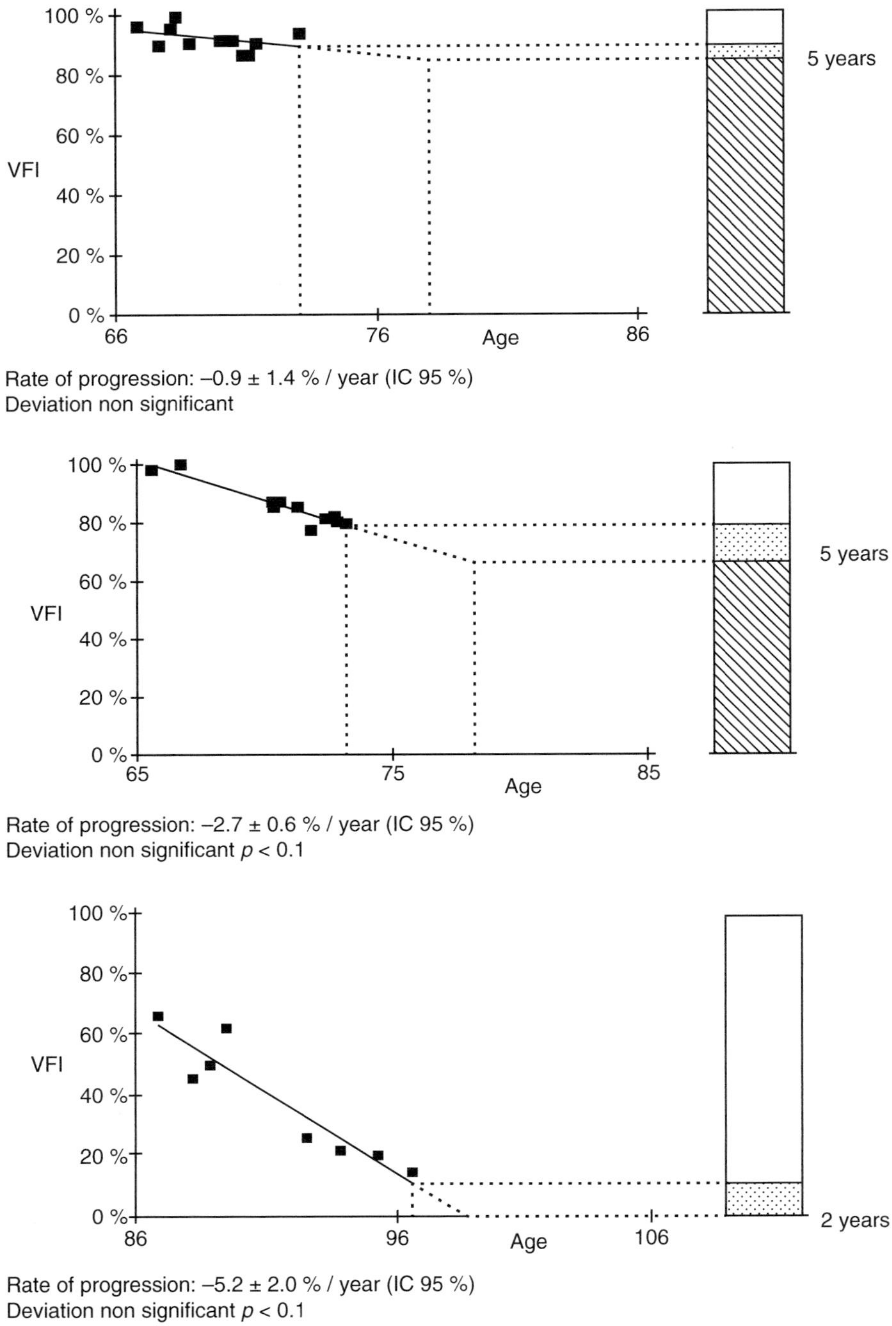

Fig. 1.14 Examples of three different VF series showing slow (*upper*) fast (*middle*) and crushing (*lower*) progression. Slow progression is represented here by a VFI rate of change of –0.9 % /year, corresponding to a MD rate of –0.3 dB/year. Note that the slope is negative but does not reach statistical significance (deviation nonsignificant). Trend in the middle case shows a VFI decay of –2.7 % or approximately –0.9 dB per year. Deviation is statistically significant. The case below progresses extremely fast, as –5.2 % or –1.7 dB per year has led to a handicapping visual loss in just 10 years

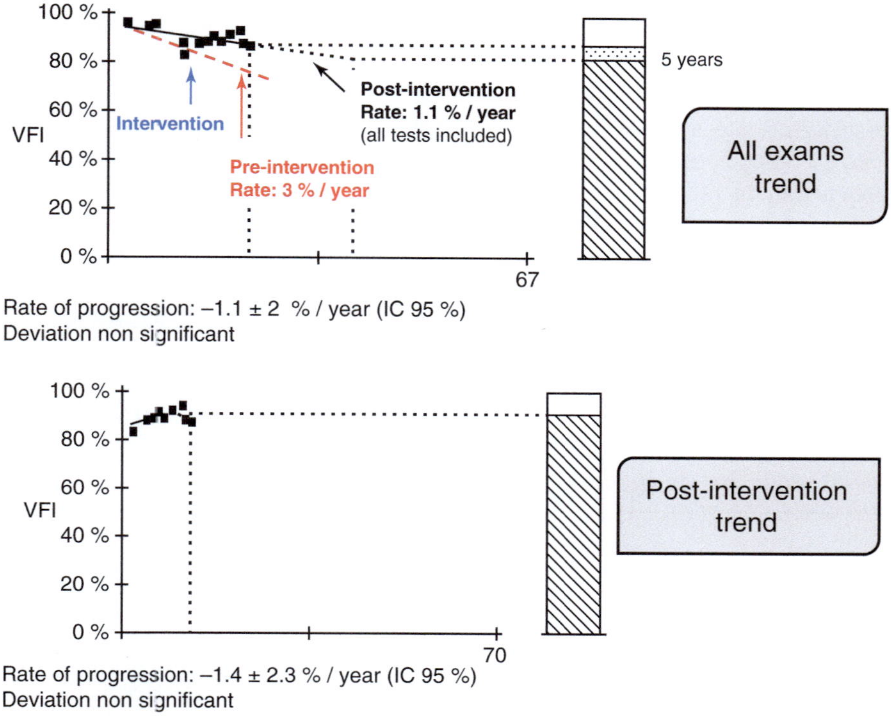

Fig. 1.15 Example of a complete (*upper graph*) and partial (*lower graph*) VF series trends of a glaucoma patient receiving a filtering surgery. The intervention was performed when the estimated ROP was −3 % per year and IOP was not controlled with maximal medical therapy. Three years later, the original trend including all tests shows a ROP of −1.1 % per year. When pre-intervention tests are excluded, a post-intervention, partial trend can be obtained showing a ROP of +1.4 % per year. In fact, sustained VF improvement can be observed after strong IOP reduction is achieved, as reported by the Collaborative Initial Glaucoma Treatment Study [35]

1.7 How Do Glaucomatous Visual Field Defects Progress?

VF defects usually progress increasing their depth and extension (Fig. 1.3). Also, new defects may appear at the same hemifield or less frequently at the opposite one [36, 37] (Fig. 1.16). Typically, progression will slowly encroach the macular VF area and in the last stages defects will invade its nasal aspect. Then, only a limited area of the central field will maintain useful visual function, the so-called *ceco-central island* of vision (Fig. 1.17). Differently, in normal tension glaucoma VF loss appears to be more localized, deeper and closer to fixation [38].

Staging VF level of damage is relevant in glaucoma management. Among the different classifications, most frequently used are those from (i) Brusini, (ii) Hodapp, Parrish, and Anderson and (iii) Mills modification of the previous one [39]. The enhanced Glaucoma Score System (eGSS) has been recommended as a better choice for its ease of use [40]. In routine clinical practice the authors classify VF loss severity according to MD level only, as early (better than 6 dB), moderate (MD between 6 and 12 dB), and advanced (worse than 12 dB).

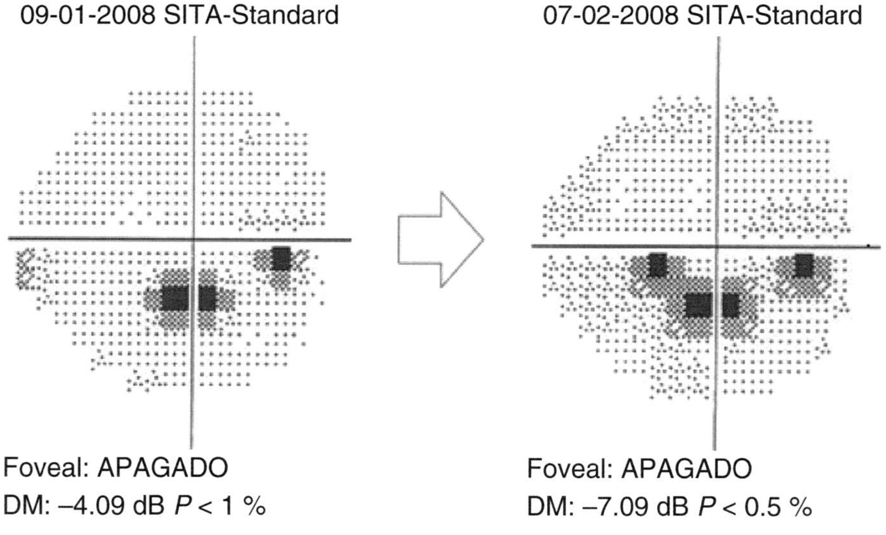

Fig. 1.16 Gray-map of a right eye VF, showing the appearance of a new scotoma on the same hemifield, just 1 month after previous test

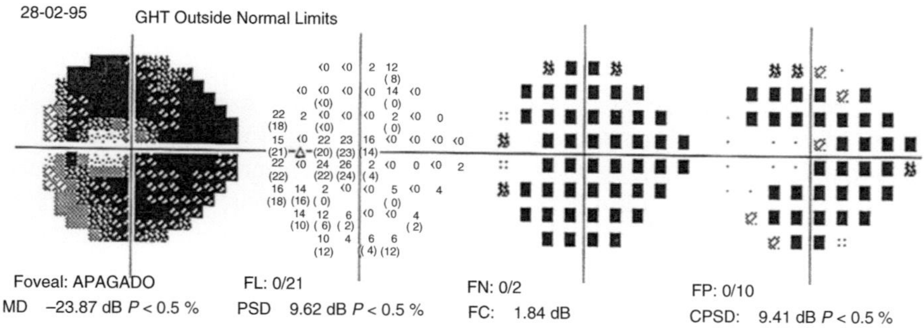

Fig. 1.17 VF example of a right eye showing typical glaucomatous advanced damage. Note that remnant light sensitivity has been measured mainly at ceco-central area and temporal row of the field, as seen at thresholds map

1.8 VF Testing in Advanced Damage

Glaucoma is quite an asymptomatic disease even at its late stages. Thus, advanced glaucoma damage at diagnosis is not an infrequent finding. Longitudinal VF testing is more challenging when light sensitivity is lower, and results show a higher variability [41], making the identification of true progression more difficult over time. When using VFI to track progression, it is important to remember that this index is calculated from the pattern deviation probability map in eyes with a MD better than 20 dB and from the total deviation probability map in eyes with a MD worse than 20 dB. In fact, a median artifactual VFI change of 15 % has been reported when the MD crosses the −20 dB boundary [42]. On the other hand, event analysis is not available in many areas of a VF showing advanced damage, as change cannot be measured anymore. It is advisable to continue examinations under standard conditions as long as possible during the course of the disease, not to lose information for comparative purposes, but in a number of cases results will be too tiring and even depressing for the patient, and meaningless for the examiner.

According to these limitations, the authors recommend to consider the use of spatial summation, selecting a size V stimulus of Goldmann, to expand the dynamic range, and/or to concentrate the examination on the macular area when significant thresholds are still detected at this region. Herein, the authors propose an algorithm to select an alternative VF testing strategy depending on results found after standard conditions (Fig. 1.18). In these cases, a new baseline can be defined and results followed over time in a similar way than for standard situations (Fig. 1.19). On the other hand, size V stimulus has shown lower test--retest variability than standard size III one in glaucoma subjects [43]. This can represent an advantage in selected cases where variability is an issue to ascertain true progression.

A number of glaucoma patients show concomitant diseases affecting the visual field. Conditions like media opacities, confluent photocoagulation in diabetic retinopathy or extensive retinal atrophy in high myopia may produce quite noisy results when using standard parameters. The authors also recommend to consider nonstandard conditions when results are repeatedly misleading or paradoxical and in cases where poor cooperation is expected. As said above, whenever nonstandard results show good thresholds apparently consistent with normality, it is advisable to return to standard conditions.

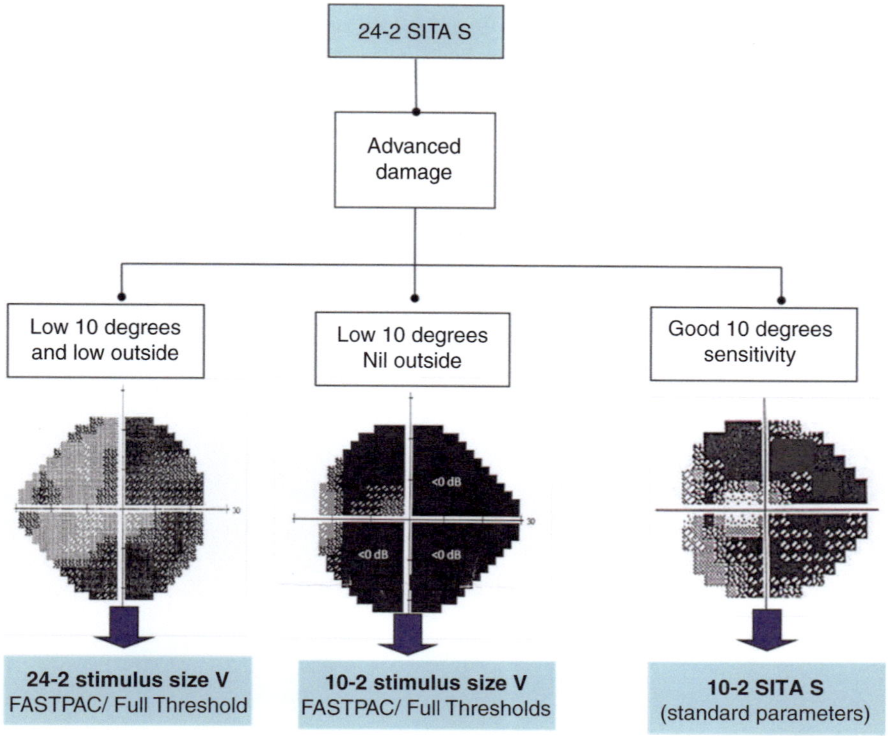

Fig. 1.18 VF examination alternatives when results under standard parameters preclude conventional follow-up. On the left, the test shows deep, diffuse depression. In this situation, the signal-to-noise ratio may be improved using a size V across the entire field. On the middle, the dynamic range is exhausted (three quadrants show thresholds <0 dB, as represented by numbers superimposed on the map) and only a remnant sensitivity may be present at the temporal superior aspect of the macula and temporally to the blind spot. If the eye still shows good fixation, as many times happens, size V stimulus concentrated at the macular area (10-2 macular grid) can help to measure some thresholds that can be monitored again. On the right, macular sensitivity is still good at the ceco-central area, and almost extinguished peripherally. Here standard conditions can be preserved, and examination be concentrated only on the macular area (only the gray-scale map is displayed for illustration)

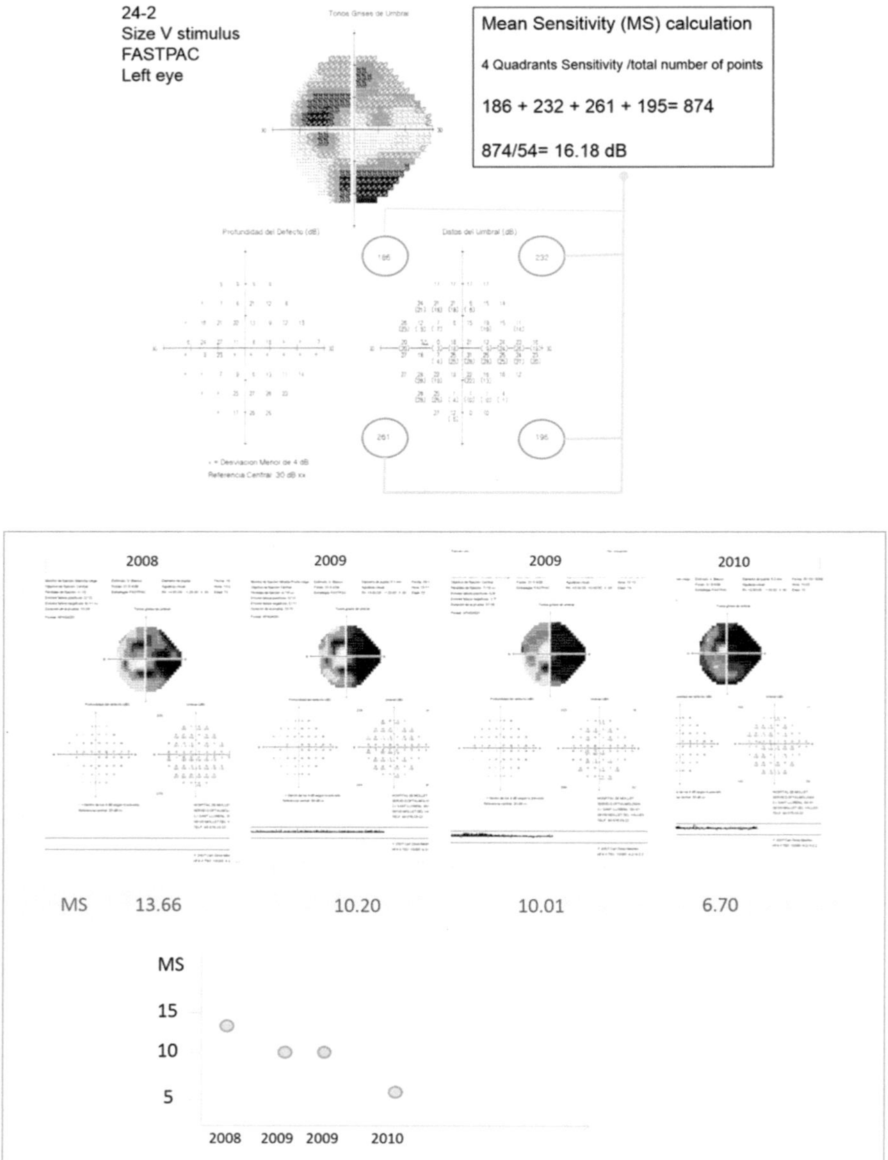

Fig. 1.19 *Upper graph:* three-in-one printout, size V stimulus, left eye. The thresholds map on the right inferior corner shows a total sensitivity value (*encircled*) for each quadrant. VF Mean sensitivity (*MS*) can be calculated dividing total sensitivity (sum of all quadrants) by the total number of points. *Lower graph:* example of a nonstandard parameters VF series. MS has been calculated for each field (*MS gray bar*) and plotted against time. Note that about 6 dB have been lost in 2 years, what can be considered a catastrophic progression

References

1. Palma C (2014) Electromagnetic radiation and astronomical observations. Course Astro 801. https://www.e-education.psu.edu/astro801/content/l3_p4.html. Accessed 20 Dec 2014
2. Flammer J (1986) The concept of visual field indices. Graefe's Arch Clin Exp Ophthalmol 224(5):389–392
3. Heijl A, Lindgren G, Olsson J (1987) Normal variability of static perimetric threshold values across the central visual field. Acta Ophthalmol 105(11):1544–1549
4. Bengtsson B, Heijl A (2008) A visual field index for calculation of glaucoma rate of progression. Am J Ophthalmol 145(2):343–353
5. Humphrey Field Analyzer II User's Guide (1994) Humphrey Instruments Inc. San Leandro
6. Newkirk MR, Gardiner SK, Demirel S et al (2006) Assessment of false positives with the Humphrey Field Analyzer II perimeter with the SITA algorithm. Invest Ophthalmol Vis Sci 47(10):4632–4637
7. Wall M, Doyle CK, Brito CF et al (2008) A comparison of catch trial methods used in standard automated perimetry in glaucoma patients. J Glaucoma 17(8):626–630
8. Caprioli J (1991) Automated perimetry in glaucoma. Am J Ophthalmol 111(2):235–239
9. Rao HL, Yadav RK, Begum VU et al (2015) Role of visual field reliability indices in ruling out glaucoma. JAMA Ophthalmol 133(1):40–44
10. Keltner JL, Johnson CA, Cello KE et al (2007) Visual field quality control in the Ocular Hypertension Treatment Study (OHTS). J Glaucoma 16(8):665–669
11. Wood JM, Wild JM, Hussey MK et al (1987) Serial examination of the normal visual field using Octopus automated projection perimetry. Evidence for a learning effect. Acta Ophthalmol (Copenh) 65(3):326–333
12. Gardiner SK, Demirel S, Johnson CA (2008) Is there evidence for continued learning over multiple years in perimetry? Optom Vis Sci 85(11):1043–1048
13. Goñi FJ; Glaucoma Progression Spanish Study Group (2012) Estudio multicéntrico Español Progress II sobre ritmos de progresión del campo visual en el glaucoma: resultados preliminares de la fase retrospectiva. Oral presentation at the 7th Spanish Glaucoma Society meeting, Alicante
14. Henson DB, Chaudry S, Artes PH et al (2000) Response variability in the visual field: comparison of optic neuritis, glaucoma, ocular hypertension and normal eyes. Invest Ophthalmol Vis Sci 41(2):417–421
15. Siderov J, Al T (1999) Variability of measurements of visual acuity in a large eye clinic. Acta Ophthalmol Scand 77:673–676
16. Chauhan BC, Tompkins JD, LeBlanc RP et al (1993) Characteristics of frequency-of-seeing curves in normal subjects, patients with suspected glaucoma and patients with glaucoma. Invest Ophthalmol Vis Sci 34(13):3534–3540
17. Heijl A, Lindgren A, Lindgren G (1989) Test-retest variability in glaucomatous visual fields. Am J Ophthalmol 108(2):130–135
18. Jansonius NM (2010) On the accuracy of measuring rates of visual field change in glaucoma. Br J Ophthalmol 94(10):1404–1405
19. Heijl A, Lundqvist L (1984) The frequency distribution of earliest glaucomatous visual field defects documented by automatic perimetry. Acta Ophthalmol (Copenh) 62(4):658–664
20. Keltner JL, Johnson CA, Quigg JM et al (2004) Invest Ophthalmol Vis Sci 45:E-Abstract 2134. Abstracts' book of 76th ARVO meeting
21. Budenz DL, Rhee P, Feuer WJ, et al (2009) Sensitivity and specificity of the Swedish interactive threshold algorithm for glaucomatous visual field defects. Ophthalmology 109(6): 1052–1058
22. Sekhar GC, Naduvilath TJ, Lakkai M et al (2000) Sensitivity of Swedish Interactive Threshold Algorithm in Humphrey visual field testing. Ophthalmology 107(7):1303–1308

23. Caprioli J, Garway-Heath DF, International Glaucoma Think Tank (2007) A critical reevaluation of current glaucoma management: International Glaucoma Think Tank, July 27-29, 2006. Ophthalmology 114(11 Suppl):S1–S41
24. Vesti E, Johnson CA, Chauhan BC (2003) Comparison of different methods for detecting glaucomatous visual field progression. Invest Ophthalmol Vis Sci 44(9):3873–3879
25. Heijl A, Leske MC, Bengtsson B et al (2002) Reduction of intraocular pressure and glaucoma progression: results from the Early Manifest Glaucoma Trial. Arch Ophthalmol 120(10): 1268–1279
26. Chauhan BC, Garway-Heath DF, Goñi FJ et al (2008) Practical recommendations for measuring rates of visual field change in glaucoma. Br J Opthalmol 92(4):569–573
27. Heijl A, Bengtson B, Hyman L et al (2009) Natural history of open angle glaucoma. Opthalmology 116(12):2271–2276
28. Chauhan BC, Mikelberg FS, Artes PH et al (2010) Canadian Glaucoma Study 3. Impact of risk factors and intraocular pressure reduction on the rates of vidual field change. Arch Opthalmol 128(10):1249–1255
29. Drance S, Anderson DR, Schulzer M, Collaborative Normal-Tension Glaucoma Study Group (2001) Risk factors for progression of visual field abnormalities in normal tension glaucoma. Am J Ophthalmol 131(6):699–708
30. AGIS investigators (2002) The Advanced Glaucoma Intervention Study (AGIS): 12. Baseline risk factors for sustained loss of visual field and visual acuity in patients with advanced glaucoma. Am J Ophthalmol 134(4):499–512
31. Wesselink C, Heeg GP, Jansonius NM (2009) Glaucoma monitoring in a clinical setting: glaucoma progression analysis vs nonparametric progression analysis in the Groningen Longitudinal glaucoma Study. Arch Ophthalmol 127(3):270–274
32. Heijl A, Buchholz P, Norrgren G et al (2013) Rates of visual field progression in clinical glaucoma care. Acta Ophthalmol 91(5):406–412
33. Chauhan BC, Malik R, Shuba LM et al (2014) Rates of glaucomatous visual field change in a large clinical population. Invest Ophthalmol Vis Sci 55(5):2885–2892
34. Artes PH, O'Leary N, Hutchison DM (2011) Properties of the statpac visual field index. Invest Ophthalmol Vis Sci 52(7):4030–4038
35. Musch DC, Gillespie BW, Palmberg PF et al (2014) Visual field improvement in the collaborative initial glaucoma treatment study. Am J Ophthalmol 158(1):96–104
36. Mikelberg FS, Drance SM (1984) The mode of progression of visual field defects in glaucoma. Am J Opththalmol 98(4):443–445
37. Boden C, Blumenthal EZ, Pascual J et al (2004) Patterns of glaucomatous visual field progression identified by three progression criteria. Am J Ophthalmol 138(6):1029–1036
38. Araie M (1995) Pattern of visual field defects in normal-tension and high-tension glaucoma. Curr Opin Ophthalmol 6(2):36–45
39. Brusini P, Johnson CA (2007) Staging functional damage in glaucoma: review of different classification methods. Surv Ophthalmol 52(2):156–179
40. Ng M, Sample PA, Pascual JP et al (2012) Comparison of visual field severity classification systems. J Glaucoma 21(9):586–589
41. Russell RA, Crabb DP, Malik R et al (2012) The relationship between variability and sensitivity in large-scale longitudinal visual field data. Invest Ophthalmol Vis Sci 53(10):5985–5990
42. Rao HL, Senthil S, Choudhari NS et al (2013) Behavior of visual field index in advanced glaucoma. Invest Ophthalmol Vis Sci 54(1):307–312
43. Wall M, Doyle CK, Eden T et al (2013) Size threshold perimetry performs as well as conventional automated perimetry with stimulus sizes III, V and VI for glaucomatous loss. Invest Ophthalmol Vis Sci 54(6):3975–3983

Chapter 2
Gonioscopy

Michele Figus, Maurizio Taloni, and Chiara Posarelli

2.1 History, Principles, and Technique

Gonioscopy is a clinical biomicroscopic technique that allows the structures in the anterior chamber angle to be visualized. The angle was first visualized by Alexios Trantas in1907 with a digital pressure with a direct ophthalmoscope using positive lens powers [1]. Salzmann introduced modern gonioscopy by the first goniolens in 1914 [2, 3]. Many other authors such as Curran, Koeppe, Troncoso, Barkan, Sugar, Schaffer, Scheie, Goldmann, and Spaeth et al. contributed to the comprehension of the angle and its role in the different types of glaucoma [4–12].

The angle of the anterior chamber cannot be visualized directly during a routine clinical examination. It can be observed only by gonioscopy, which is based on an optical phenomenon called "total internal reflection" (Fig. 2.1). It occurs when the angle of incidence of the light is so great that the light will be completely reflected (critical angle). When light crosses a boundary between materials with different refractive indices, the light beam is partially reflected and partially refracted (Fig. 2.2). But if the angle of incidence is greater than the critical angle the light is totally reflected back [13].

In the eye the critical angle is 46° at the air-cornea interface. The use of a goniolens eliminates total internal reflection by replacing the tear film-air interface with a new tear film-goniolens interface. Direct gonioscopy provides a direct view of the angle. Indirect gonioscopy provides a mirror image of the opposite angle.

This method utilizes a dome-shaped lens, which provides a panoramic view and direct visualization of the angle structures with a hand-held microscope and with

M. Figus, MD, PhD (✉) • C. Posarelli, MD
Department of Surgical, Medical and Molecular Pathology and Critical Care Medicine, U.O.Oculistica Universitaria, Azienda Ospedaliero-Universitaria Pisana, University of Pisa, Pisa, Italy
e-mail: figus@ocupisa.it

M. Taloni, MD
Department of Neurosciences, U.O.Oculistica, Azienda Ospedaliera San Camillo-Forlanini, Rome, Italy

A. Ferreras (ed.), *Glaucoma Imaging*, DOI 10.1007/978-3-319-18959-8_2

the patient in supine position. The lenses commonly used for direct gonioscopy have been realized by Koeppe (Fig. 2.3) and Swan-Jacob. The patient lies in a supine position. The lens is placed on the cornea, and a saline or viscous solution is used to bridge the gap between the lens and the cornea. The angle is examined using a counterbalanced hand-held binocular microscope and an illuminator. An operating microscope can also be used. The advantages of this technique are the panoramic view, an erect image, the binocularity and the possibility to examine both eyes simultaneously. The disadvantages include a deeper angle due to the supine position, poor details, and special equipment. Direct gonioscopy is employed mainly in congenital glaucoma surgery.

This technique utilizes some lenses called gonioprisms. These lenses may have 1–6 mirrors with angles ranging from 59° to 64° to the horizontal (Fig. 2.4). The light reflected from the angle of the anterior chamber passes into the lens and is reflected by a mirror onto the examiner (Fig. 2.5). The examination is performed at the slit lamp with the patient in sitting position. This method provides the clearest visualization of the anterior chamber angle structures while the illumination and magnification is provided by the slit lamp. Indirect gonioscopy can be divided into two sections: static gonioscopy and dynamic gonioscopy.

Static gonioscopy can be performed by scleral type lenses. They have a broad area of contact and a steep convex surface. A viscous methylcellulose fluid is used as coupling substance between the lens and the corneal surface. There are a lot of lenses available for static gonioscopy, the most commonly used is the Goldmann three mirror lens (Fig. 2.6). This lens has the following features: a mirror inclined at 59°, a posterior diameter of 12 mm and a posterior radius of curvature of 7.38 mm. Many other lenses by Goldmann (1–6 mirrors), Ritch, Latina, Karickhoff, and Russel-Fankhauser (Fig. 2.7) etc. can be used.

The anterior chamber angle width should be evaluated with the lens located centrally on the cornea; indentation should be avoided because of the narrowing of the angle; inadvertent pressure of the lens can also determine corneal folds (Fig. 2.8), or blood to reflux into the Schlemm's canal. If the iris profile is convex and the structures of the angle cannot clearly be visualized, a more tangential viewing is necessary. In this case there are two options to look "over the hill": moving the mirror toward the angle being viewed (Fig. 2.9), or asking the patient to look in the direction of the mirror (Fig. 2.10).

Dynamic gonioscopy can be performed by corneal type 4 mirror lenses (Sussmann, Posner, Zeiss). The Zeiss lens (Fig. 2.11) has a posterior diameter of 9 mm and a posterior radius of curvature of 7.72. This allows usage of the lens without a coupling fluid, obtaining a central depression of the corneal surface and a posterior displacement of the iris root (Figs. 2.12 and 2.13).

In narrow angles, performing dynamic gonioscopy is crucial (Fig. 2.14). The corneal indentation displaces the aqueous humor peripherally and the iris root posteriorly. If the angle is not visible there is a synechial angle closure, otherwise there is an appositional closure that is reversible and the angle structures become visible with indentation. An anteriorly displaced lens or a larger diameter lens can also be involved in the angle closure mechanism (Fig. 2.15).

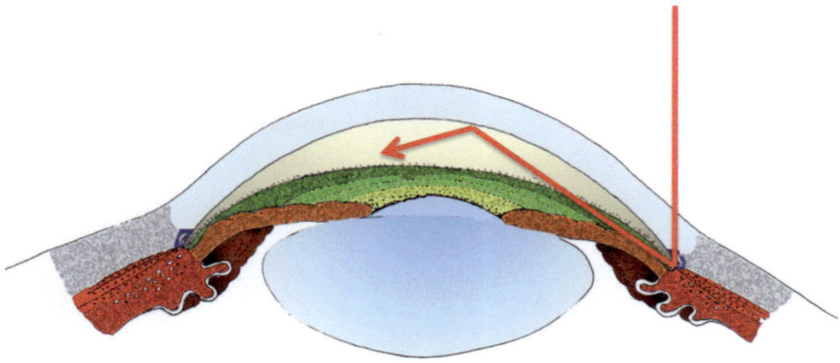

Fig. 2.1 Total internal reflection phenomenon

Fig. 2.2 The principle of total internal reflection

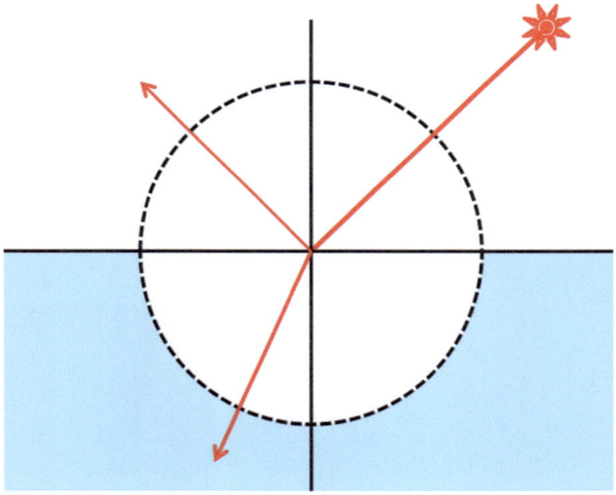

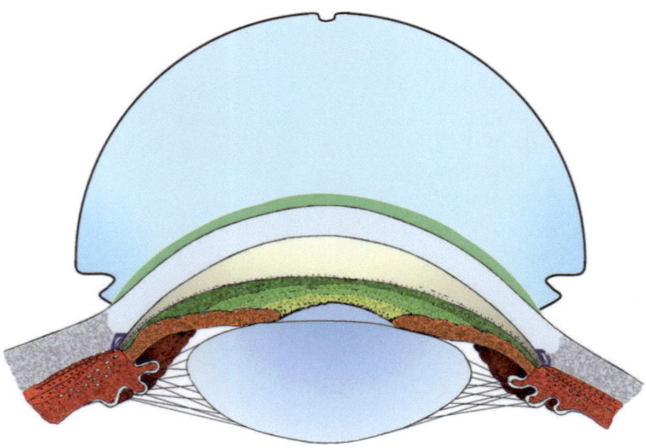

Fig. 2.3 Direct gonioscopy by the Koeppe lens

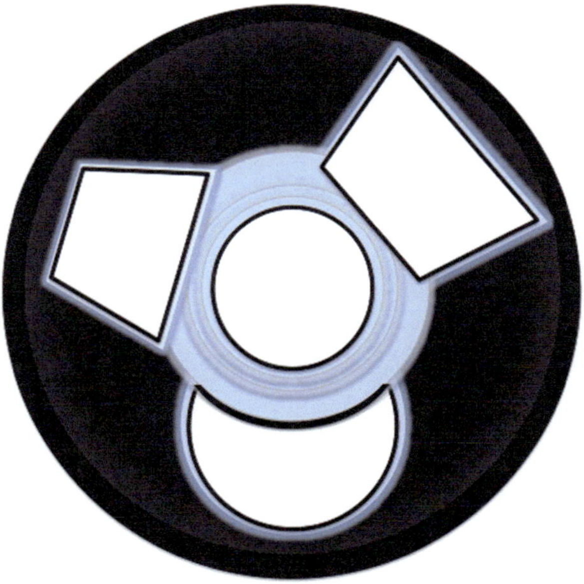

Fig. 2.4 A scheme of the Goldmann three mirror lens

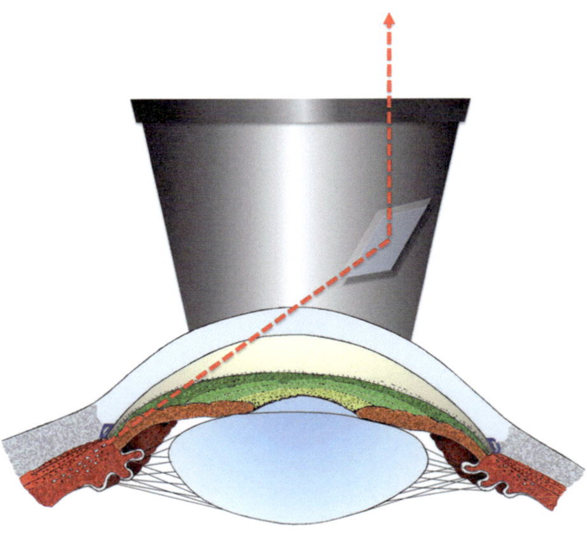

Fig. 2.5 The mirror reflects the light from the angle to the examiner

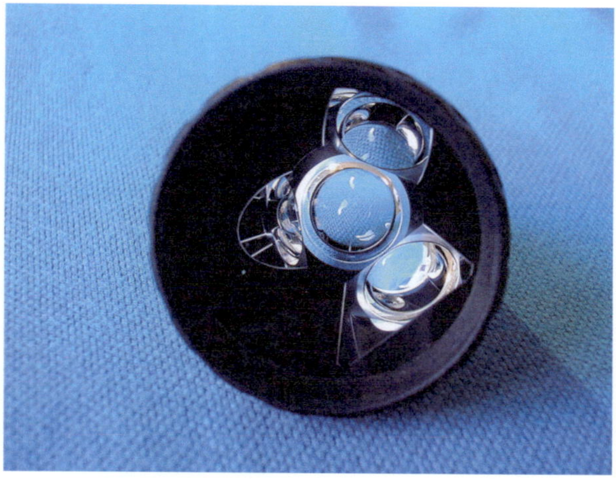

Fig. 2.6 The Goldmann three mirror lens

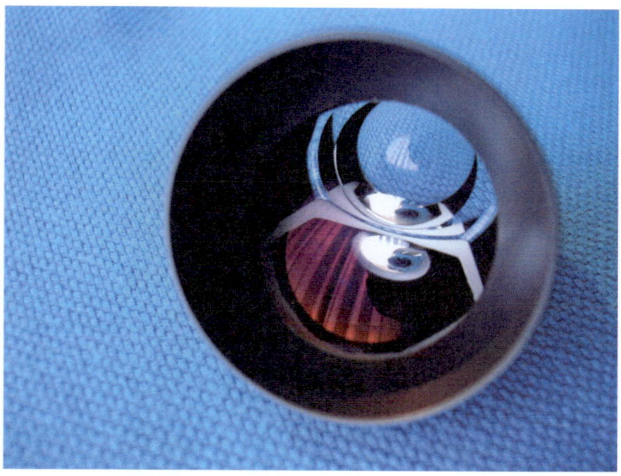

Fig. 2.7 The Russel-Fankhauser single mirror lens

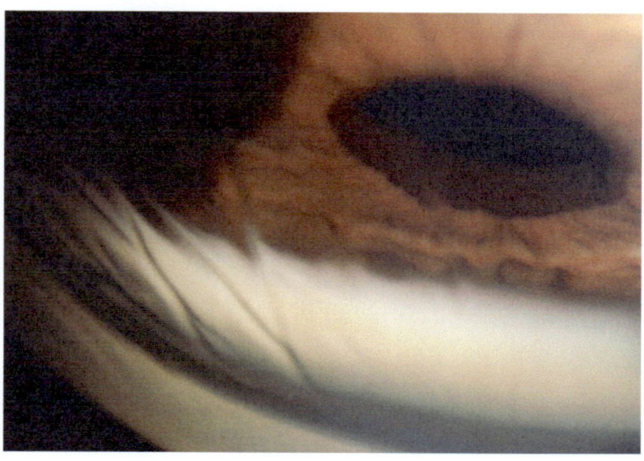

Fig. 2.8 Corneal folds induced by an excessive pressure on the lens. The angle cannot be visualized in detail

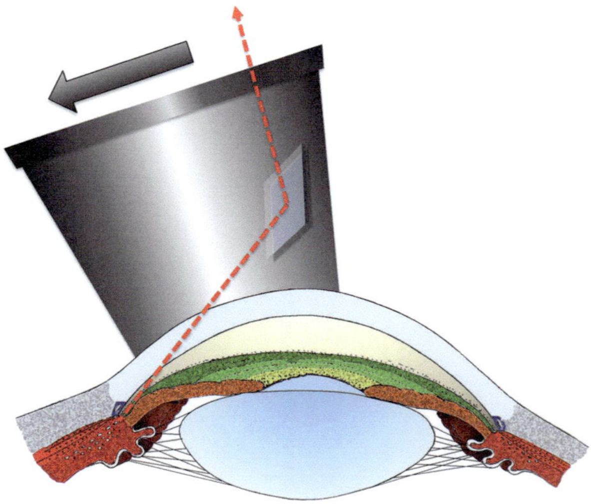

Fig. 2.9 In narrow angles, it is possible to move the mirror toward the angle to study the anatomy

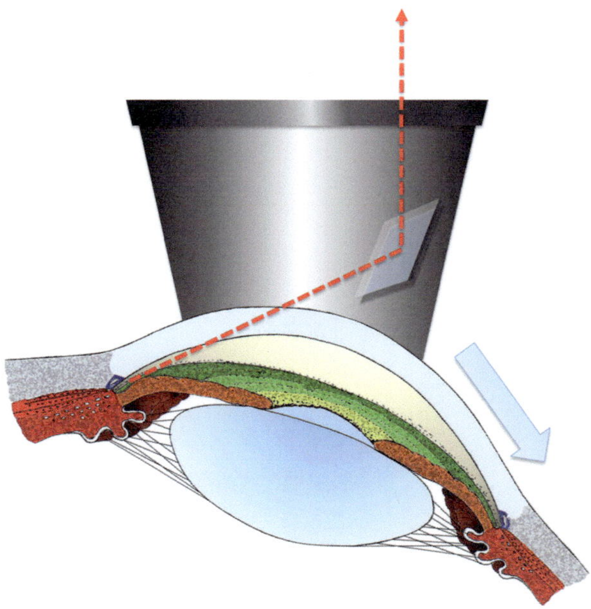

Fig. 2.10 Alternatively, in narrow angles it is possible to ask the patient to look at the mirror we are looking at

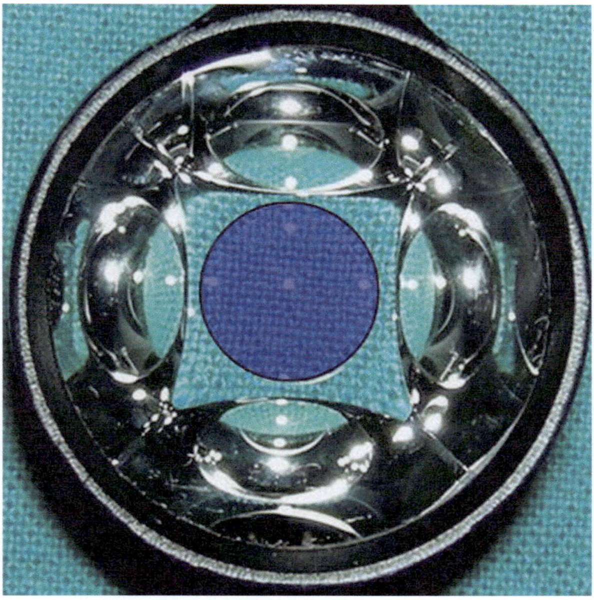

Fig. 2.11 The Zeiss four mirror lens

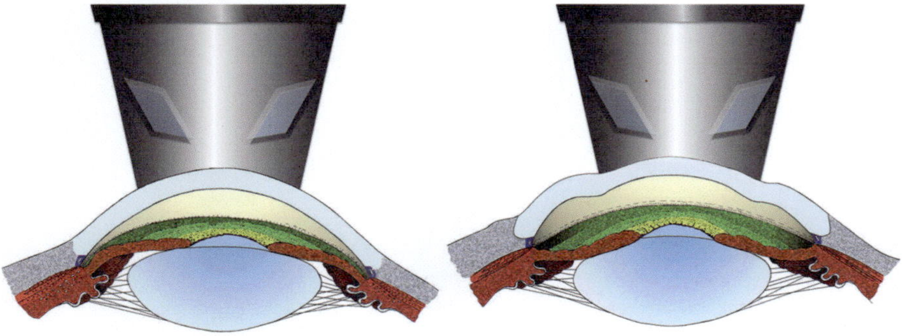

Fig. 2.12 The central depression of the corneal surface causes a peripheral displacement of the aqueous humor and a posterior displacement of the iris root

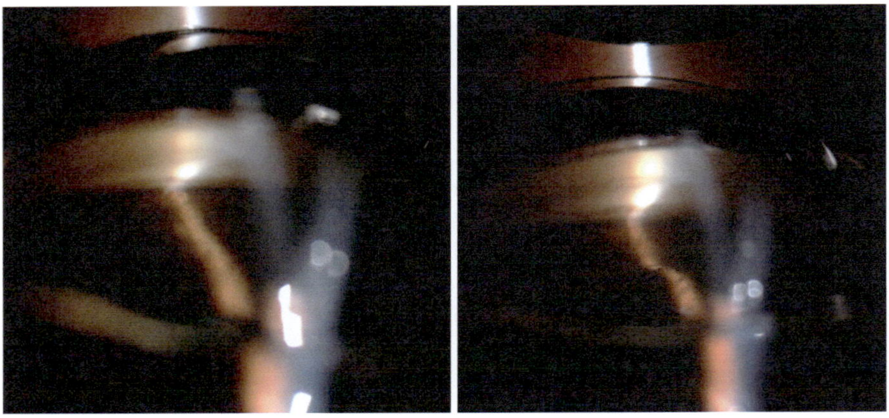

Fig. 2.13 Dynamic gonioscopy in a narrow angle. The posterior displacement of the iris opens the angle

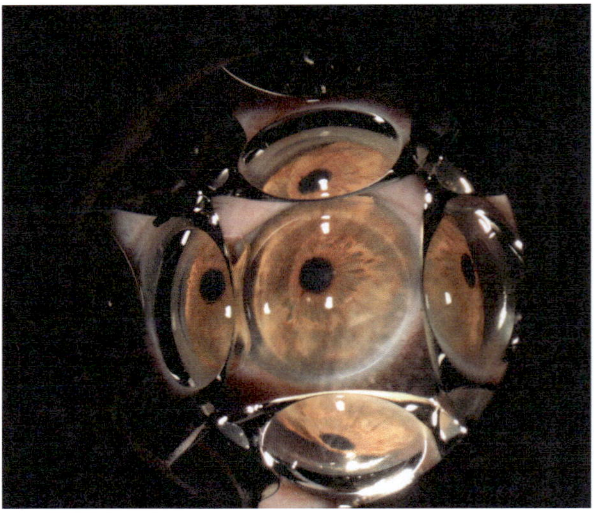

Fig. 2.14 Dynamic gonioscopy in a narrow angle with a convex iris profile. Visualization before performing central corneal indentation

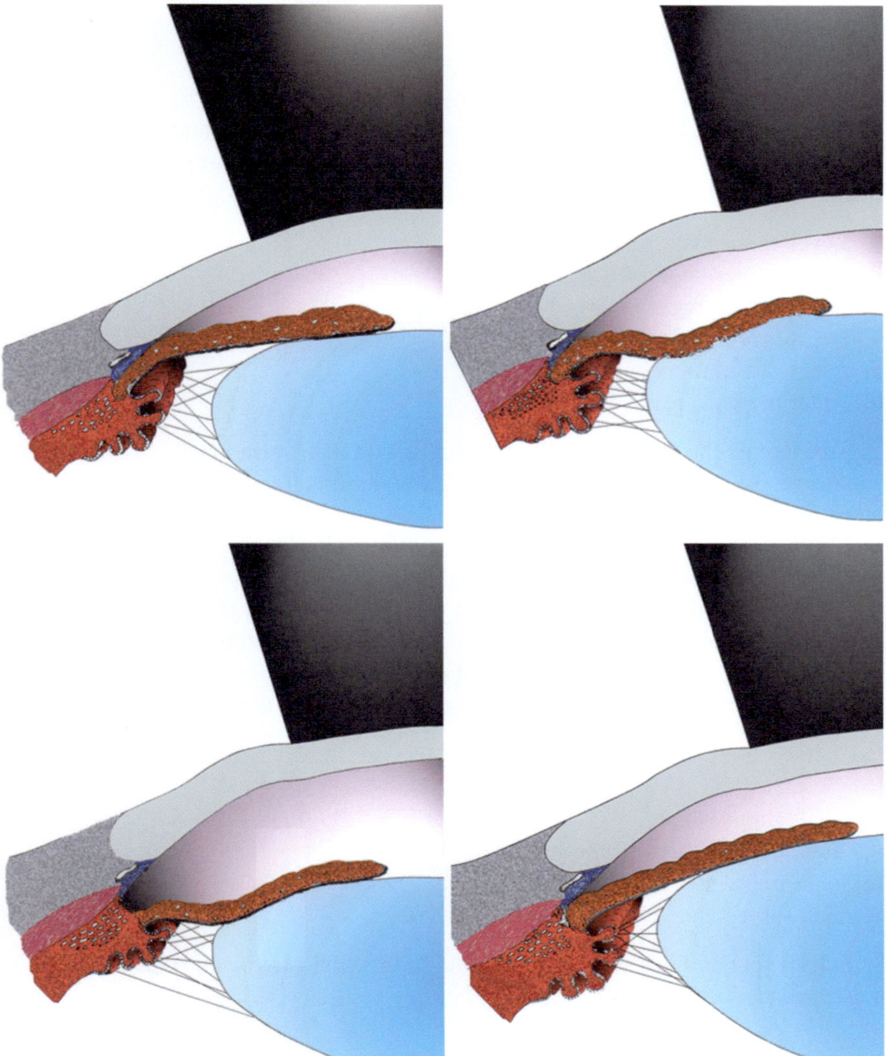

Fig. 2.15 Mechanism of dynamic gonioscopy. Indentation can open appositional angle closures, but it does not work in chronic or synechial angle closures. Sometimes an increased lens also could not allow the opening of the angle

2.2 Anatomy

Gonioscopy allows evaluation of the normal anatomy of the anterior chamber angle. Looking at the angle to understand the normal anatomy is important to recognize the angle landmarks. The following structures should be identified during the angle examination in primary gaze and on manipulation or indentation:

1. Level of iris insertion
2. Shape of peripheral iris profile
3. Width of the angle recess
4. Degree of trabecular pigmentation
5. Areas of iridotrabecular apposition
6. Anterior synechiae

To examine the angle direct focal illumination is necessary, and a narrow beam should be used to evaluate the width of the angle. It is important to avoid pupillary constriction, which can open the angle recess and deepen the anterior chamber. Sometimes, to identify the scleral spur retro-illumination is necessary. A fixation light may be used to maintain ocular alignment.

At first, the inferior quadrant should be examined because of its greater depth and pigmentation, so that it is easier to identify the structures mentioned above. Then in a clockwise direction, all the other quadrants can be observed. The following structures are present in a normal angle starting from the iris root (Fig. 2.16):

(a) Ciliary body band
(b) Scleral spur
(c) Schlemm's canal
(d) Pigmented trabecular meshwork
(e) Non-pigmented trabecular meshwork
(f) Schwalbe's line

Scleral spur and Schwalbe's line should be identified at first and then all the other structures can be recognized [14].

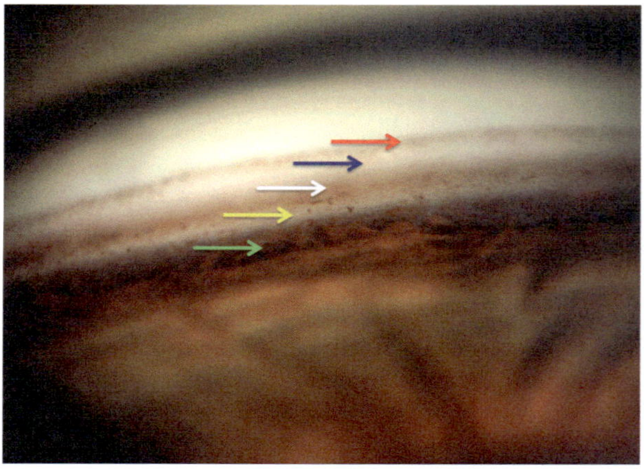

Fig. 2.16 Normal anatomy of an anterior chamber angle visible by gonioscopy. The following landmarks can be recognized: Schwalbe's line (*red arrow*), non-pigmented trabecular meshwork (*blue arrow*), pigmented trabecular meshwork (*white arrow*), Schlemm's canal, scleral spur (*yellow arrow*), ciliary body band (*green arrow*)

2.2.1 *Schwalbe's Line*

The Schwalbe's line appears as an opaque translucent line that represents the peripheral termination of Descemet's membrane and the anterior limit of the trabeculum. It marks the transition between the endothelium of the cornea and the trabecular meshwork. Sometimes, it may be prominent and anteriorly displaced (posterior embryotoxon) (Fig. 2.17), or heavy pigmented; pigmentation anterior to the Schwalbe's line constitutes the Sampaolesi's line (Fig. 2.18), and this is often disposed noisily, resembling salt and pepper.

The parallelepiped or the corneal wedge technique can be used to identify the exact position of the Schwalbe's line (Figs. 2.19, 2.20, and 2.21). By using a thin slit of light inclined 10–15° from the angle of the oculars, two separate corneal reflections can be seen, one from the inner surface of the cornea, and one from the outer surface. These two reflections meet at Schwalbe's line, which extends in a perpendicular direction across the trabecular meshwork and marks the anterior border of the trabecular meshwork itself. This technique is very useful in lightly pigmented angles and in angles with a confusing anatomy (Fig. 2.22). In the superior and inferior quadrant, it is easiest to generate a vertical slit and to identify the corneal wedge.

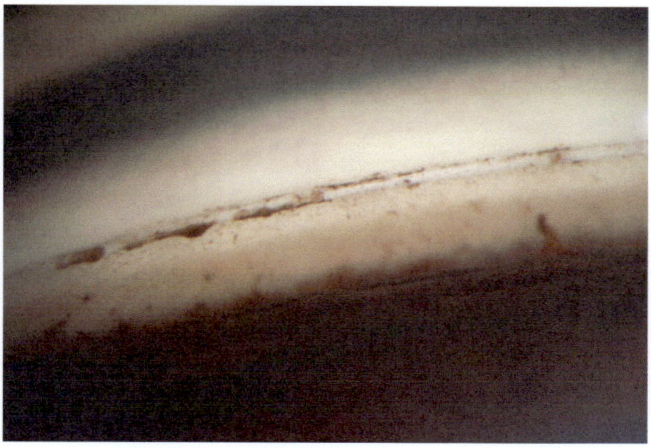

Fig. 2.17 A prominent anteriorly displaced Schwalbe's line

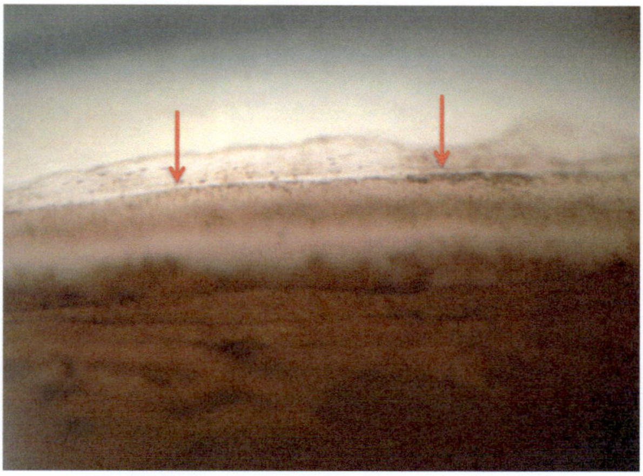

Fig. 2.18 Pigment distribution anterior to the Schwalbe's line (*red arrows*) to constitute the Sampaolesi's line

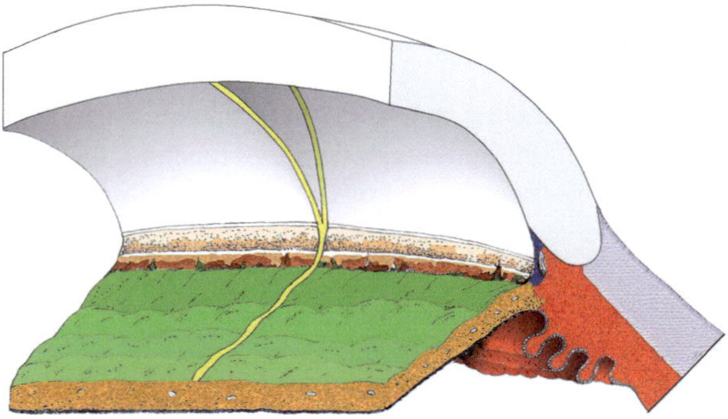

Fig. 2.19 The corneal wedge technique

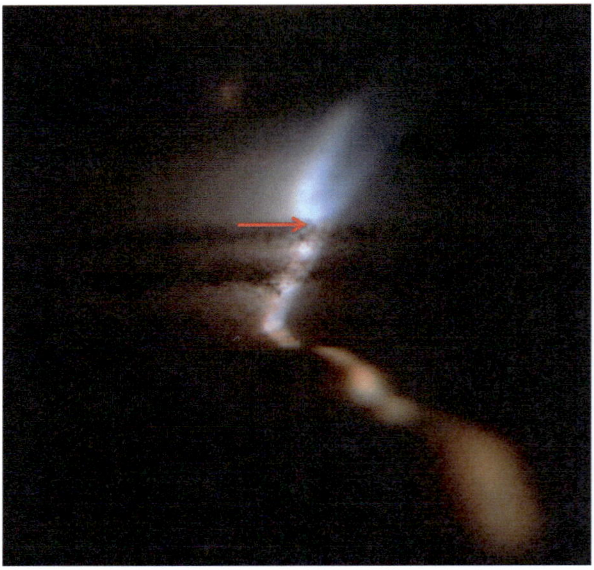

Fig. 2.20 The two light reflections, respectively, from the inner and the outer surface of the cornea, meet at Schwalbe's line (*red arrow*)

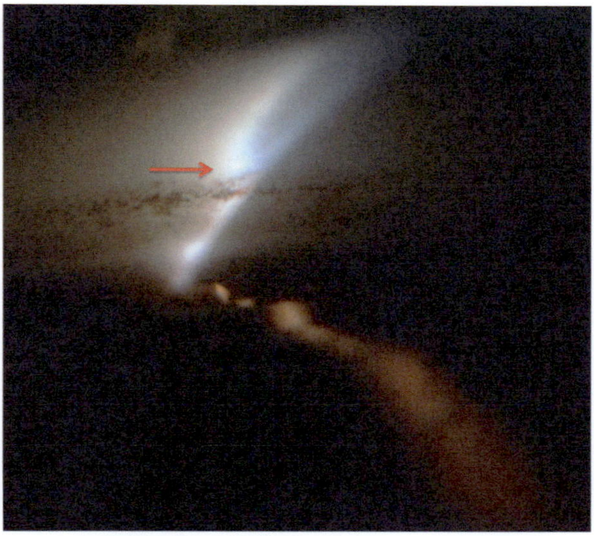

Fig. 2.21 Corneal wedge technique in a lightly pigmented angle. The apex indicates the Schwalbe's line (*red arrow*)

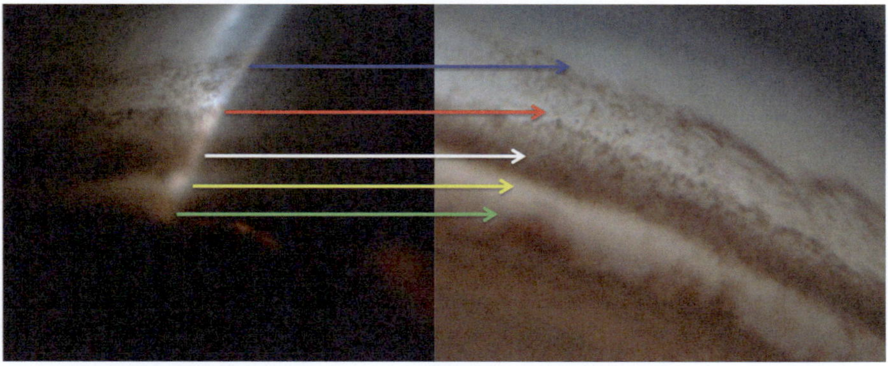

Fig. 2.22 An easiest representation of the angle's landmarks: Sampaolesi's line (*blue arrow*), Schwalbe's line (*red arrow*), trabecular meshwork (*white arrow*), scleral spur (*yellow arrow*), ciliary body band (*green arrow*)

2.2.2 Trabecular Meshwork

This extends posteriorly from the Schwalbe's line to the scleral spur. It is possible to distinguish an anterior nonfunctional part next to the Schwalbe's line with a whitish color; and a posterior functional part adjacent to the scleral spur, which is pigmented (Fig. 2.23). Trabecular pigmentation increases with age and is accentuated in the inferior quadrant due to gravitational setting and aqueous circulation; an increase in the pigmentation of the angle could be related to pathological conditions such as exfoliation syndrome, pigment dispersion syndrome, or inflammation. Pigmentation has little relation to skin or hair color. At gonioscopy, it appears with an irregular and rough surface; the trabecular meshwork band appears as 5 mm wide at the slit-lamp examination.

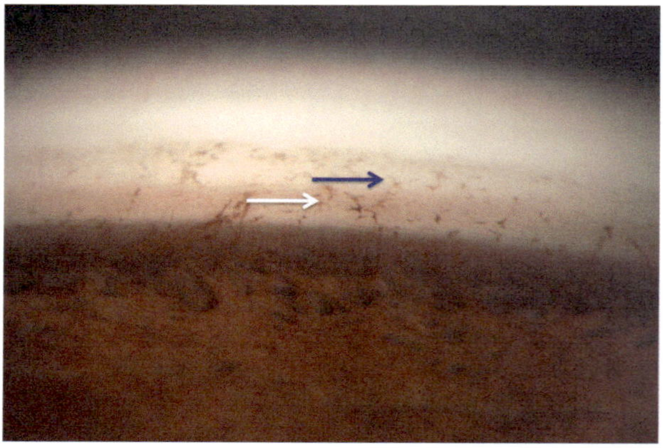

Fig. 2.23 The trabecular meshwork. It can be divided into two parts: a lightly or non-pigmented anterior (*blue arrow*) trabecular meshwork and a pigmented posterior (*white arrow*) trabecular meshwork

2.2.3 Scleral Spur

Going posteriorly between the trabecular meshwork and the ciliary body there is the scleral spur, which appears as a narrow whitish band that marks the posterior border of the trabecular meshwork (Fig. 2.24). Sometimes it is not visible because of an anterior iris insertion, iris processes (Fig. 2.25), excessive pigmentation (Fig. 2.26), or peripheral anterior synechiae (PAS).

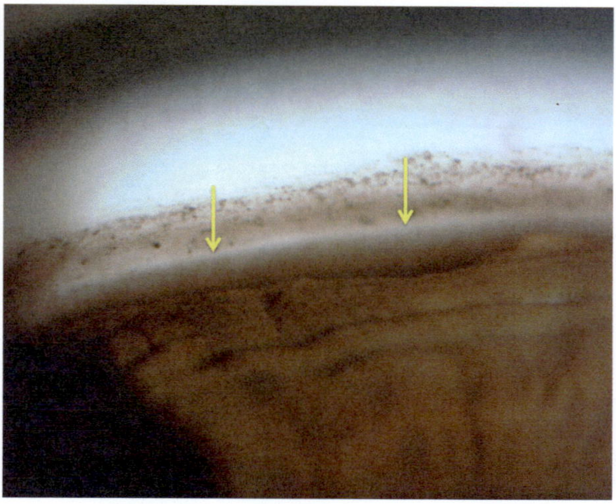

Fig. 2.24 The scleral spur (*yellow arrows*)

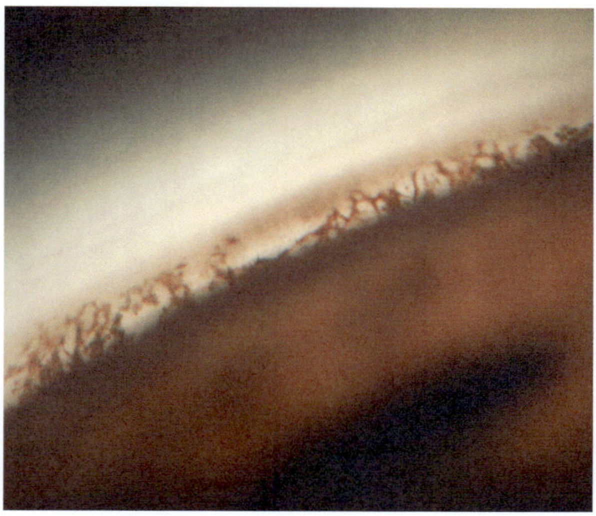

Fig. 2.25 Iris processes may obscure the scleral spur

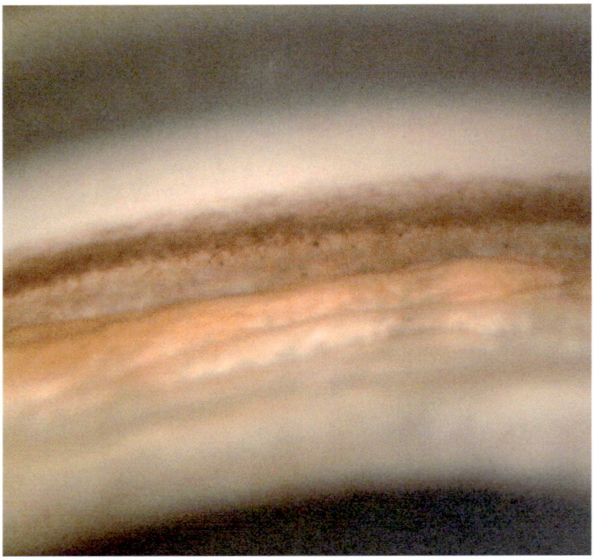

Fig. 2.26 The scleral spur is not visible due to an excessive pigmentation

2.2.4 Ciliary Body Band

Anterior to the iris insertion, a portion of the ciliary body is visible (Fig. 2.27). The width of the band depends on the position of the iris insertion, and it may be wide in myopia or following trauma, but it also can be narrow in hyperopia and anterior insertion of the iris. The band appears as gray or dark brown at gonioscopic examination. Before commenting on any abnormality, the width of the band must be compared between the two eyes.

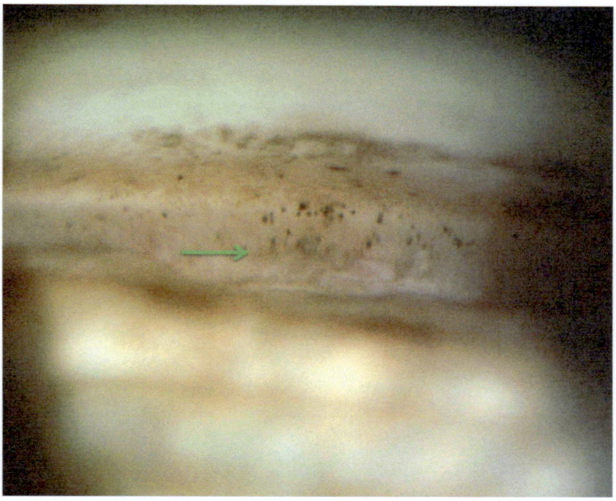

Fig. 2.27 A wide ciliary body band (*green arrow*)

2.2.5 *Iris and Iris Process*

The iris insertion is usually at the anterior face of the ciliary body, and normally the iris has radial markings with crypts. Three features are really important to determine the angle anatomy: the contour of the iris (convex, concave, or flat), the site, and the way of the iris insertion. It is important during the examination of the iris to notice the presence of nevi, tumors, atrophy, iridodonesis, and abnormal pigmentation. The peripheral iris configuration may provide important clues to the presence of pigment dispersion syndrome, plateau iris, or pupillary block.

Iris processes are small extensions of the anterior surface of the iris, which insert at the level of the scleral spur (Figs. 2.25 and 2.28). The iris processes are more frequent in young patients and in brown eyes. They appear as gray or brown finger-like extensions of the peripheral iris at gonioscopy and do not block the iris movements during indentation gonioscopy.

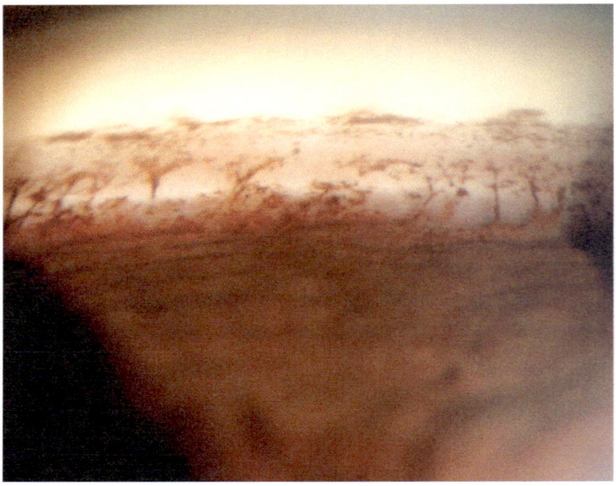

Fig. 2.28 Iris processes between the peripheral iris and the scleral spur

2.2.6 Schlemm's Canal

Schlemm's canal is not normally visible, it is located within the posterior trabecular meshwork and is anterior to the scleral spur. It may be seen when there is blood inside the canal for example, if the goniolens compresses the episcleral veins such that the episcleral venous pressure exceeds the intraocular pressure (IOP) (Fig. 2.29).

At gonioscopic examination it is seen deep in the posterior half of the trabecular meshwork as a red discontinuous line (Figs. 2.30 and 2.31). The pressure of the episcleral veins may be high also in different conditions: carotid-cavernous fistula, in Sturge-Weber syndrome, venous compression, ocular hypotony, or sickle cell disease.

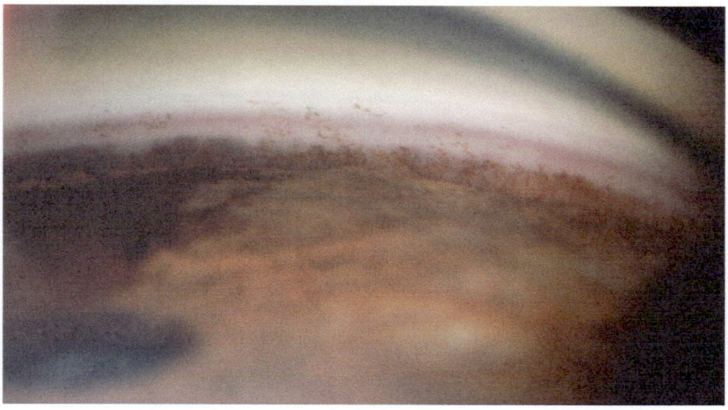

Fig. 2.29 The Schlemm's canal can be visualized as a red discontinuous line

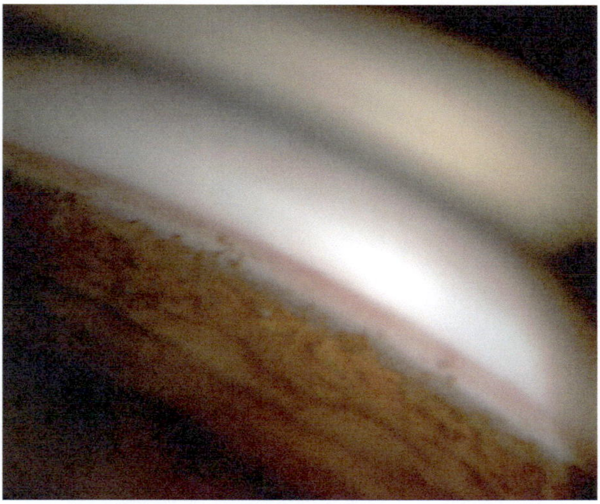

Fig. 2.30 The Schlemm's canal can be visualized if there is blood inside

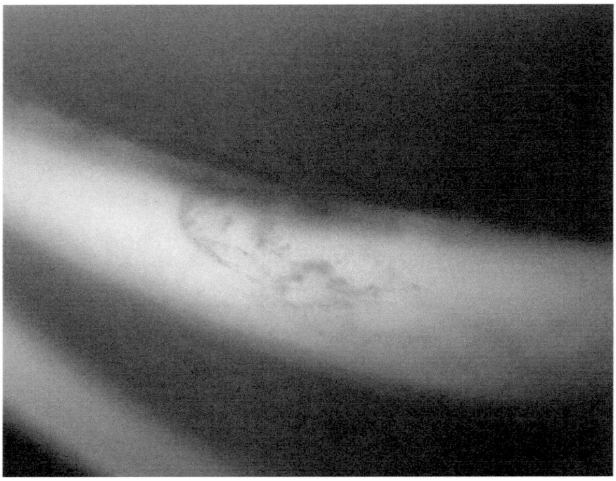

Fig. 2.31 Bleeding from the Schlemm's canal

2.2.7 *Blood Vessels*

Blood vessels may be visible in the normal anterior chamber angle (Fig. 2.32). They are more visible in blue eyes rather than in dark eyes. Normally the vessels run in a radial pattern at the base of the angle recess or perpendicular to the iris plane deep in the ciliary body. Normal vessels as a rule do not cross the scleral spur, are large and have a radial or circumferential orientation (Figs. 2.33 and 2.34). Pathological vessels are usually thinner, have a disordered orientation with anastamoses, and may run across the scleral spur.

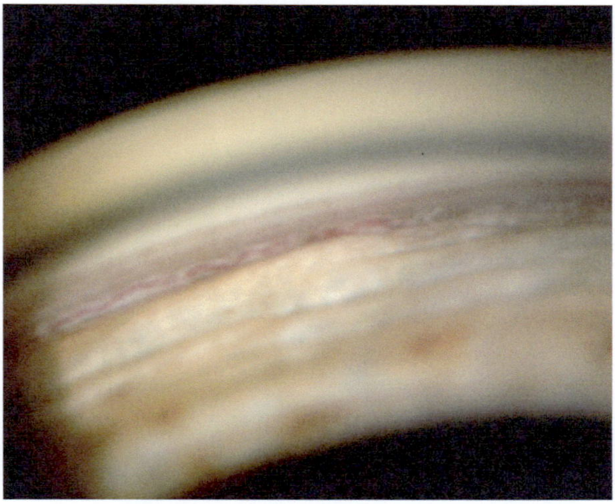

Fig. 2.32 Blood vessels may be visible in a normal angle

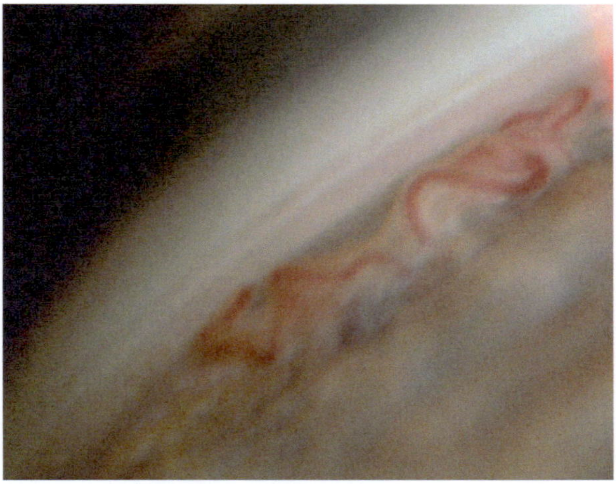

Fig. 2.33 Large vessels in a normal angle

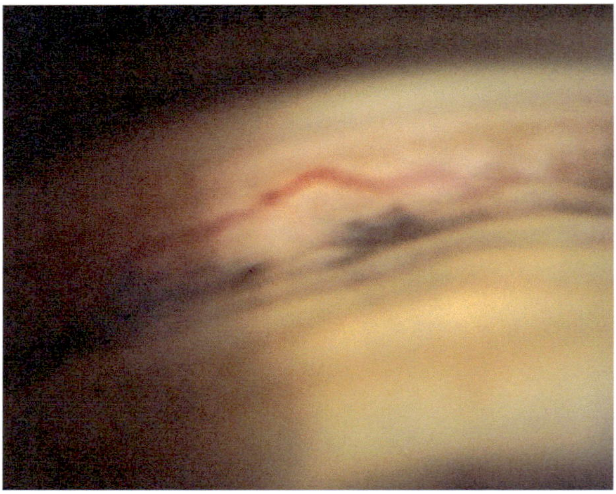

Fig. 2.34 Circumferential normal vessel not crossing the scleral spur

2.3 Gonioscopy Grading Systems

Determination of the angle width is really important in order to understand the functional status of the angle, the degree of angle closure, and the risk of future closure.

Grading of the angle can be obtained by the Van Herick method or by a gonioscopic grading system.

The Van Herick technique is used to assess the limbal anterior chamber depth. A narrow beam of light is directed perpendicularly at the temporal limbus, and the depth of the anterior chamber is evaluated as a fraction of the adjacent corneal thickness (Fig. 2.35) [15].

The width of the angle is determined by the insertion of the iris root on the ciliary body, the convexity of the iris, the prominence of the peripheral iris roll and the pupillary size.

Gonioscopy provides a subjective assessment of the angle width, but grading of the angle is essential for a systematic approach in the evaluation of the angle anatomy.

The use of a grading system allows comparison of findings at different times in the same patient, or to classify different patients.

There are three grading systems currently in use:

1. Shaffer
2. Spaeth
3. Scheie

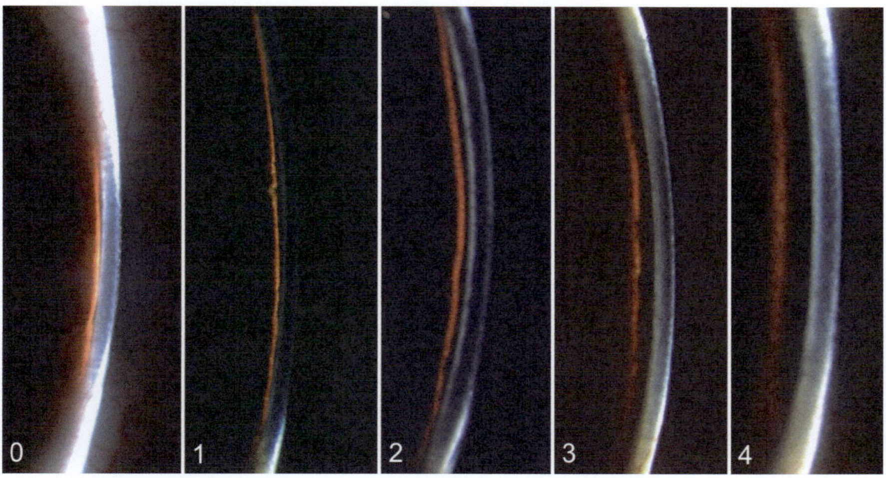

Fig. 2.35 The Van Herick method. *Grade 0*: iridocorneal contact (angle closed). *Grade 1*: the space between the iris and corneal endothelium is <¼ of corneal thickness (angle closure likely). *Grade 2*: the space is >¼ – <1/2 of corneal thickness (angle occludable). *Grade 3*: the space is >1/2 of corneal thickness (angle not occludable). *Grade 4*: the space is equal to the corneal thickness (open angle)

2.3.1 Shaffer's System

The Shaffer's system describes the angle between the iris and the trabecular meshwork [9].

The angle is recorded in degrees of arc subtended by two imaginary tangential lines: a line tangential to the inner surface of the trabeculum and the other line tangential to the iris surface about one-third of the distance from its periphery. In practice, the angle is graded according to the visibility of various angle structures. Angle >20° is considered open. The system assigns a numerical grade (4-0) to each angle with associated anatomical description, angle width in degrees, and implied clinical interpretation (Fig. 2.36).

- *Grade 4* (35-45°) is the widest angle in which the ciliary body can be visualized, closure is impossible
- *Grade 3* (20–35°) is an open angle in which the scleral spur can be identified, closure is impossible.
- *Grade 2* (20°) is a moderately narrow angle in which only the trabeculum can be identified; angle closure is possible but unlikely.
- *Grade 1* (10°) is a very narrow angle in which only Schwalbe's line can be identified; there is a high risk of angle closure.
- *Slit angle* no angle structures can be identified; this angle has the danger of imminent closure.
- *Grade 0* (0°) is a closed angle; there is iridocorneal contact, and it is not possible to recognize the apex of the corneal wedge.

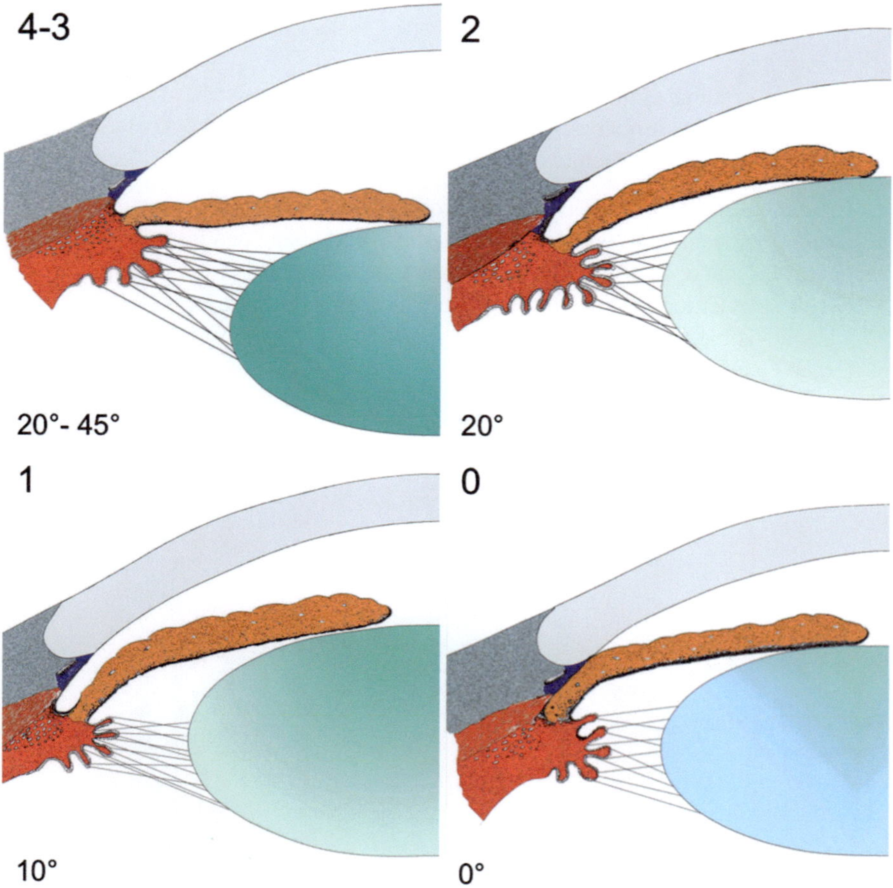

Fig. 2.36 The Shaffer's System

2.3.2 *Scheie Grading System*

The Scheie grading system describes with Roman numerals the degree of angle closure, with larger numbers signifying a narrower angle; the system is based on the extent of visible angle structures (Fig. 2.37) [10].

- *Grade 0* the widest angle in which the ciliary body can be seen.
- *Grade I* wide angle in which a narrow ciliary body band can be seen.
- *Grade II* is an open angle in which at least the scleral spur can be identified.
- *Grade III* is a moderate narrow angle in which only the anterior trabecular meshwork is visible.
- *Grade IV* angle is closed.

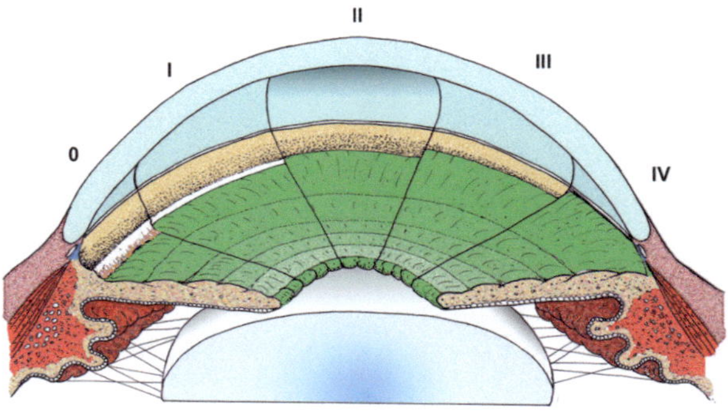

Fig. 2.37 The Scheie grading system

2.3.3 *Spaeth System*

The Spaeth system grades three aspects of angle configuration [12]:

2.3.3.1 Angular Width of Angle Recess

The examiner estimates the width of the angle, considering the angle between a line tangential to the trabecular meshwork and a line tangential to the iris surface about one-third of the way from the periphery (Fig. 2.38).

(a) Slit
(b) 10° Narrow
(c) 20°
(d) 30° Wide
(e) 40°

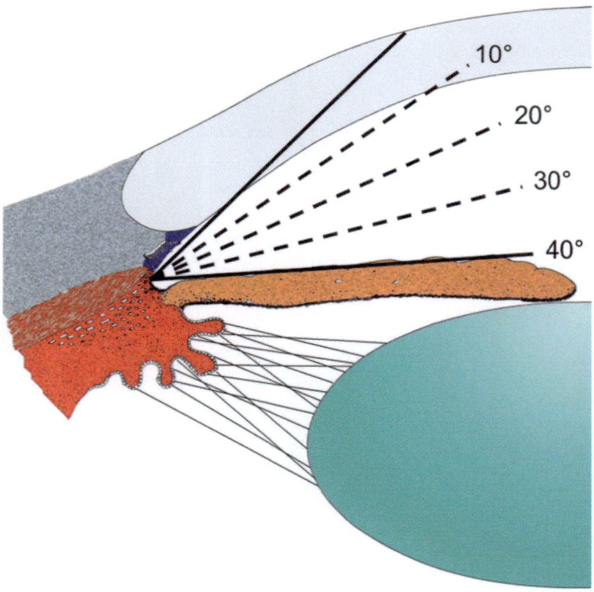

Fig. 2.38 The Spaeth System: angular width of angle recess

2.3.3.2 Level of Iris Insertion (Fig. 2.39)

(a) Anterior: iris insertion anterior to the Schwalbe's line
(b) Behind Schwalbe's line: iris insertion behind the Schwalbe's line
(c) Centered on sclera: on the scleral spur
(d) Deep to scleral spur: behind the scleral spur
(e) Extremely deep: on the ciliary band

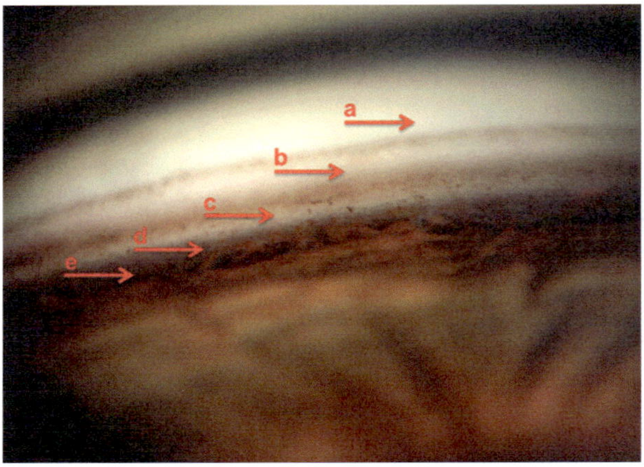

Fig. 2.39 The Spaeth System: level of iris insertion. The letters on the (*arrows*) identifies the level of the iris insertion (Anterior, Behind Schwalbe's line, Centered on the sclera, Deep to scleral spur, Extremely deep)

2.3.3.3 Iris Configuration (Fig. 2.40)

s: steep, anteriorly convex
r: regular or flat
q: queer, anteriorly concave.

It also considers the grade of *trabecular meshwork pigmentation (TMP)* from 1 (minimal) to 4 (dense) (Fig. 2.41).

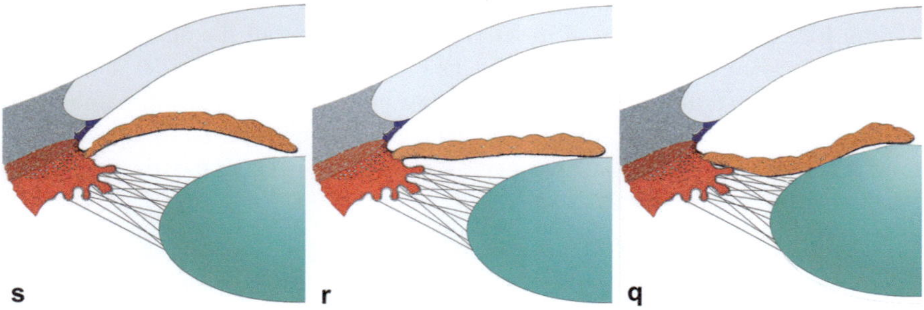

Fig. 2.40 The Spaeth System: iris configuration

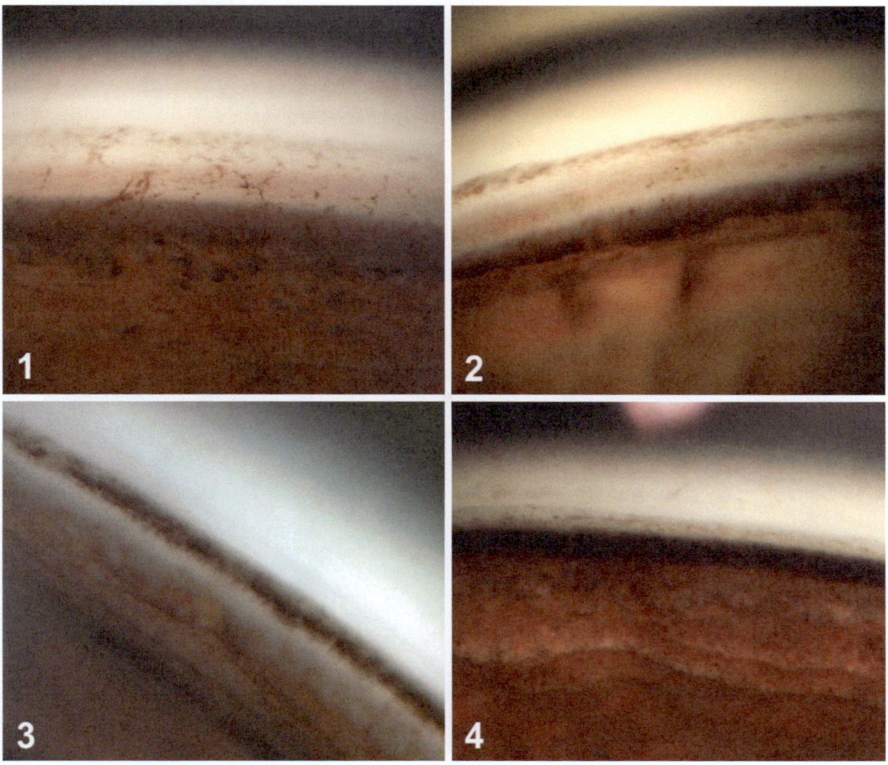

Fig. 2.41 The Spaeth System: trabecular meshwork pigmentation

2.4 Pathology

2.4.1 Congenital and Developmental Glaucoma

In infants gonioscopy is performed using Koeppe lens or the Swan-Jacob lens; the baby could be sedated for the examination on the operating microscope; but the examination could also be performed at the office. Gonioscopy distinguishes primary congenital glaucoma from secondary glaucoma and is really helpful in planning surgery. Congenital glaucoma presents at birth or between 1 month and 2 years of age. It is the consequence of the developmental arrest of the anterior chamber angle tissue; the trabeculo-dysgenesis is the only ocular anomaly in 50 % of cases; with a higher insertion of the iris and ciliary body onto the posterior trabecular beams which causes their compression and creates an obstruction to aqueous outflow. It is typical to observe an open angle with high insertion of the iris root, which forms a line with small curves.

(a) The iris insertion could be at or anterior to the scleral spur (Fig. 2.42), and the ciliary body is covered by this insertion and is not visible (in normal infants the iris inserts flatly on the ciliary body face). The appearance of the trabecular meshwork is orange peel and the iris stroma may be thin and may expose radial blood vessels.
(b) The iris insertion could be into the chamber angle. The plane of the iris is posterior to the scleral spur, but the anterior stroma inserts just behind the Schwalbe's line.

Usually, abnormal tissue with a glistening appearance is seen in the angle and seems to pull the peripheral iris anteriorly. Above the iris root loops of vessels from the major arterial circle are sometimes visible, and there could be a fine tissue covering the peripheral iris, which usually is thinner and flatter.

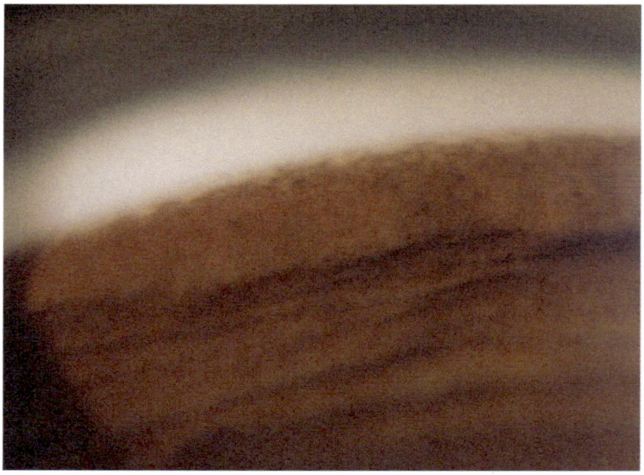

Fig. 2.42 Congenital glaucoma. The iris insertion is at the Schwalbe's line

2.4.1.1 Axenfeld-Rieger Syndrome

Axenfeld-Rieger Syndrome is a set of diseases, which includes Axenfeld anomaly (posterior embryotoxon associated with iridocorneal adhesions) (Fig. 2.43); Axenfeld syndrome (Axenfeld anomaly with glaucoma) (Fig. 2.44); Rieger anomaly (Axenfeld anomaly, iris stromal thinning, iris hole, corectopia); and Rieger Syndrome (Rieger anomaly with systemic developmental anomalies) (Fig. 2.45) [16].

Glaucoma originates from the developmental arrest of the anterior segment tissue derived from the neural crest cells.

Typical gonioscopic features are:

1. Anteriorly displaced Schwalbe's line (posterior embryotoxon) (Fig. 2.17); sometimes the line is suspended from the cornea by a thin membrane.
2. Tissue strands in the anterior chamber angle; similar in color and texture to the iris (Fig. 2.46).
3. Open angle.
4. The scleral spur is covered by the iris insertion.

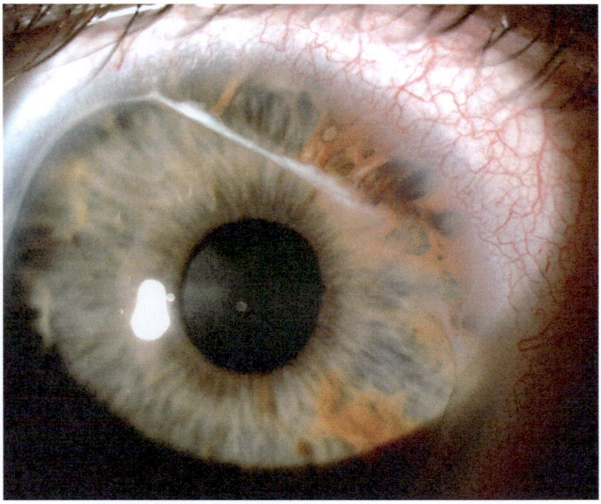

Fig. 2.43 Axenfeld syndrome. Irido-corneal adhesions at biomicroscopy

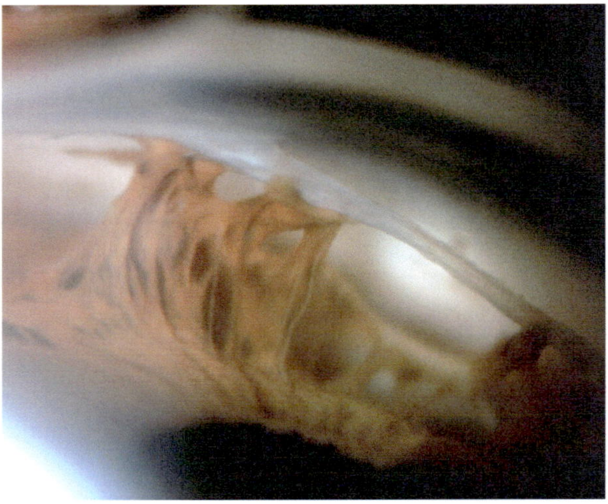

Fig. 2.44 Gonioscopy of the same patient. Tissue strands in the anterior chamber

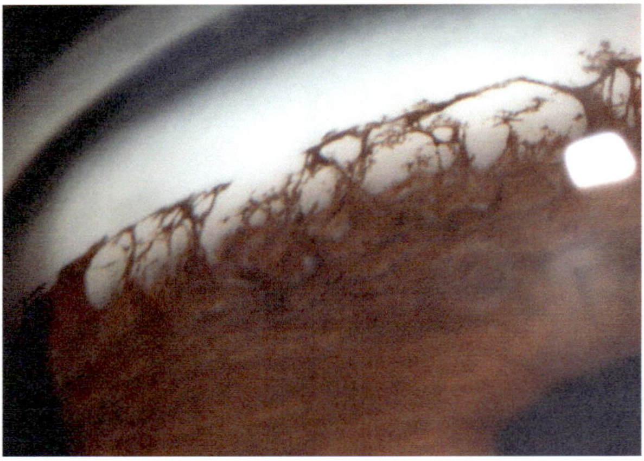

Fig. 2.45 Rieger syndrome

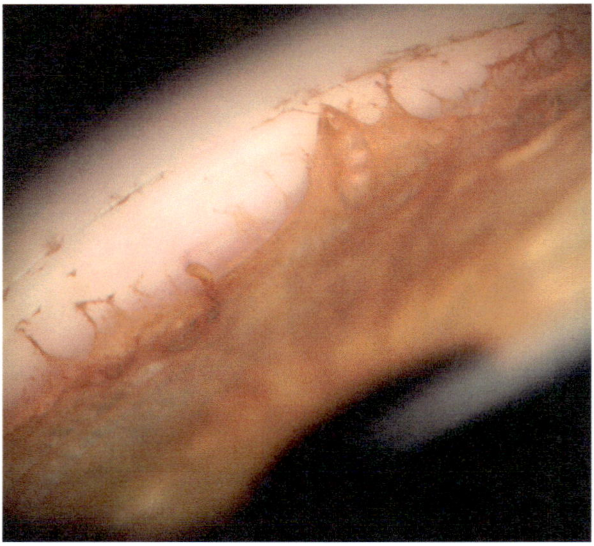

Fig. 2.46 Axenfeld syndrome. Tissue strands in the anterior chamber angle

2.4.1.2 Aniridia

Aniridia is characterized by the absence of the iris; even if at gonioscopy a rudimentary stump of the iris is usually present (Figs. 2.47 and 2.48) [17]. The angle is open and sometimes strands of tissue in the angle with fine blood vessels extending from the iris root to the trabecular meshwork are visible. In 10–15 years the angle progressively closes and the iris comes to lie over the trabecular meshwork.

Gonioscopy can demonstrate anomaly of the angle in primary and secondary developmental glaucoma. It is possible to observe anterior iris insertion, prominent iris process, and featureless angle. Iris processes are the remnants of normal development of angle and can be a normal variation.

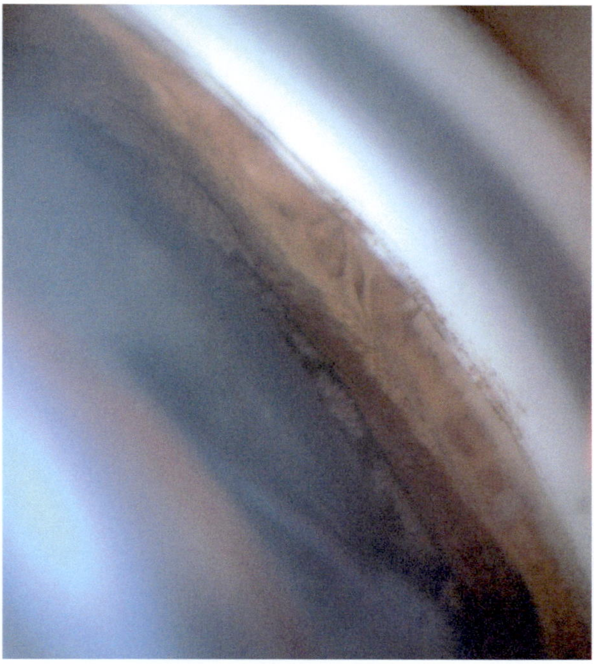

Fig. 2.47 Aniridia. A small part of the iris is visible

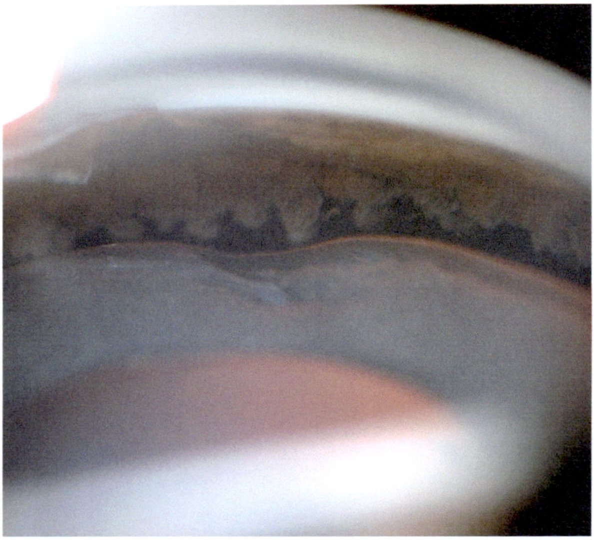

Fig. 2.48 Aniridia. The ciliary body is visible. It is visible also a blue loop of the IOL in the bag

2.4.2 *Open Angle Glaucomas*

2.4.2.1 Pseudoexfoliation Syndrome

The deposition of fibrillar protein matrix throughout the anterior segment (on the lens, the angle, the iris, the corneal endothelium, the zonula and the ciliary body) is the main feature of this syndrome. In these patients the IOP can increase to higher values than in POAG patients. It is very important to observe the angle to recognize the syndrome [18] even if the severity of the material deposition cannot be related to an increased risk of glaucoma development. It is possible to observe flecks of exfoliation material adherent to the trabecular meshwork (Fig. 2.49) and pigmentation may be increased with a discontinuous segmental distribution (Fig. 2.50) [19]. A scalloped band of pigment running anterior to the Schwalbe's line (Sampaolesi's line) is frequent (Figs. 2.51 and 2.52).

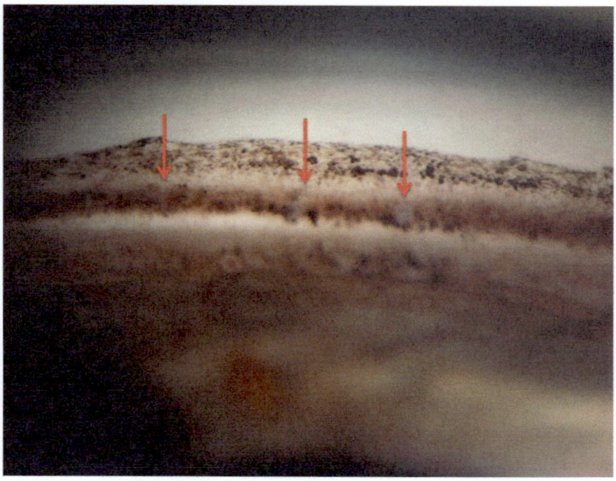

Fig. 2.49 Flecks of exfoliation material adherent to the trabecular meshwork (*red arrows*) in pseudoexfoliation syndrome

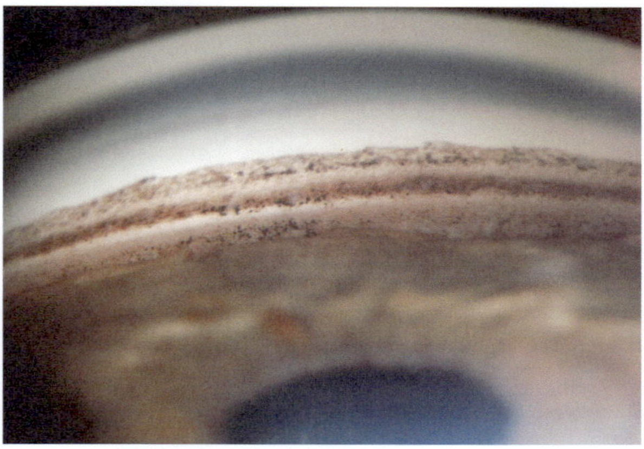

Fig. 2.50 The discontinuous distribution of the pigment throughout the angle in pseudoexfoliative glaucoma

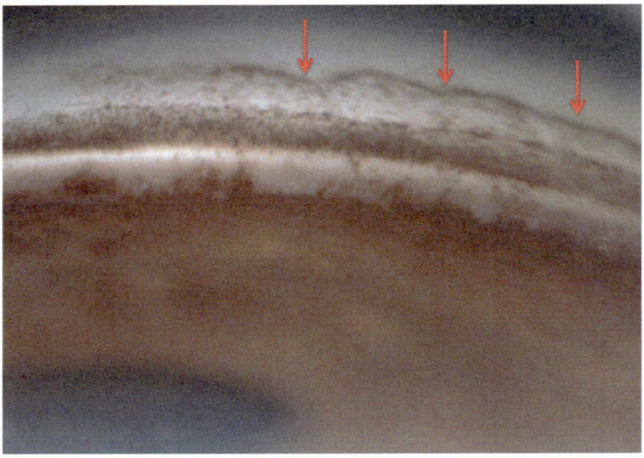

Fig. 2.51 The Sampaolesi's line (*red arrow*) above the Schwalbe's line

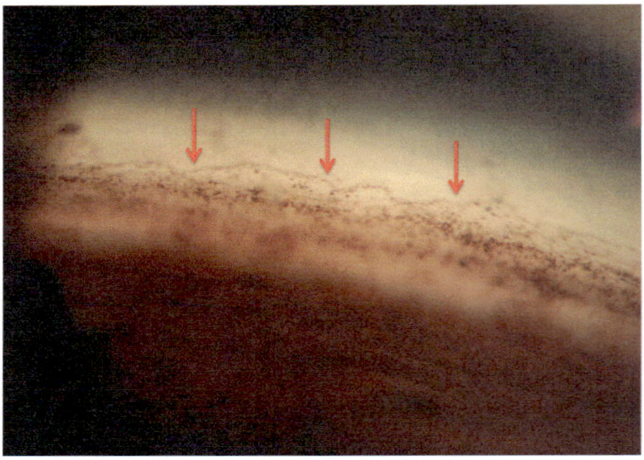

Fig. 2.52 The Sampaolesi's line (*red arrow*) in pseudoexfoliative glaucoma

2.4.2.2 Pigment Dispersion Syndrome

Pigment dispersion syndrome is usually a bilateral disorder characterized by the liberation of pigment granules from the iris pigment epithelium and their deposition throughout the anterior segment, mainly in the trabecular meshwork. The diagnosis is possible by the slit-lamp observing mid-peripheral iris trans-illumination defects, diffuse and dense brownish pigmentation of the angle, and pigment granules on the corneal endothelium (Krukenberg spindle) [20]. The angle is open with a deeper anterior chamber both because the iris could be more posterior inserted or the iris stroma could be floppy. The iris has a marked concave configuration in the mid periphery (Fig. 2.53). The pigment distribution can be positioned over all the angle structures (Fig. 2.54), even if usually a homogeneous dense, very dark band covering the trabecular meshwork can be observed (Figs. 2.55, 2.56, and 2.57) [21].

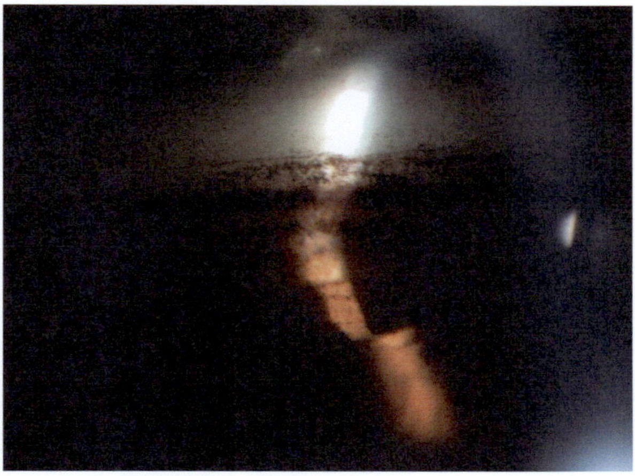

Fig. 2.53 In pigment dispersion syndrome there is a wide concavity of the iris profile

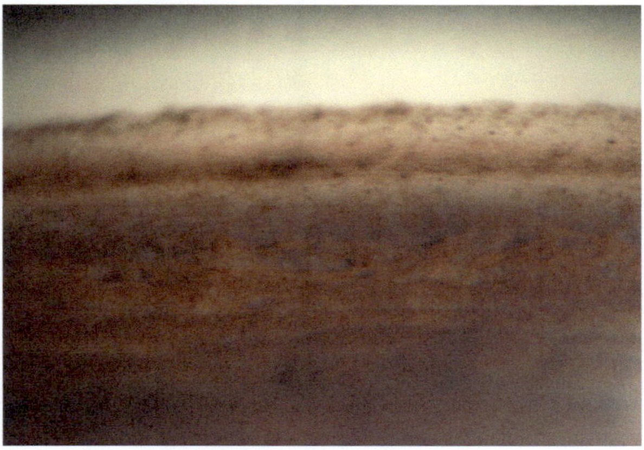

Fig. 2.54 Deposition of pigment all over the angle structures

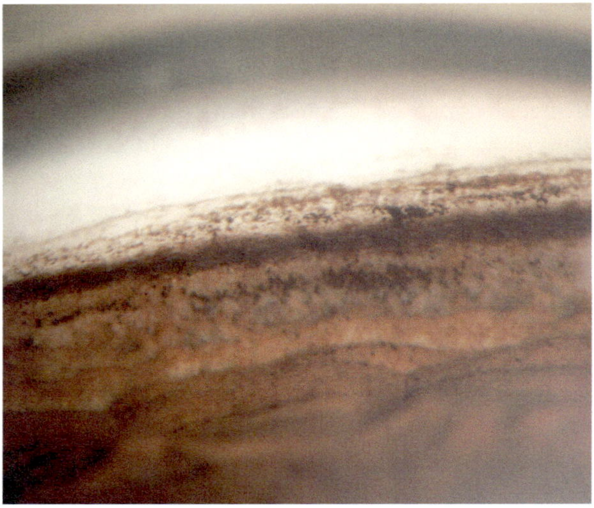

Fig. 2.55 Pigmentary glaucoma. Deposition of pigment mainly on the trabecular meshwork

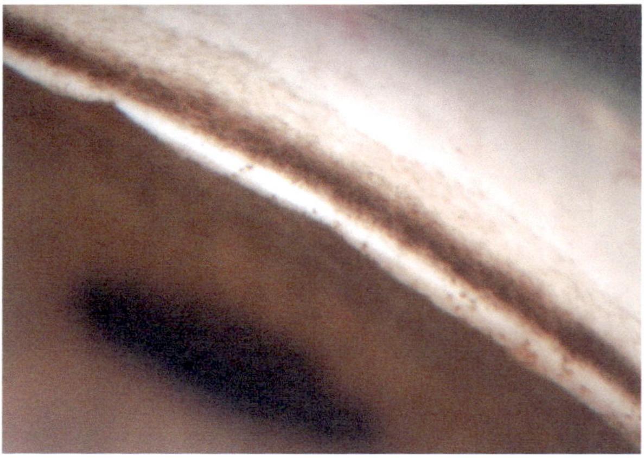

Fig. 2.56 Deposition of pigment over the trabecular meshwork. The Sampaolesi's line and the scleral spur are visible

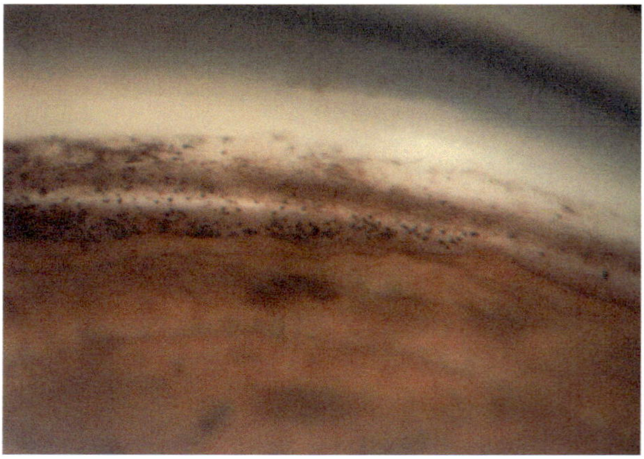

Fig. 2.57 Pigment granules in the angle

2.4.2.3 Post-traumatic Glaucoma

Gonioscopy must be performed in every patient with unexplained unilateral glaucoma or in patients with a history of ocular trauma, even after many years [22]. Many different signs may be observed after a blunt trauma. A bleeding vessel may be noted (Fig. 2.30), a blood clot may obscure the angle structures (Fig. 2.58) or blood may be present in the Schlemm's canal (Figs. 2.29 and 2.30). An increased irregular pigmentation after anterior inflammation (Fig. 2.59) or peripheral anterior synechiae (Figs. 2.60 and 2.61) may be observed. The posterior displacement of the iris root, the angle recession (Fig. 2.62), or an iridodialysis (Figs. 2.63 and 2.64) could lead more frequently to a post-traumatic glaucoma. An irregularly broadened ciliary body band must be compared with the fellow eye to diagnose an angle recession.

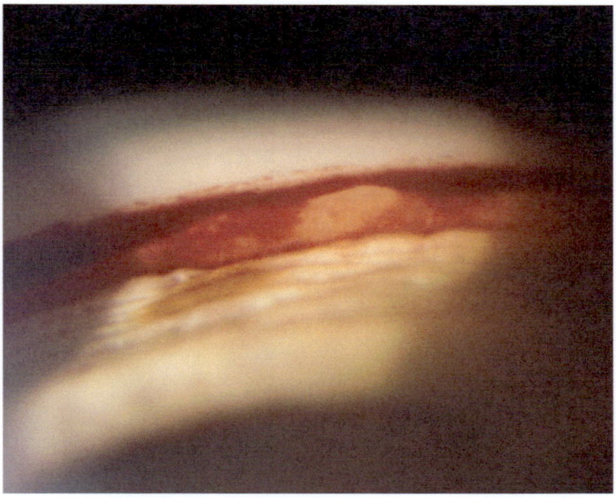

Fig. 2.58 Post-traumatic hyphema covering the angle landmarks

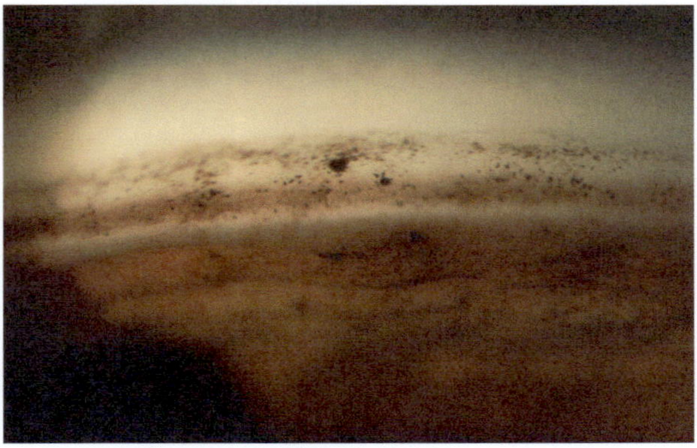

Fig. 2.59 Pigment granules in the angle after an iridociclitis

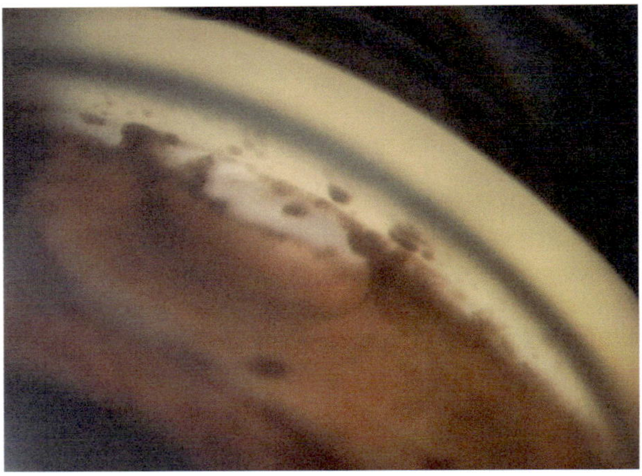

Fig. 2.60 Wide angular synechiae and precipitates in anterior uveitis

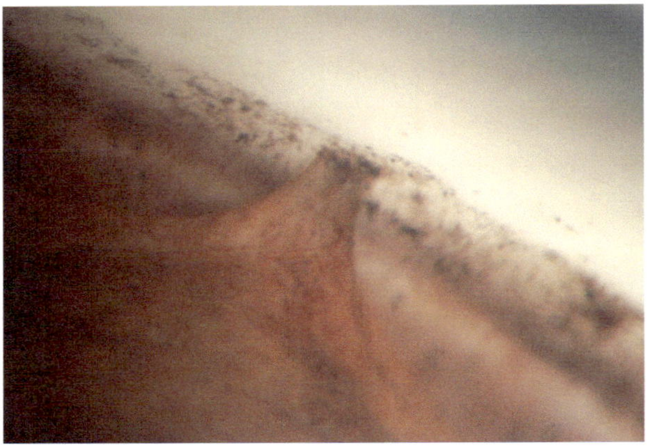

Fig. 2.61 A peripheral anterior synechia

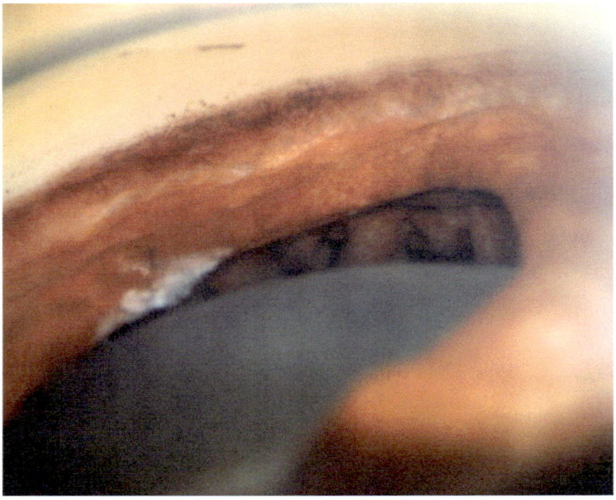

Fig. 2.62 A post-traumatic angle recession, mydriasis, lens subluxation, and ciliary body visualization

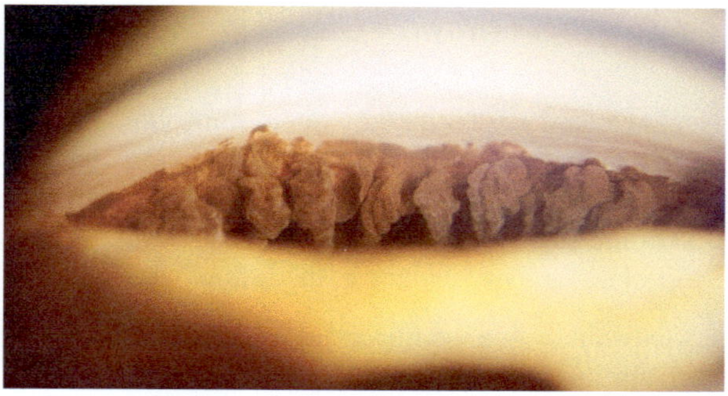

Fig. 2.63 A wide iridodialysis with visualization of the ciliary processes

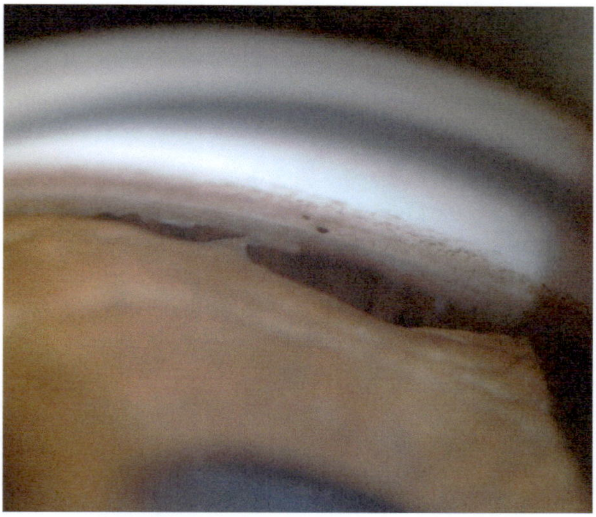

Fig. 2.64 Iridodyalisis

2.4.3 *Angle Closure Glaucomas*

Angle closure is identified by gonioscopy, the "reference standard" diagnostic procedure. A narrow angle recess, usually narrower than 20°, characterizes primary angle closure. Fundamental during gonioscopy is the manipulation and the indentation of the angle to establish if the closure is appositional or synechial.

Looking at a narrow angle, the following features should be evaluated [4, 23]

1. Schwalbe's line visible or not; if not the angle is closed (Fig. 2.65).
2. Trabecular meshwork visible or not; if not in at least three quadrants in primary position without manipulation, the angle can be classified as occludable (Fig. 2.66).
3. Evidence of a previous angle closure attack: goniosynechiae, peripheral anterior synechiae, glaukomflecken, iris atrophy, increased or pattern pigmentation.
4. Symmetry of gonioscopic findings between the two eyes and between the superior and inferior quadrants of the same eye (Figs. 2.67 and 2.68).

Primary angle closure may become chronic after an acute attack or due to the long-term use of miotics [24]. The angle is permanently closed and PAS can be easily identified by indentation gonioscopy [25]. Laser iridotomy is mandatory in angle closure glaucoma and gonioscopy should be repeated at least every 6 months to identify any possible change even if there is a patent iridotomy. Irido-trabecular apposition after iridotomy suggests a secondary mechanism of angle closure; mechanisms of secondary angle closure include disorders of the ciliary body, lens-induced angle closure (phacomorphic glaucoma) or malignant glaucoma with a misdirection of the aqueous humor [26]. The treatment of all these types of glaucoma is related to the identification of the underlying pathophysiology.

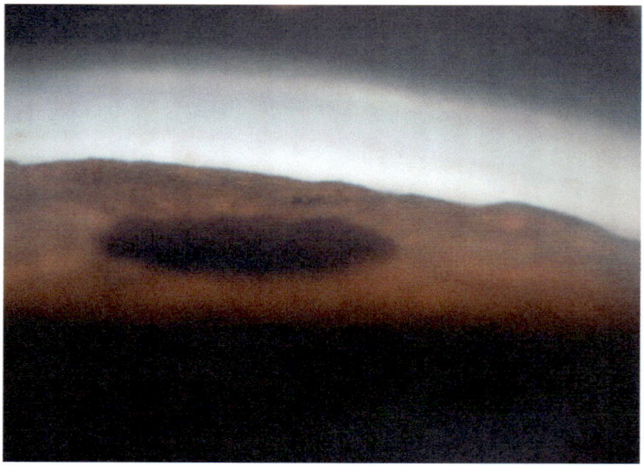

Fig. 2.65 Angle closure. The Schwalbe's line is not visible

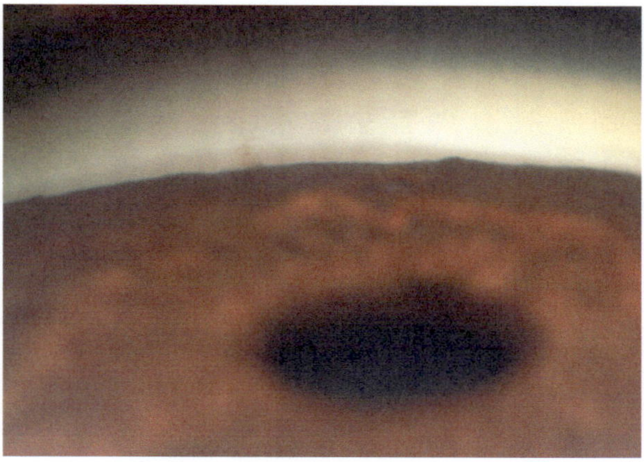

Fig. 2.66 Occludable angle. The trabecular meshwork is visible under the Schwalbe's line

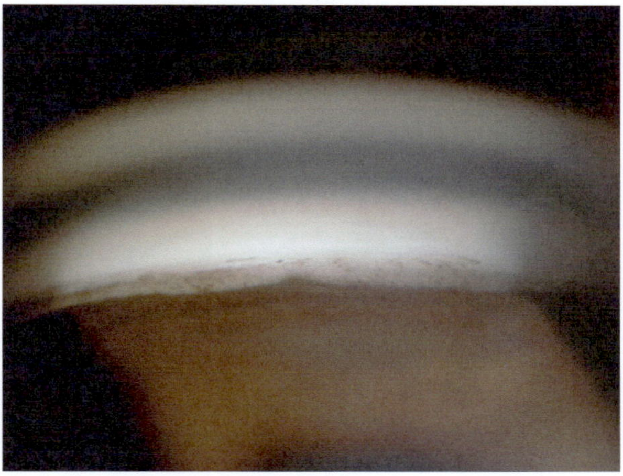

Fig. 2.67 The inferior sector of an angle. The Schwalbe's line and the trabecular meshwork are visible

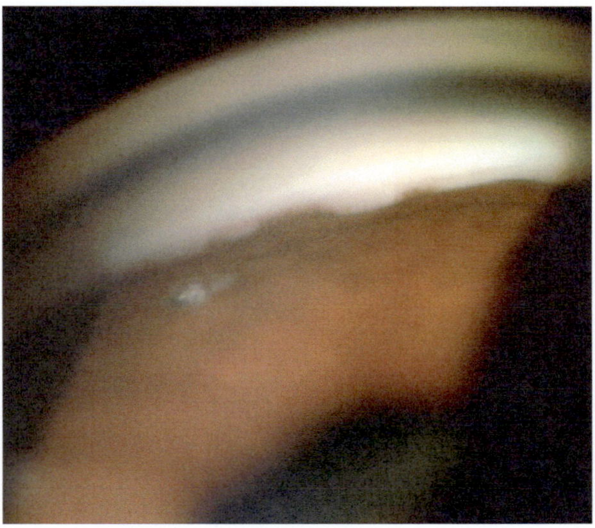

Fig. 2.68 The superior sector of the same eye. Some synechiae are visible and the angle is partially closed. An iridotomy is also visible

2.4.3.1 Iridocorneal Endothelial (Ice) Syndrome

ICE syndrome is a rare disorder, more frequent in young to middle-aged females, characterized by unilateral angle closure glaucoma. There are some typical features of these groups of disorders, first of all an abnormal physiology of the endothelium, then corneal edema and progressive iris atrophy. There are three types of the disease:

- Chandler's syndrome (corneal edema predominates)
- Iris Nevus/Cogan Reese Syndrome (nodular iris lesions are present associated with corneal and iris defects)
- Progressive iris atrophy (iris changes predominate with corectopia, atrophy, and hole formation).

Peripheral anterior synechiae are common findings at gonioscopic examination; PAS usually extends anterior to the Shwalbe's line [16]. These result from contraction of endothelial cell layers and fibrous tissue that extends from the corneal endothelium onto the trabecular meshwork and the iris (Fig. 2.69).

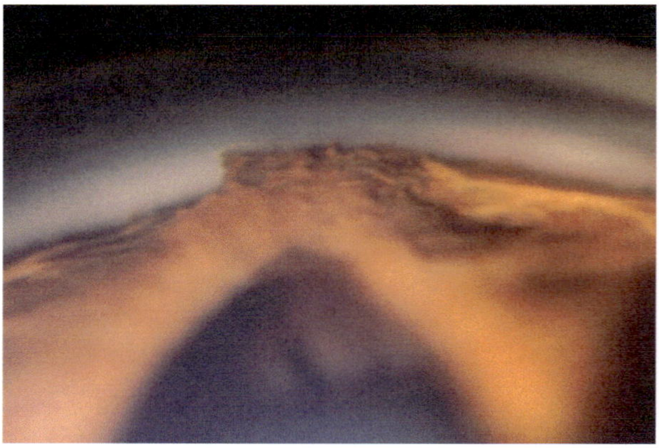

Fig. 2.69 Irido-corneal-endothelial syndrome. A wide goniosynechia is visible

2.4.3.2 Uveitic Glaucoma

Inflammation in uveitis leads to hypersecretion of aqueous humor and to obstruction of the trabecular meshwork by serum components and inflammatory precipitates (Fig. 2.70), trabeculitis, scarring of trabecular meshwork and peripheral anterior synechiae formation. As a consequence, the intraocular pressure rises and glaucoma develops. In uveitic glaucoma the angle can be open or closed. Closed angle glaucoma is related to several mechanisms: pupillary block, iris bombe, PAS (Fig. 2.60), anterior rotation of lens iris diaphragm or neovascularization. The IOP rise can develop both during the acute phase of the inflammation for trabecular obstruction or later on, due to the scarring of the trabecular meshwork. Observing the anterior chamber angle after iridocyclitis, a typical clod deposition of pigment may be noted (Fig. 2.59). Other frequent findings after inflammation are the anterior peripheral synechiae that can be small or tent-shaped and the angle that remains open (Figs. 2.61 and 2.71). But PAS can also be larger, causing a secondary angle closure (Fig. 2.72).

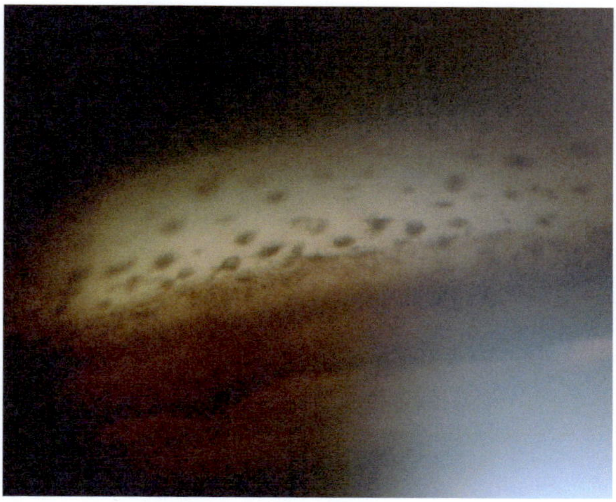

Fig. 2.70 Acute anterior uveitis. Endothelial inflammatory precipitates

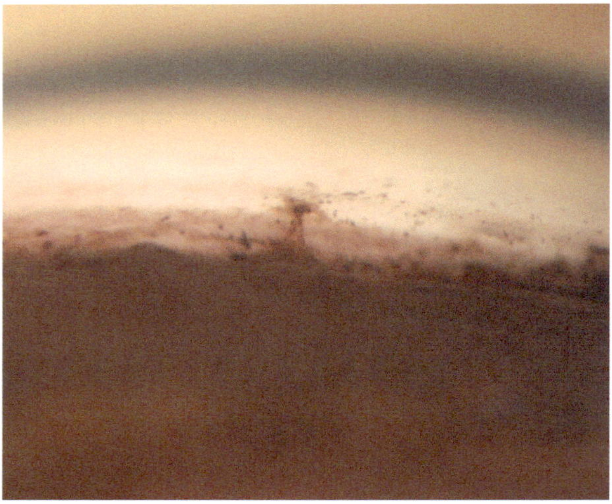

Fig. 2.71 Anterior synechia adherent to the Schwalbe's line

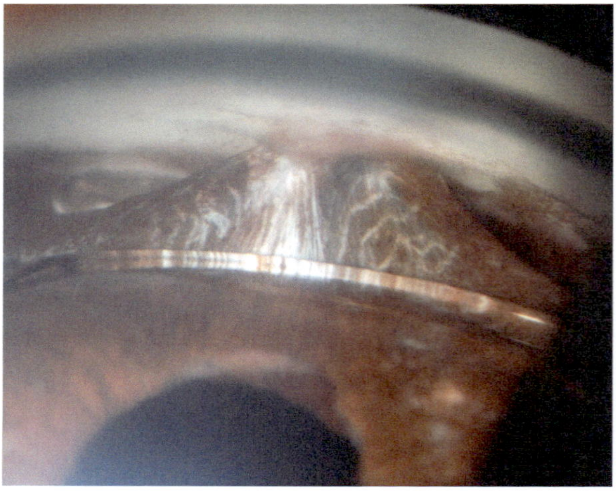

Fig. 2.72 A wide anterior sinechia. The edge of an anterior chamber IOL is visible

2.4.3.3 Neovascular Glaucoma

Retinal ischemia may lead to a neovascularization of the angle till the development of a neovascular glaucoma. This disease has a pre-glaucoma stage, an open angle glaucoma stage and an angle closure glaucoma stage. In the first stage, neovascularization appears on the pupillary margin or in the angle. Vascular trunks may cross the scleral spur and arborize irregularly on the trabecular meshwork. In the second stage, there is a fine fibrous membrane, invisible on gonioscopy, obstructing the aqueous flow [27] (Fig. 2.73). In the angle closure stage, the fibrovascular membrane pulls the iris toward the trabecular meshwork with peripheral anterior synechiae formation [28] (Fig. 2.74).

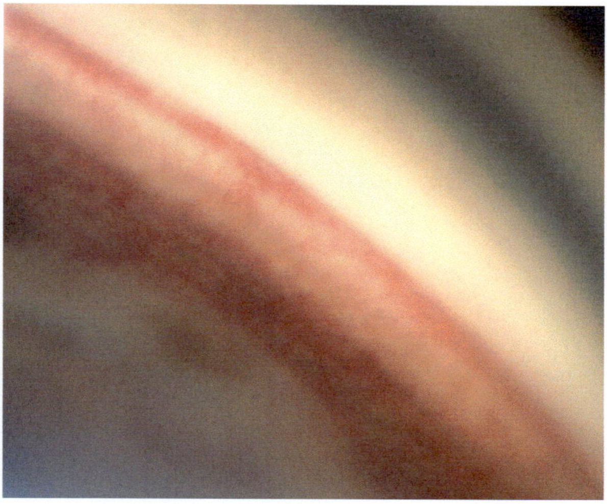

Fig. 2.73 Neovascular glaucoma. Vascular trunks cross the scleral spur. The Schlemm's canal also is filled with blood

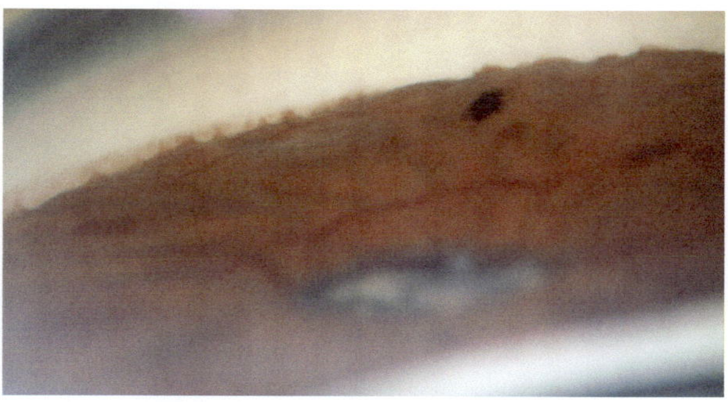

Fig. 2.74 New vessels on the iris surface. A secondary angle closure is present

2.4.4 Post-surgical Evaluation of the Anterior Chamber Angle

After filtering surgery gonioscopy is critical to understand the outcome of the surgery. Trabeculectomy represents the gold standard for glaucoma surgery (Fig. 2.75), and with gonioscopy it is possible to study the site where the trabecular tissue is removed during surgery and the site of iridectomy. Sometimes, a rise in IOP can be due to the obstruction of this site by anterior synechiae or any other material (Figs. 2.76, 2.77, and 2.78).

Vitreoretinal surgery sometimes can cause glaucoma; a rise of intraocular pressure may be observed in early postoperative period due to overfilling of the posterior chamber with silicon oil or gas. But also secondary glaucoma may develop for the obstruction of the trabecular meshwork by emulsified silicon oil (Fig. 2.79). Sometimes, perfluorocarbon liquid bubbles can also be observed in the inferior sector as a remnant of intraoperative tamponade to lay down the retina (Fig. 2.80).

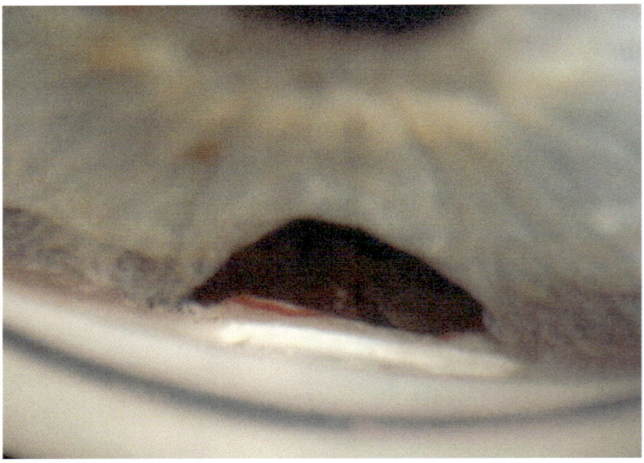

Fig. 2.75 Trabeculectomy. A large vessel is visible in the sclerostomy site

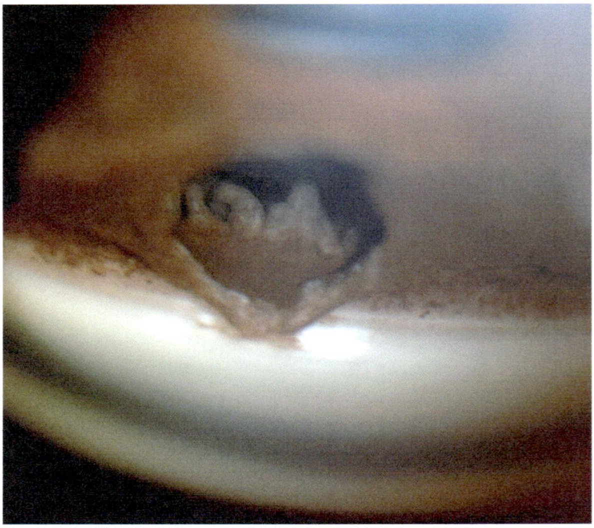

Fig. 2.76 Partially closed trabeculectomy by a basal synechia due to a too central iridectomy

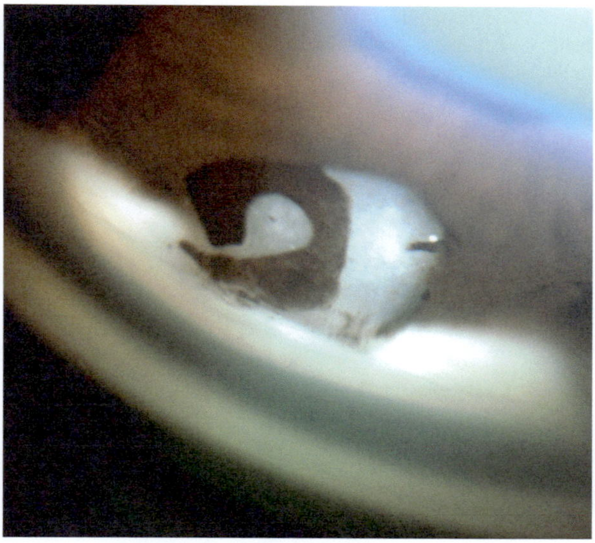

Fig. 2.77 Remnant of a cataract occluding the iridectomy and the trabeculectomy

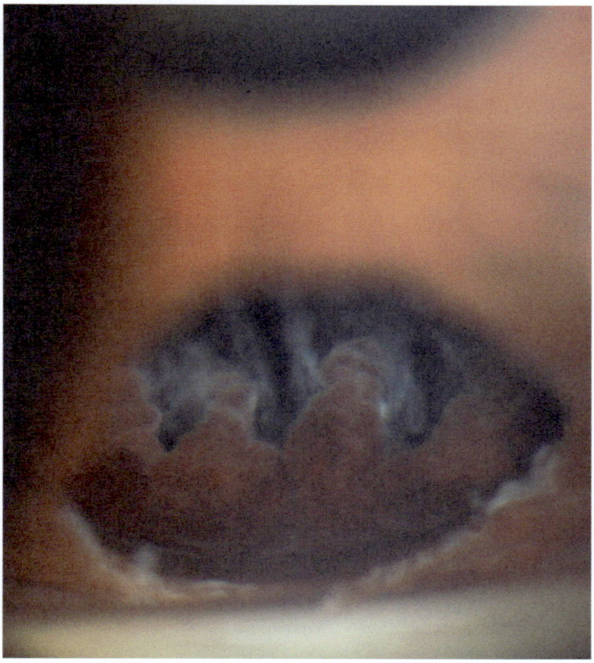

Fig. 2.78 Through the iridectomy, it is possible to observe the ciliary body and exfoliative material over the ciliary processes

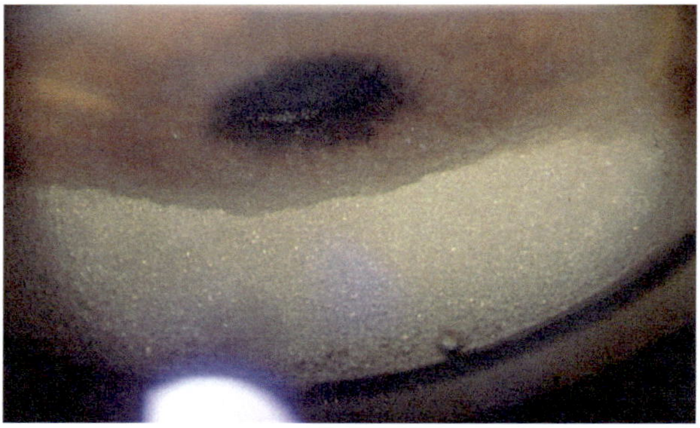

Fig. 2.79 Silicon oil bubbles occlude the angle in the superior sector

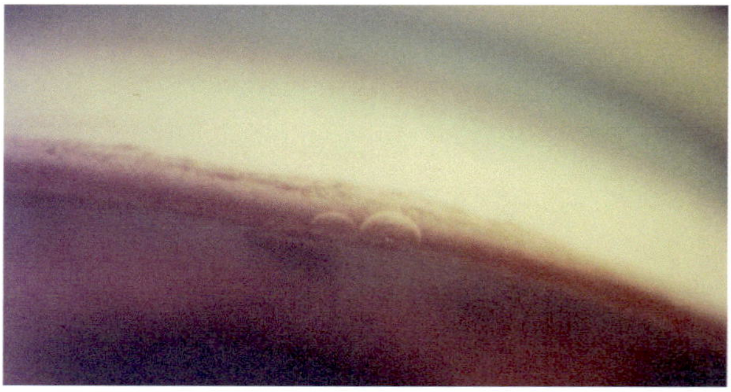

Fig. 2.80 Perfluorocarbon liquid bubbles in the inferior sector as remnant of vitreous surgery

References

1. Trantas A (1918) L'ophthalmoscopie de l'angle irido-cornéen (gonioscopie). Arch Ophthalmol 36:257–276
2. Salzmann M (1914) Die Ophthalmoskopie der Kammberbucht. Z Augenheilk 31:1–19
3. Salzmann M (1915) Nachtrag zu Ophthalmoskopie der Kammberbucht. Z Augenheilk 34:160–162
4. Curran EJ (1920) A new operation for glaucoma involving a new principle in the etiology and treatment of chronic primary glaucoma. Arch Ophthalmol 49:131
5. Koeppe A (1920) Das stereo-mikroskopische Bild des lebenden Kammerwinkels an der Nernstspaltlampe bein Glaukom. Klin Monatsbl Augenheilk 65:389–391
6. Troncoso MU (1925) Gonioscopy and its clinical applications. Am J Ophthalmol 8:433–439
7. Barkan O, Boyle SF, Maisler S (1936) On the genesis of glaucoma. An improved method based on slit lamp microscopy of the angle of the anterior chamber. Am J Ophthalmol 19:209–215
8. Sugar HS (1949) Newer conceptions in the classification of the glaucomas. Am J Ophthalmol 32:425–433
9. Shaffer RN, Tour RL (1956) A comparative study of gonioscopic methods. Am J Ophthalmol 41:256–265
10. Scheie HG (1957) Width and pigmentation of the angle of the anterior chamber; a system of grading by gonioscopy. Arch Ophthalmol 58:510–512
11. Goldmann H (1968) Biomicroscopy of the eye. Am J Ophthalmol 66:789–804
12. Spaeth GL (1971) The normal development of the human anterior chamber angle: a new system of descriptive grading. Trans Ophthalmol Soc UK 91:709–739
13. Dada T, Sharma R, Sobti A (2013) Gonioscopy. A text and atlas. Jaipee Borthers, New Delhi
14. Fish BM (1993) Gonioscopy of the glaucomas. Butterworth-Heineman, Boston
15. Van Herick W, Shaffer RN, Schwartz A (1969) Estimation of width of angle of anterior chamber. Incidence and significance of the narrow angle. Am J Ophthalmol 68:626–629
16. Schields MB (1983) Axenfeld-Rieger syndrome: a theory of mechanism and distinctions from the iridocorneal endothelial syndrome. Trans Am Ophthalmol Soc 81:736–784
17. Grant WM, Walton DS (1974) Progressive changes in the angle in congenital aniridia with development of glaucoma. Am J Ophthalmol 78:842–847
18. Prince AM, Streeten BW, Ritch R, Dark AJ, Sperling M (1987) Preclinical diagnosis of pseudoexfoliation syndrome. Arch Ophthalmol 105:1076–1082
19. Ritch R (1994) Exfoliation syndrome and occludable angles. Trans Am Ophthalmol Soc 92:845–944
20. Lehto I, Vesti E (1998) Diagnosis and management of pigmentary glaucoma. Curr Opin Ophthalmol 9:61–64
21. Lichter PR, Shaffer RN (1970) Iris processes and glaucoma. Am J Ophthalmol 70:905–911
22. Blanton FM (1964) Anterior chamber angle recession and secondary glaucoma. A study of the aftereffects of traumatic hyphemas. Arch Ophthalmol 72:39–43
23. Chandler PA (1952) Narrow-angle glaucoma. Arch Ophthalmol 35:1696
24. Pollack IP (1971) Chronic angle-closure glaucoma; diagnosis and treatment in patients with angles that appear open. Arch Ophthalmol 85:676–689
25. Forbes M (1966) Gonioscopy with corneal indentation. A method for distinguishing between appositional closure and synechial closure. Arch Ophthalmol 76:488–492
26. Ritch R (1982) Argon laser treatment for medically unresponsive attacks of angle-closure glaucoma. Am J Ophthalmol 94:197–204
27. Schulze RR (1967) Rubeosis iridis. Am J Ophthalmol 63:487–495
28. John T, Sassani JW, Eagle RC Jr (1983) The myofibroblastic component of rubeosis iridis. Ophthalmology 90:721–728

Chapter 3
Measurement of Intraocular Pressure with Goldmann Applanation Tonometry, Dynamic-Contour Tonometry, and Ocular Response Analyzer

Paolo Fogagnolo, Maurizio Digiuni, and Luca Rossetti

Intraocular pressure (IOP) is an eye parameter of fundamental importance for the diagnosis of several eye conditions, including glaucoma, ocular hypertension, uveitis, and trauma.

Ideally IOP could be directly *measured* only be means of manometry. This technique consists on the cannulation of the anterior chamber using a needle with a double-cutting edge connected to a bottle of sterile saline and to a reference sensor which measures the IOP value as steady state and pulse amplitude.

In clinical settings, manometry is used very rarely – in general only on patients requiring eye surgery for other reasons.

The standard for IOP measurement is tonometry, which consists on the IOP *estimation.*

Several instruments are available to measure IOP, and different classifications have been used for them. Tonometries can be divided on contact and non-contact based on the presence or absence of eye contact to measure IOP. A second classification is based on the mechanism to evaluate IOP (applanation, indentation, applanation-indentation, rebound, dynamic-contour tonometry).

The aim of this chapter is to review the characteristics and clinical advantages and limitations of three tonometries, i.e., Goldmann applanation tonometry, dynamic-contour tonometry, and Ocular Response Analyzer.

P. Fogagnolo (✉) • M. Digiuni • L. Rossetti
Department of Medicine, Surgery and Odontoiatry, Eye Clinic, Ospedale San Paolo, University of Milan, Milan, Italy
e-mail: fogagnolopaolo@googlemail.com

A. Ferreras (ed.), *Glaucoma Imaging*, DOI 10.1007/978-3-319-18959-8_3

3.1 Goldmann Applanation Tonometry

Goldmann applanation tonometry (GAT) is the standard for IOP assessment in clinical settings and it has been used to measure IOP on the vast majority of clinical trials on glaucoma. Most of the knowledge on glaucoma management derives from GAT data.

Applanation tonometry is based on Imbert-Fick's law, which is a modification of Newton's third law of motion:

$$P = F / S$$

where P is pressure, F is force, and S is surface.

In applanation tonometry, IOP is inferred by keeping a constant flattening area (fixed-area applanation tonometry) or force (fixed-force applanation tonometry) and by respectively modulating force or area.

GAT is a fixed-area applanation tonometry: applanated area is a circle with diameter of 3.06 mm; the force exerted to the eyeball is variable. An image of GAT is given in Fig. 3.1.

A prism is mounted on the tonometer head and then placed against the cornea. Because the probe makes contact with the cornea, anesthetic eyedrop is required.

The correct procedure to measure IOP by GAT is reported below.

The examiner puts fluorescein into the conjunctival fornex in order to mark the lacrimal film. A cobalt blue filter is used to view two green semicircles. The force applied to the tonometer head is then adjusted using a dial connected to a variable tension spring until the inner edges of the green semicircles in the viewfinder meet (Fig. 3.2). Figure 3.3 is an example of the process to achieve a correct reading when the tonometer and the eye are correctly positioned, but applanation is not correct and it must be modified by rotating the dial. Figure 3.4 shows errors in probe positioning and their correction.

The amount of fluorescein is directly related to a correct IOP measurement (Fig. 3.5). If fluorescein staining is low, measures tend to be underestimated by 1.5–9.5 mmHg [1]. If fluorescein staining is adequate but there is excessive tearing, semicircles will be broader than normal, and this may cause an overestimation of IOP by 2–4.5 mmHg [2].

Measuring IOP without fluorescein is associated with an underestimation up to 5.5 mmHg [3].

GAT can be influenced by a number of factors, including sclerocorneal characteristics, blepharospasm, and episcleral venous pressure (which may be affected by factors such as ties or tight collars).

Scleral thickness is known to significantly affect ocular hysteresis, but this is not measurable.

On the other hand, the effects of corneal characteristics have been well investigated and it has been confirmed that IOP is affected by the following corneal factors:

(a) Central corneal thickness (CCT)
(b) Astigmatism
(c) Corneal curvature
(d) Corneal edema

(a) Theoretical assumptions of GAT are based on corneas of normal thickness, i.e., 520 μm. CCT affects IOP in the sense that higher CCT is associated with IOP overestimation and vice versa, as shown in the case of Fig. 3.6.

    When evaluating patients' IOP, it is crucially important to know CCT, in order not to misdiagnose patients with low IOP and thin corneas, or subjects with thick corneas and high IOP.

(b) The effect of astigmatism is shown in Fig. 3.7. When regular astigmatism is present, an elliptical contact with tonometer head occurs. This results in an underestimation of IOP in with-the-rule astigmatism and an over estimation with against-the-rule astigmatism. The error may range between –2.5 and +2.5 mmHg [4].

    In order to reduce this error, three options can be used:

    1. Align tonometer head at 43° to axis of astigmatism (in negative cylinder).
    2. Average IOP readings at 0 and 90°.
    3. Average IOP readings at the two main corneal axes.

(c) The effect of corneal curvature is summarized in Fig. 3.8. Steeper corneas give IOP overestimation, as they need to be indented more (i.e., they require more force) to produce the standard area of contact. In contrast, flatter corneas are more easily applanated and this is associated with underestimation. IOP error due to corneal curvature does not exceed 3 mmHg for corneas ranging between 40 and 49 diopters [5].
(d) Corneal edema, particularly epithelial edema, is associated with gross errors in IOP measurement. Edematous epithelium is much easier to indent than normal epithelium, and this may lead to errors ranging from 10 to 30 mmHg [6].

Other limits of GAT are inter-operator variability, which is known to vary up to 2–3 mmHg, and manual reading.

Due to the high number of possible sources of errors, it has been claimed that newer tonometries may be more reliable than GAT. Though this may be true in theory, in practice it should be kept in mind that most glaucoma literatures (and in particular prospective randomized controlled studies) are based only on GAT.

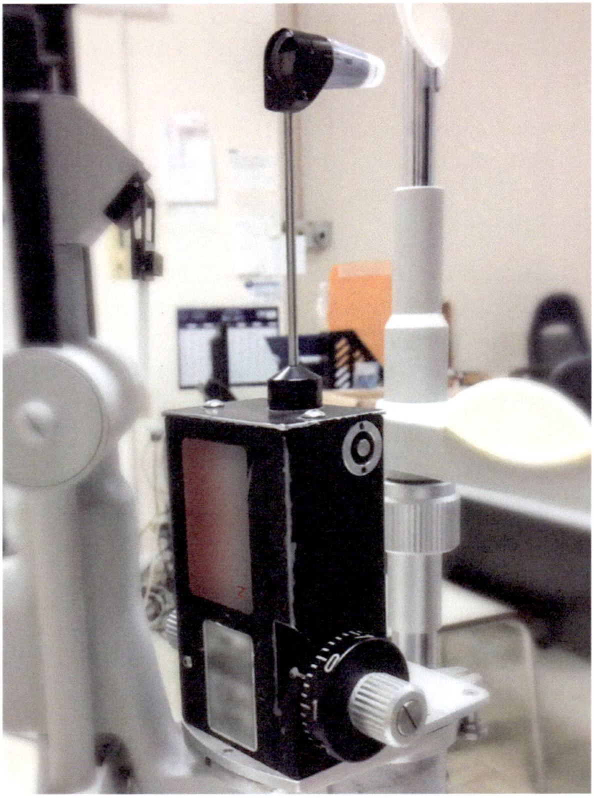

Fig. 3.1 Goldmann applanation tonometer

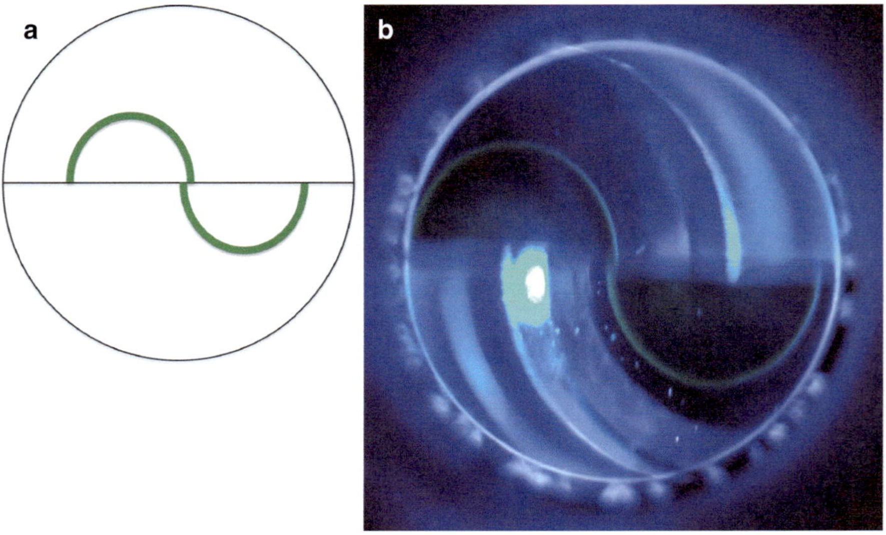

Fig. 3.2 Diagram (**a**) and correct view (**b**) of the semicircles. The correct reading is achieved when the inner edges of the green semicircles in the viewfinder meet

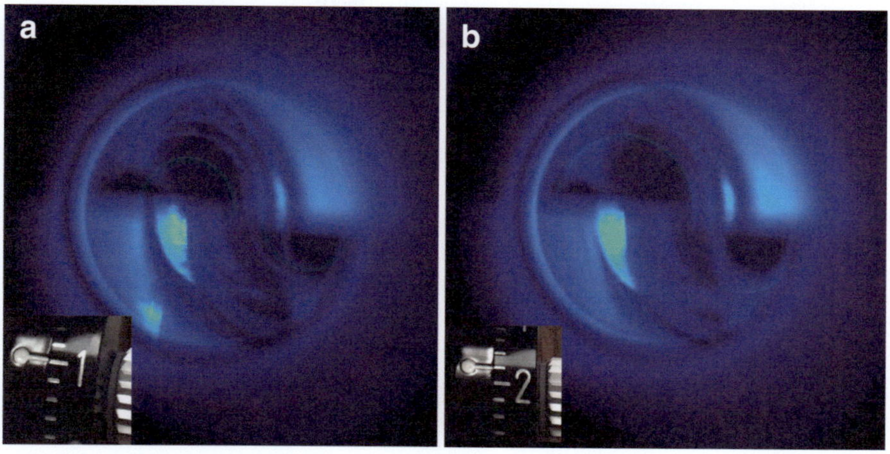

Fig. 3.3 Examples of wrong measurement of IOP. This patient had IOP of 15 mmHg. (**a**) If the tonometer is positioned at 10 mmHg, the two semicircles are too distant. (**b**) If the tonometer is positioned at 18 mmHg, the two semicircles are too close. The correct position to be obtained is the one of Fig. 3.2

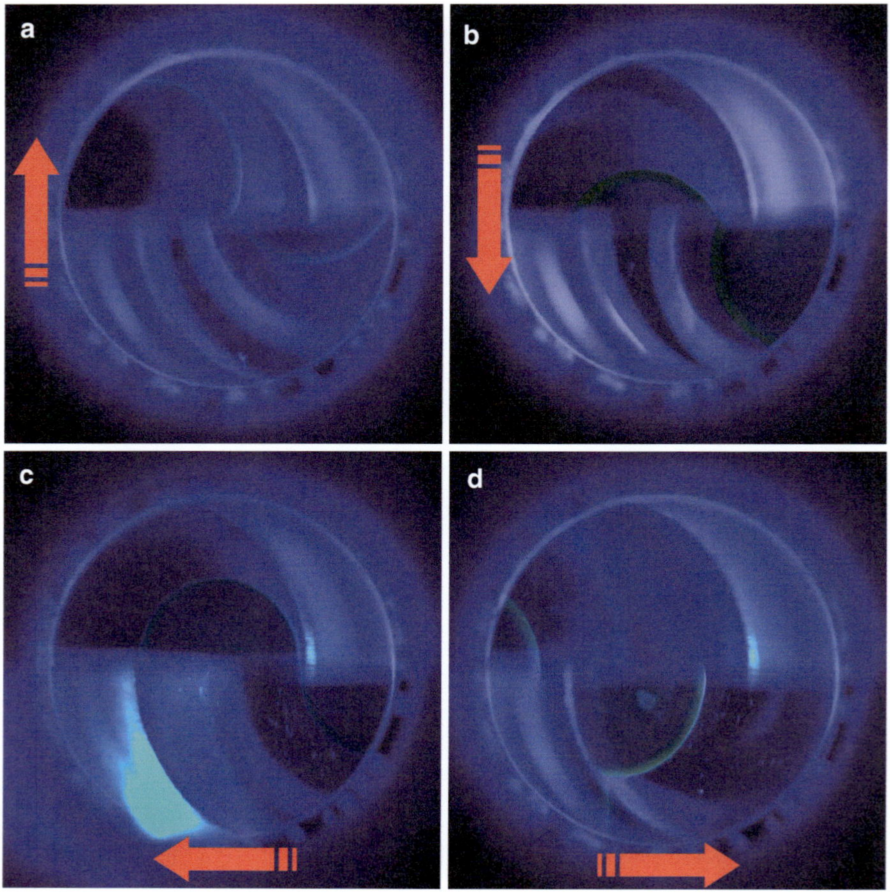

Fig. 3.4 Examples of wrong positioning of the probe. (**a**) The two semicircles are not symmetric: the superior is larger than the inferior. It is necessary to move the tonometer up. (**b**) The two semicircles are not symmetric: the inferior is larger than the superior. It is necessary to move the tonometer down. (**c**) The two semicircles are not symmetric: the left is larger than the right. It is necessary to move the tonometer to the left. (**d**) The two semicircles are not symmetric: the right is larger than the left. It is necessary to move the tonometer to the right

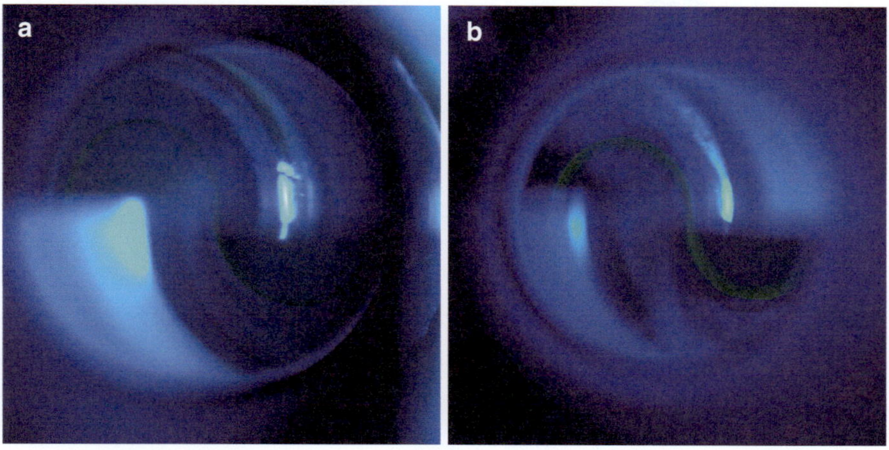

Fig. 3.5 Examples of errors in measurement. (**a**) Inadequate, and (**b**) excessive quantity of fluorescein

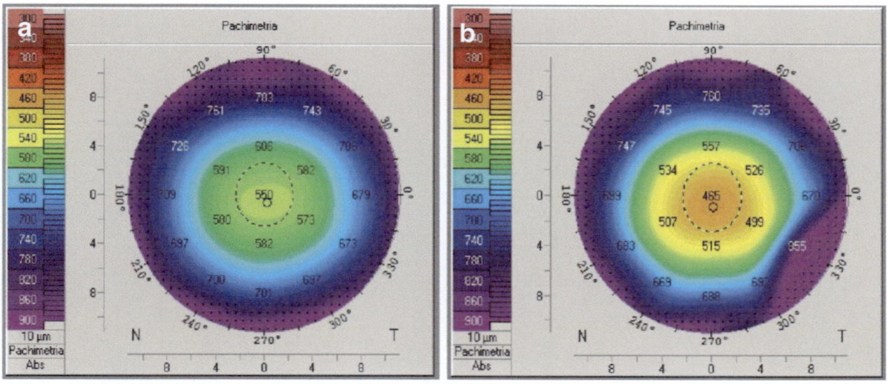

Fig. 3.6 The effects of CCT on IOP readings. A normal subject received photorefractive keratectomy to treat a myopia of −6.5 D; preoperative and postoperative pachimetric maps are given in (**a**, **b**), respectively. A change of 85 μm was induced by treatment, and IOP dropped from 20 mmHg before surgery to 15 mmHg due to the reduction of corneal thickness, with facilitates indentation. In the presence of high-tension glaucoma, such a CCT reduction may confound diagnosis

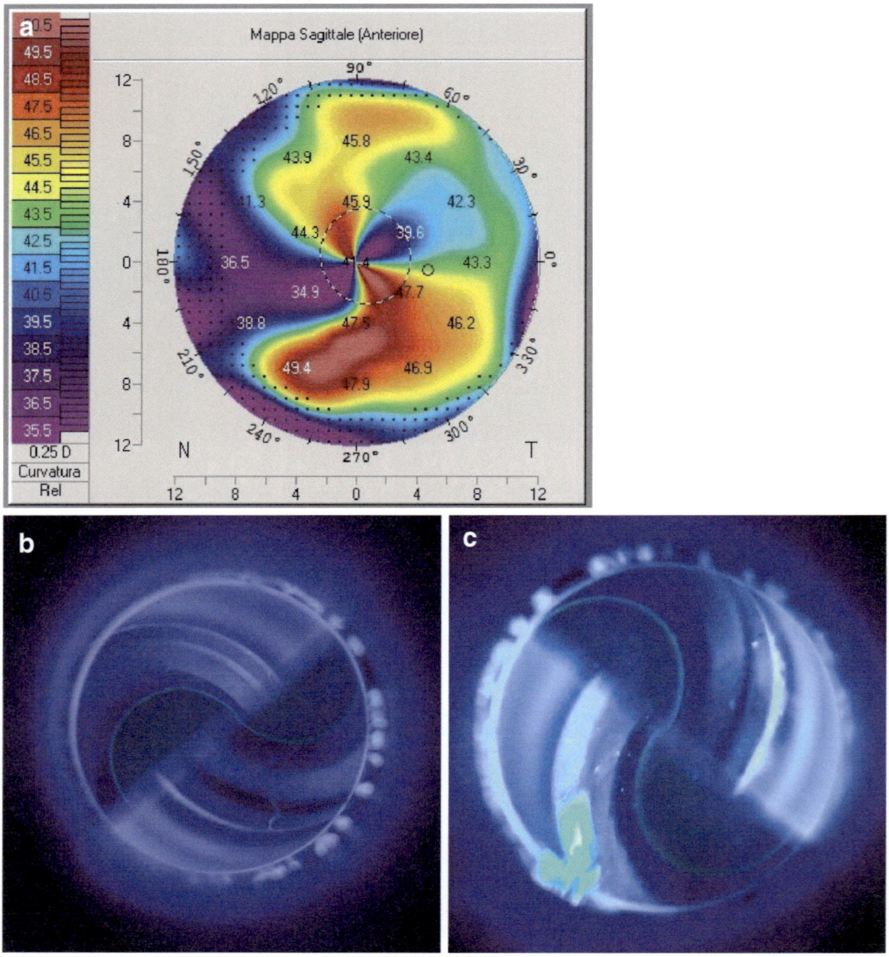

Fig. 3.7 (**a**) Corneal astigmatism can significantly affect IOP. This patient had a corneal astigmatism of 13 diopters due to severe pterygium, as shown by corneal topography. (**b**) IOP measurement showed a difference of 5 mmHg when the prism is positioned at 45°, and (**c**) 135°; the steeper meridian is the one with the highest reading, as explained in Fig. 3.8. In the case of high astigmatism, the most precise IOP reading is the mean of those obtained on the two main meridians

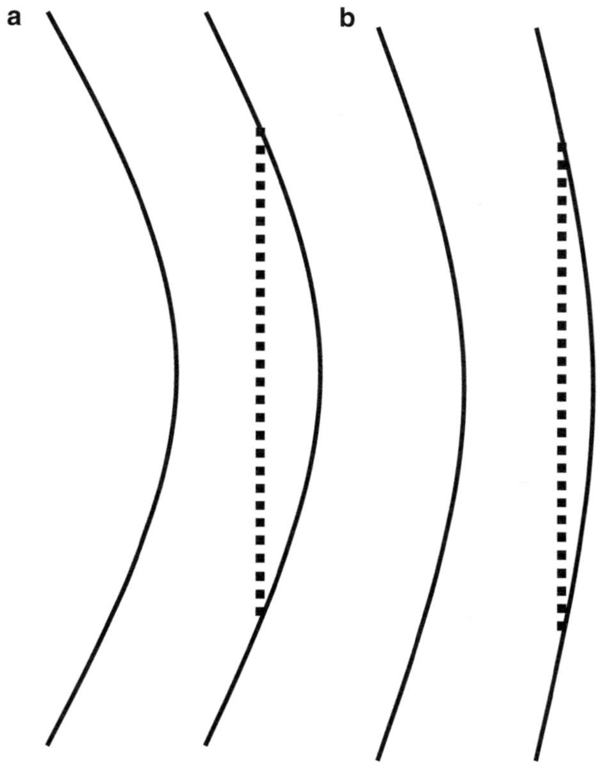

Fig. 3.8 The effect of corneal curvature. (**a**) Steeper corneas give IOP overestimation, as to produce the standard area of contact; they have to be indented more than normal. (**b**) Flatter corneas give IOP underestimation as they are more easily applanated

3.2 Dynamic-Contour Tonometry

The Pascal dynamic-contour tonometer (DCT, Swiss Microtechnology AG, Port, Switzerland; Fig. 3.9) is a recent tonometer designed to provide IOP measurements that are not affected by corneal properties.

The measurement is based on the interface forces between the tip and the cornea that counterbalance the force distribution generated by the IOP. When contact between these two structures is obtained, a sensor embedded in the tip (Fig. 3.10) provides IOP measurements transcorneally [7]. The matching between cornea and tonometer tip is obtained thanks to the shape of the silicon cover, which matches the contour of the cornea causing minimal distortion while taking the IOP readings.

The small interference between the tonometer and the eye is responsible of a very small tonometric effect (0.6 ± 1.6 mmHg; Fig. 3.11) [8] found with DCT (compared with 2 mmHg with GAT).

Studies on human cadaver eyes have shown that DCT provided a better accuracy than GAT, and similar findings have also been reported in patients who underwent corneal refractive surgery. A well-conducted study also showed that DCT measurements have a good concordance with the "true" manometric IOP taken by intracameral cannulation during cataract surgery [9].

In addition to IOP measurements, during the period of contact between the tonometer and eye, DCT also provides an ocular pulse amplitude (OPA; Fig. 3.12), which is the difference between systolic and diastolic IOP (whereas IOP is defined as the mean of systolic and diastolic values). OPA is indicative of ocular blood flow and might be a parameter to evaluate when managing glaucoma patients [10, 11].

In a population of normal subjects, OPA has been found to be 3.0 ± 1.2 mmHg, which was similar to a glaucoma population (3.2 ± 1.4 mmHg) [8].

A recent paper addressed the test-retest variability of DCT and found it out to be almost perfect for IOP (intraclass coefficient of variability had a range of 0.74–0.95) and good for OPA (0.64–0.84). Coefficient of variability was about 5 % for IOP and 10 % for OPA (Fig. 3.13). Compared with GAT, DCT tended to overestimate both a population of normal subjects and glaucoma patients by 2.3 and 2.5 mmHg (Figs. 3.14 and 3.15) [8].

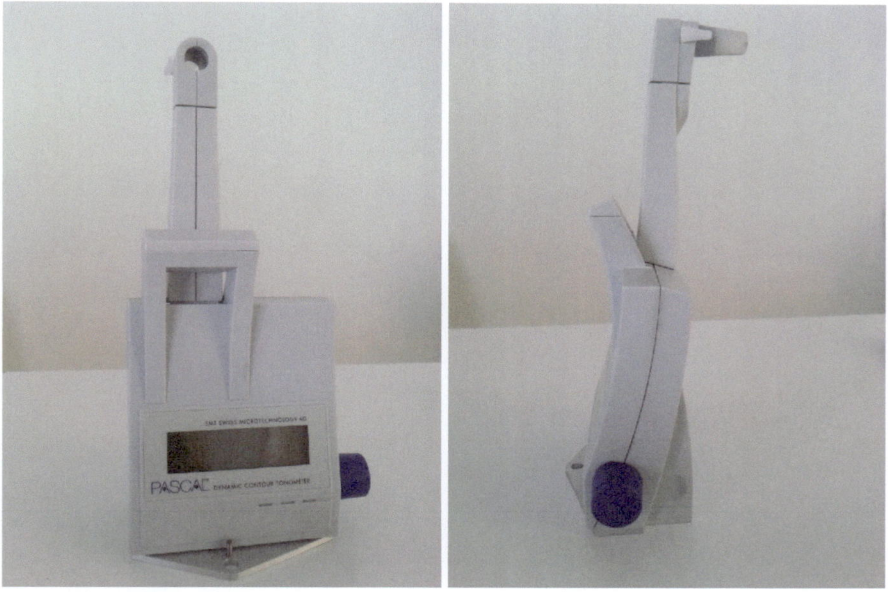

Fig. 3.9 Dynamic-contour tonometry (Courtesy of Matteo Pelagatti)

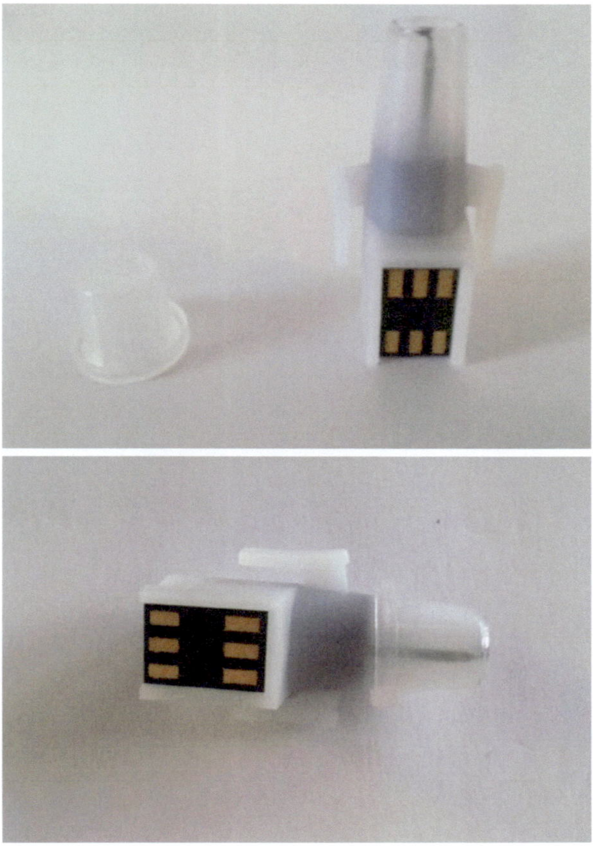

Fig. 3.10 DCT silicon tip with transducer (Courtesy of Matteo Pelagatti)

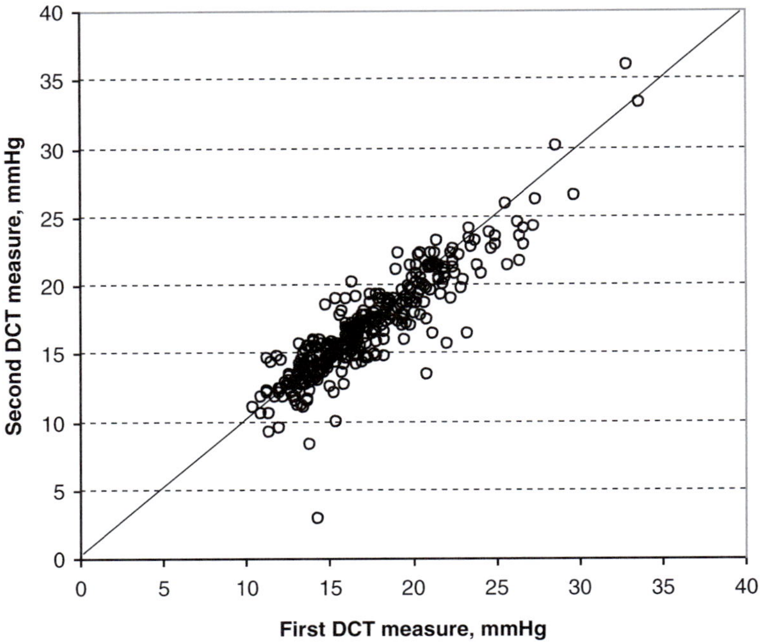

Fig. 3.11 Test-retest variability of DCT. The tonometric effect consists on a lowering of IOP during serial measurements (mostly due to a displacement of aqueous from the eye). On two consecutive DCT measurements, this effect is overall small, as most of the points are close to the identity line

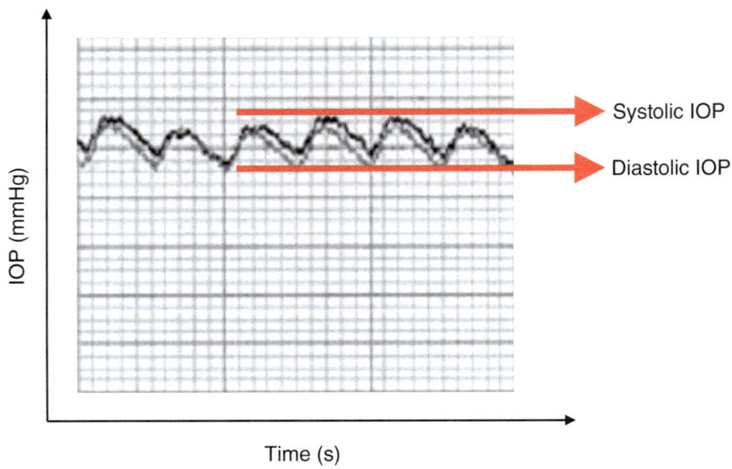

Fig. 3.12 Diagram of ocular pulse amplitude (OPA). IOP is not static, but pulsing. Pulse reflects heart pulse, so that systolic and diastolic values can be found. IOP is the mean of these two values, whereas OPA is the difference of the two

Fig. 3.13 Coefficient of variability for DCT. This parameter was 5 % for IOP (range 0 %-) and 10 % for OPA

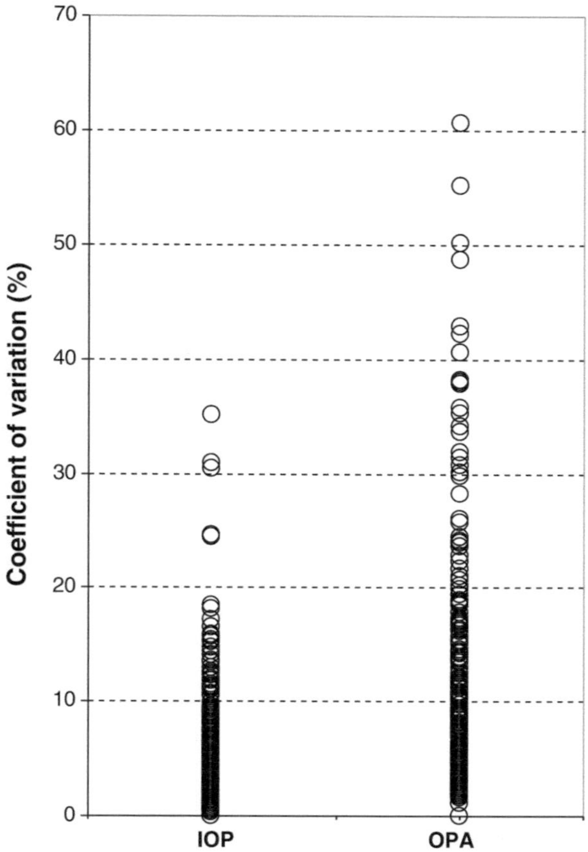

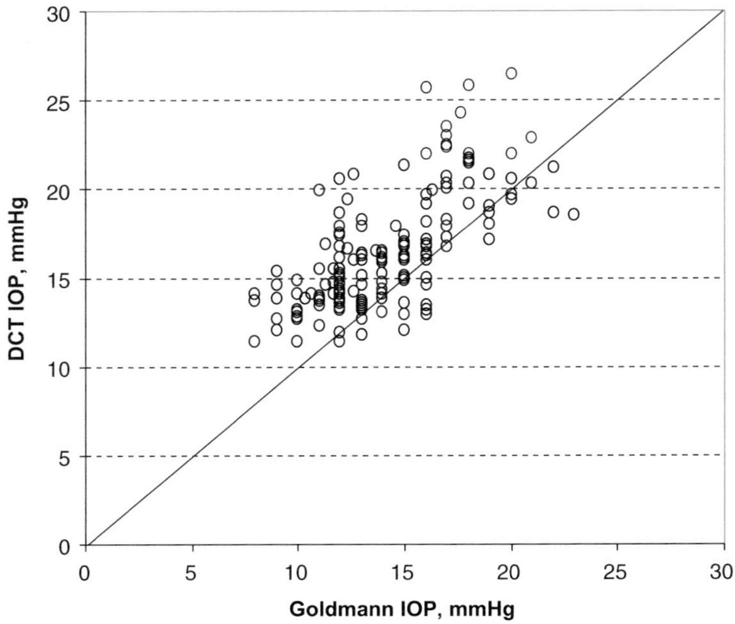

Fig. 3.14 Comparison of Goldmann and DCT measurements in normal subjects. DCT gave IOP values higher than GAT by a mean of +2.27 mmHg (2.27 ± 2.50 mmHg, range −4.5; +9.6 mmHg)

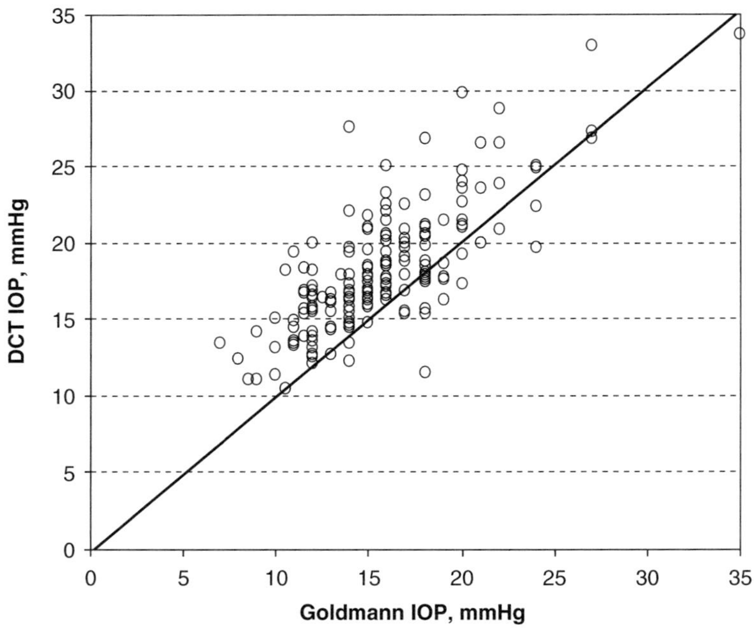

Fig. 3.15 Comparison of Goldmann and DCT measurements in glaucoma subjects. DCT gave IOP values higher than GAT by a mean of +2.49 mmHg (2.49 ± 2.75 mmHg, range −6.5; +13.5 mmHg)

3.3 Ocular Response Analyzer

The Reichert Ocular Response Analyzer (ORA; Fig. 3.16) is a novel non-contact tonometer which measures IOP and also gives an estimation of ocular hysteresis.

Figure 3.17 shows a typical ORA diagram. The tonometer uses air to give an applanation of the central 3 mm of the cornea. After the first applanation (Fig. 3.18a), air pressure is maintained to indent the cornea (Fig. 3.18b), and a second applanation is finally obtained (Figs. 3.18c).

The reading of IOP is obtained twice as two applanations occur. The difference between these two values is defined as corneal hysteresis, and their mean is GAT-correlated IOP.

ORA has the advantage of being a non-contact tonometer providing automated readings; therefore, it is not operator-dependent and it is not a source of potential infections as contact tonometers. The reproducibility of the instrument is high, ranging from 0.78 to 0.93.

Despite these advantages, the instrument is more useful for research rather than for clinical use. The possibility to measure hysteresis (as well as cornea-compensated IOP values) has in fact gained scientists' attention. Thanks to ORA, it has been shown that hysteresis is a parameter independent from axial length, corneal curvature, and IOP; it is also poorly correlated with central corneal thickness and it tends to reduce with age.

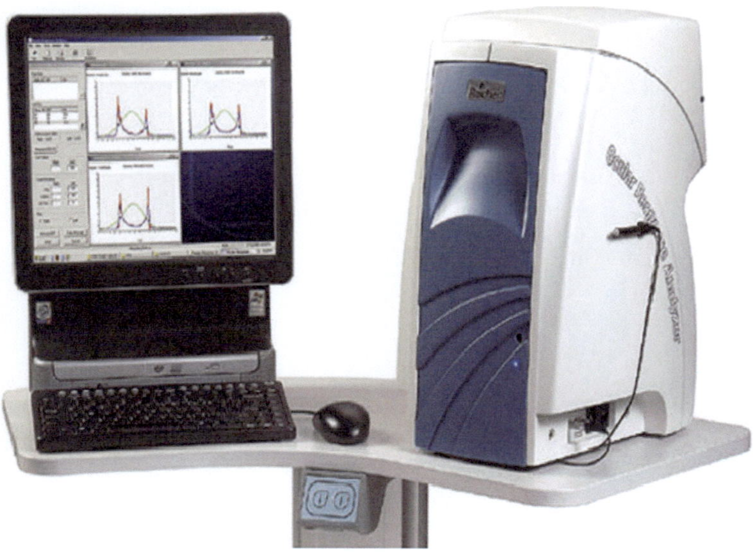

Fig. 3.16 Ocular Response Analyzer (ORA)

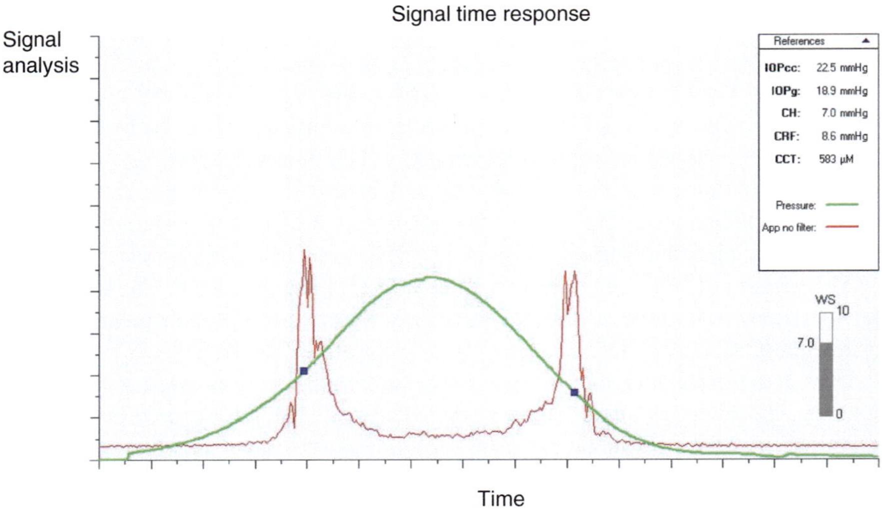

Fig. 3.17 Example of ORA printout. The green curve shows air pulse pressure, the red diagram is the applanation signal. IOP is read at the intersection of the two diagrams (*blue squares*). As two applanations are done, two IOP values are available. The difference between the two values is corneal hysteresis (*CH*), and their mean is GAT-correlated IOP (*IOPg*). Corneal resistance factor (*CRF*) and corneal-compensated IOP (*IOPcc*) are also given (Courtesy of Francesco Oddone)

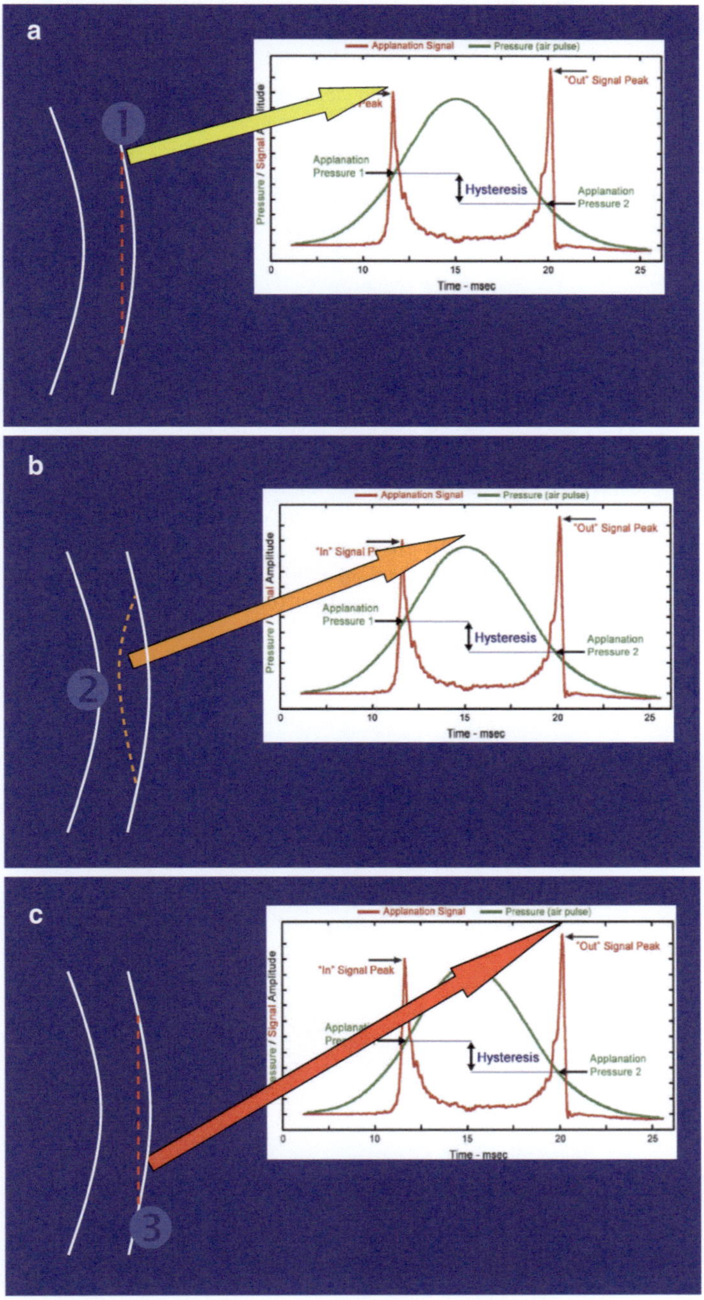

Fig. 3.18 The three determinants of ORA measurements. (**a**) First applanation. When the first applanation is obtained, an "in" signal peak is recorded. (**b**) Corneal indentation. After the first applanation, the instruments continue to provide pressure to the central cornea up to a plateau, corresponding to the value of maximum indentation of the cornea. (**c**) Second applanation. After indentation, the pressure to the eye is reduced and the cornea returns to its natural shape, passing through a second applanation, when an "out" signal peak is recorded

References

1. Moses RA (1960) Fluorescein in applanation tonometry. Am J Ophthalmol 49:1149–1155
2. Goldmann H, Schmidt T (1961) Uber applanations tonometrie. Ophthalmologica 141:441–446
3. Hoffer KJ (1979) Applanation tonometry without fluorescein. Correspondence. Am J Ophthalmol 88:798
4. Kaufman HE, Wind CA, Waltman SR (1970) Validity of Mackay- Marg electronis applanation tonometer in patients with Scarred irregular corneas. Am J Ophthalmol 69:1003–1007
5. Mark HH (1973) Corneal curvature in applanation tonometry. Am J Ophthalmol 76:223–224
6. Kaufman HE (1972) Pressure measurement: which tonometer? Invest Ophthalmol 11:80–85
7. Kanngiesser HE, Kniestedt C, Robert YC (2005) Dynamic contour tonometry: presentation of a new tonometer. J Glaucoma 14:344e50
8. Fogagnolo P, Figus M, Frezzotti P (2010) Test-retest variability of intraocular pressure and ocular pulse amplitude for Dynamic Contour Tonometry: a multicenter study. Br J Ophthalmol 94:419–423
9. Boehm AG, Weber A, Pillunat LE, Koch R, Spoerl E (2008) Dynamic contour tonometry in comparison to intracameral IOP measurements. Invest Ophthalmol Vis Sci 49:2472–2477
10. Punjabi OS, Ho HK, Kniestedt C, Bostrom AG, Stamper RL, Lin SC (2006) Intraocular pressure and ocular pulse amplitude comparisons in different types of glaucoma using dynamic contour tonometry. Curr Eye Res 31:851–862
11. Weizer JS, Asrani S, Stinnett SS, Herndon LW (2007) The clinical utility of dynamic contour tonometry and ocular pulse amplitude. J Glaucoma 16:700–703

Chapter 4
Ultrasound Biomicroscopy in Glaucoma

Julián García-Feijoo, Carmen Méndez-Hernández, José María Martínez de la Casa, Federico Sáenz-Francés, Rubén Sánchez-Jean, and Julián García-Sánchez

Currently, there are several methods that can image the anterior segment of the eye, such as ultrasound biomicroscopy (UBM), confocal microscopy, or optical coherence tomography (OCT). OCT is an excellent imaging tool, but uses optical waves and therefore its penetration and capacity of imaging structures behind the pigmented epithelium or deep sclera is limited.

UBM is a high-resolution ultrasound technique developed in the 1980s. This technology uses ultrasound frequencies in the 35–100 MHz range, which allows noninvasive in vivo imaging of the anterior ocular segment [1]. It is capable of direct visualization of anterior ocular structures. High-frequency UBM provides high-resolution (approximately 25–35 μm axially and 50 μm laterally depending on the transducer frequency) images of the internal microstructures of the anterior chamber of the eye with an imaging depth of approximately 5 mm, which is suitable to characterize not only the angle but deeper structures. It also provides information on filtering blebs and suprachoroidal drainage following glaucoma surgery and can be of use in the postsurgical management of the patients [2, 3].

The introduction of this technique in ophthalmology has improved the study of the structures of the anterior segment. It shows excellent images of the anterior chamber, angle, and the ciliary body. It also allows a good reference to see causes of obstruction of aqueous flow and is of help in the etiological diagnosis of suspected secondary glaucoma.

J. García-Feijoo, MD, PhD (✉) • C. Méndez-Hernández, MD, PhD
J.M.M. de la Casa, MD, PhD • F. Sáenz-Francés, MD, PhD • R. Sánchez-Jean, OD
J. García-Sánchez, MD, PhD
Servicio de Oftalmología, Hospital Clínico San Carlos, Madrid, Spain

Departamento de Oftalmología y ORL, Facultad de Medicina,
Universidad Complutense de Madrid, Instituto de Investigación Sanitaria del Hospital Clínico San Carlos (IdISSC), Madrid, Spain

Cooperative Research Network on Age-Related Ocular Pathology,
Visual and Life Quality, Instituto de Salud Carlos III, Madrid, Spain
e-mail: jgarciafeijoo@hotmail.com

A. Ferreras (ed.), *Glaucoma Imaging*, DOI 10.1007/978-3-319-18959-8_4

4.1 Technique

In 1990s, the first UBM instrument for clinical use with a 50-MHz transducer was developed [4]; since then UBM examination technique has not evolved much and a water bath or the use of some sort of coupling media is needed.

UBM provides higher image resolution (50-MHz transducer axial resolution: approximately 35 μm) than conventional B-scan due to the higher transducer frequency of the UBM, but it is not able to image as deeply as a conventional B-scan because of the reduced penetration depth of the ultrasonic beam (approximately 5 mm for a 50-MHz UBM instrument). Also the scanning area width ranges from 5 to 11 mm depending on the transducer characteristics (linear, arc scan).

The examination can be done with the patient in the supine or sitting position under topical anesthesia. Different plastic or silicone eyecups or shells have been proposed and should be used to create a small water bath with saline (Open Systems) [5]. Saline or 1 or 2 % methylcellulose solution can be used as the coupling fluid [6]. Some devices use a closed probe; the transducer is located inside a cylinder filled with sterile water and then covered and sealed. However, the use of an eyecup filled with a coupling fluid or a probe cover (such as the ClearScan) is still necessary to obtain quality scans. With the open-systems, scanning is performed with the ultrasound transducer oscillating within the coupling solution.

The transducer should be oriented perpendicularly to maximize the detection of reflected signals. It is possible to perform UBM in the prone and sitting positions that allows the examiner to determine alterations in anatomic relationships among anterior segment structures in these positions [7].

4.2 Clinical Uses in Glaucoma

With the UBM iris, ciliary body and scleral spur can be recognized [8] (Figs. 4.1 and 4.2) and it is possible to determine the mechanism of elevated intraocular pressure by analyzing the relationship between the structures of the angle.

Imaging of the anterior segment structures is possible in eyes with corneal edema or corneal opacification. UBM can be also used to evaluate the iris insertion and its relationship with the trabecular meshwork. It is possible to identify ciliary processes pushing the lens and iris forward in angle closure glaucoma or iris cysts pushing the iris against the cornea. The angle opening distance (AOD), trabecular iris angle (TIA), iris thickness, and iris curvature can be easily measured (Figs. 4.3 and 4.4).

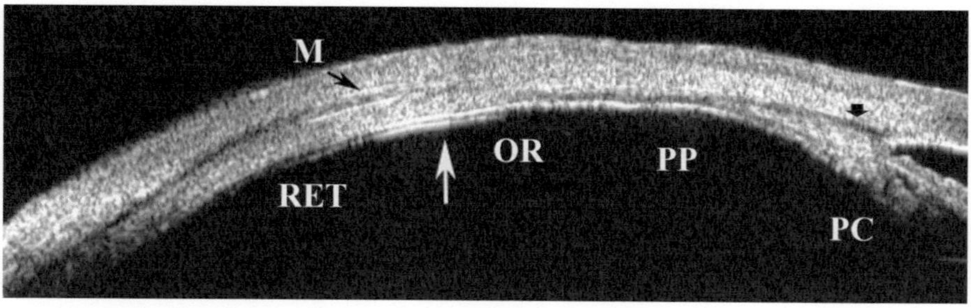

Fig. 4.1 UBM of the angle, ciliary body, and peripheral retina. Reconstruction from four consecutive radial scans. Note the hipoecogenic band in the superficial area of the ciliary body (*Black arrow*). *M* lateral muscle, *RET and white arrow* retina, *OR* ora serrata, *PP* ciliary body *pars plana*, *PC* ciliary body *pars plicata*

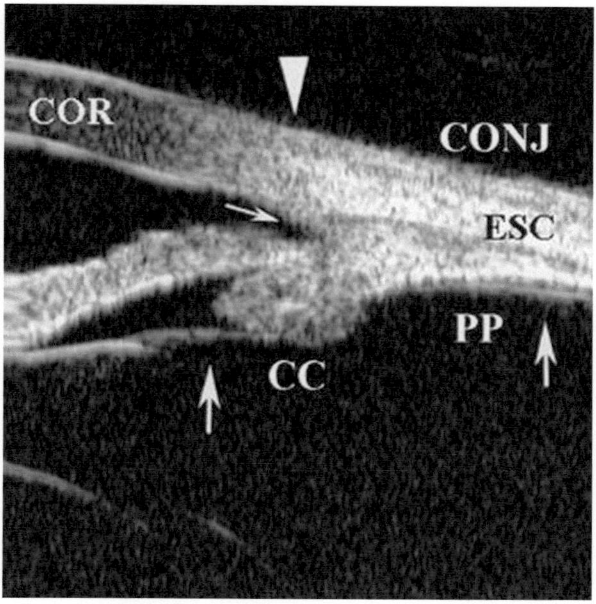

Fig. 4.2 Angle structures. *COR* cornea, *ESC* sclera, *CC* ciliary body, *PP* ciliary body *pars plana. Small arrow* scleral spur, *arrowhead* corneal limbus, *two arrows* zonular fibers

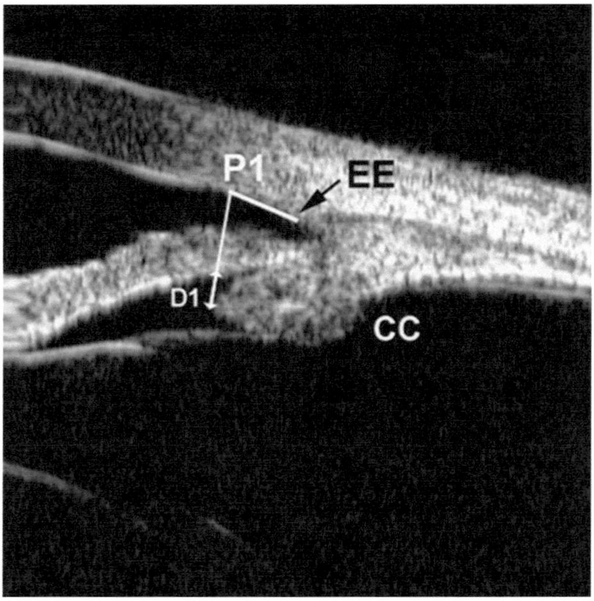

Fig. 4.3 Sulcus opening and (*D1*) and trabecular Meshwork (*white line* from P1 to scleral spur: EE). *CC* ciliary body

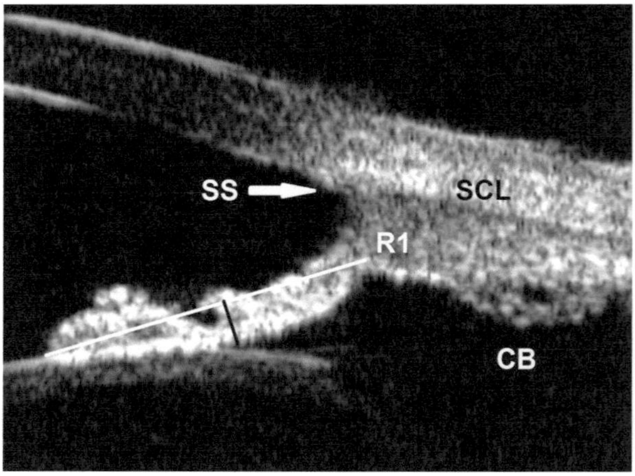

Fig. 4.4 Iris curvature. Distance between the posterior iris surface (pigment epithelium) and a line from the posterior iris root (end of the iris pigment epithelium: R1) to the first point of contact between the iris and lens. The largest perpendicular distance from this line to the iris epithelium is then measured (*Black line*; convex: positive, concave: negative). *SCL* sclera, *CB* ciliary body, *SS* scleral spur

4.3 Pigmentary Glaucoma

In the pigment dispersion syndrome, a wide open angle and posterior bowing of the peripheral iris causing reverse pupillary block can be observed by UBM (Figs. 4.5 and 4.6) [9–11]. Mendez-Hernandez et al. [12] studied the effect of Nd:YAG iridotomy (LI) on iris configuration in pigmentary glaucoma. They found that LI rectified the posterior bowing of the iris and reduced the drugs required to control IOP. Pillunat et al. [13] evaluated the effect of Nd:YAG LPI on anterior segment structures and IOP. They showed that iridozonular contact does not exist in every patient with pigmentary glaucoma. In this study, only in patients with iridozonular contact did laser iridotomy significantly reduce intraocular pressure.

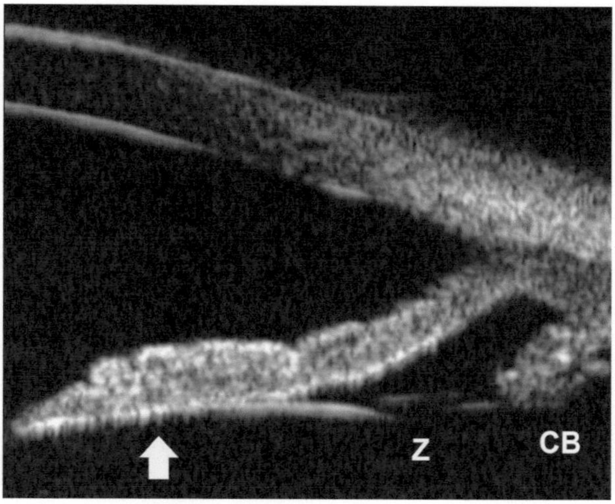

Fig. 4.5 Posterior bowing of peripheral iris in pigmentary glaucoma. Increased area of iris--lens contact (*arrow*). The proximity of the zonules (*Z*) to the posterior iris surface can also be seen. *CB* ciliary body

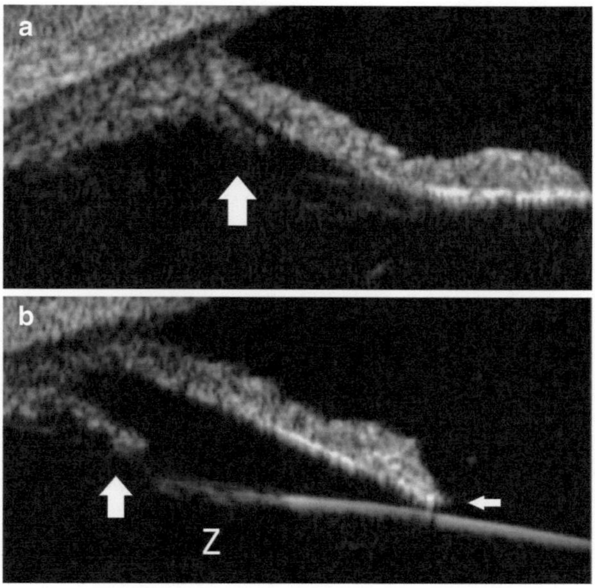

Fig. 4.6 Iris morphology pre (**a**) and after LI (**b**). Note the rectification and anterior displacement of the iris. See also the absence of iridozonular contact and even of irido-lens contact (*small arrow*); *Z* zonula, *big arrows* ciliary body

4.4 Iris Plateau

In plateau iris syndrome, UBM usually reveals an anterior angulation of the peripheral iris and anterior insertion of the iris on to the ciliary body [14, 15] (Fig. 4.7). In some cases, a thickening of the peripheral iris with or without anterior rotation of the ciliary body can be observed (Fig. 4.8). Garudadri et al. [16] evaluated the presence of plateau iris in eyes with PACG after LI by gonioscopy and UBM. Among the PACG eyes after LI, 40 % had an open angle and 60 % had a narrow angle. They found that anteriorly directed ciliary processes were seen in eyes with plateau iris as well as in eyes with PACG that had deep anterior chambers after iridotomy. Thus, the presence of anteriorly directed ciliary processes alone was insufficient to diagnose plateau iris syndrome.

Kumar et al. [17] found that about 30 % of PACG eyes with a patent laser peripheral iridotomy had plateau iris on UBM, highlighting the importance of nonpupil block mechanisms in Asian individuals. Parc et al. [18] compared optical coherence tomography (OCT) and UBM for detection of plateau iris configuration and confirmation of plateau iris syndrome. Whereas UBM directly identified the iris root indentation caused by the ciliary body, OCT only picked up indirect signs of plateau iris configuration.

Diniz Filho et al. [19, 21] reported that the biometric parameters were completely different between normal eyes and the eyes with plateau iris configuration found in 10 % of the open angle and narrow angle glaucoma. Eyes with plateau iris configuration have significantly shorter axial length and higher central corneal thickness than eyes with primary open-angle glaucoma with narrow angles [20].

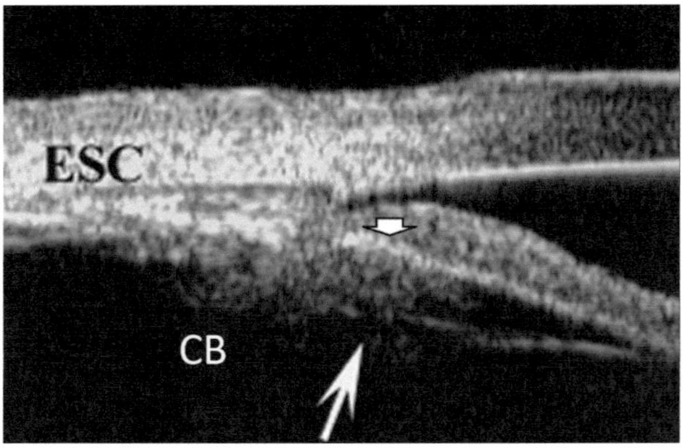

Fig. 4.7 Plateau iris syndrome. The ciliary body (CB, big arrow) is rotated and anteriorly located (small arrow). With the CB in this position the ciliary sulcus is closed and prevents the iris from falling away after iridotomy (small arrow). ESC: sclera

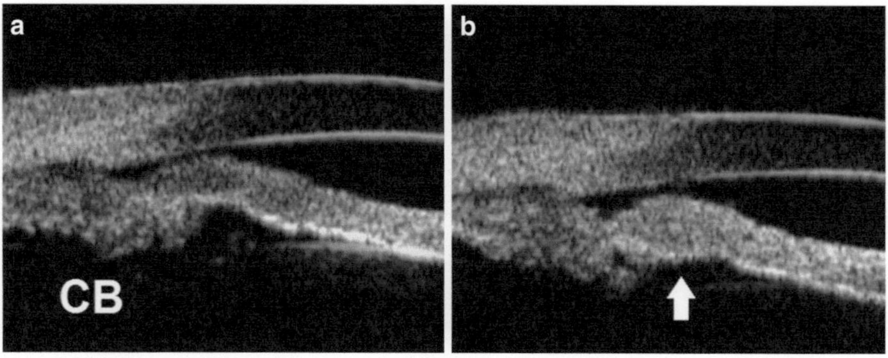

Fig. 4.8 Plateau iris syndrome. In some patients the ciliary body/iris (**a**, *CB*) configuration is not typical. In this patient UBM shows not only the CB anterior displacement but also displaced iris root and thickening peripheral iris (**b**, *arrow*). UBM after iridotomy

4.5 Other Conditions

As mentioned before, UBM can be used to assess and measure the angle opening and configuration in angle closure glaucoma and pupillary block, and to visualize the underlying mechanisms involved and analyze the changes after peripheral iridotomy (Fig. 4.9) [21, 22]. It can show the extent of peripheral anterior synechiae even if the cornea is hazy or opaque (Fig. 4.10). UBM has been able to differentiate between primary angle closure and secondary angle closure caused by lens dislocation, hemorrhagic choroidal detachment pushing the lens and iris anteriorly or cysts in the iridociliary sulcus (Figs. 4.11 and 4.12).

In patients with aniridia, UBM shows the iris and ciliary body hypoplasia [23] (Fig. 4.13).

In Sturge-Weber syndrome-associated glaucoma, UBM findings such as intrascleral vessels and supraciliary fluid support the hypothesis of increased episcleral venous pressure as the cause of elevated intraocular pressure in this condition [24] (Fig. 4.14).

Zhang et al. [25] compared UBM findings in normal subjects with three clinical types of iridocorneal endothelial (ICE) syndrome: progressive iris atrophy, Chandler syndrome, and Cogan-Reese syndrome. UBM was found to be more effective in detecting peripheral anterior synechiae and iris atrophy than slit lamp biomicroscopy and gonioscopy, mainly because of corneal edema. Different subtypes of ICE syndrome may have different UBM manifestations. UBM also helps to identify angle closure in the fellow eye of unilateral ICE syndromes.

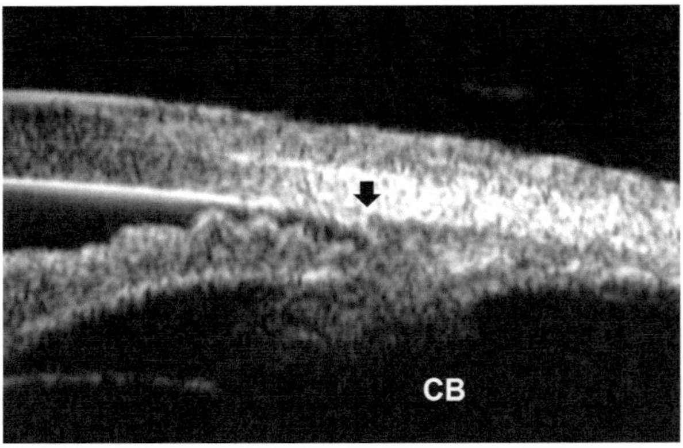

Fig. 4.9 Angle Closure Glaucoma. Note the iris convexity before iris iridotomy was performed. The sulcus is opened and no iris--trabecular meshwork contact is seen in this scan (UBM scan taken with lights on) (scleral spur: *black arrow*). *CB* ciliary body

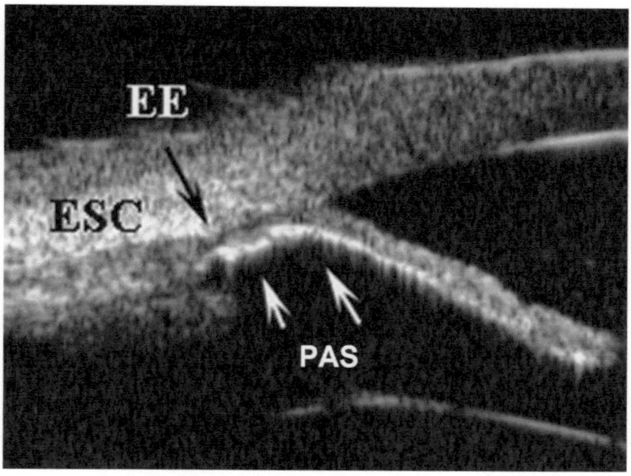

Fig. 4.10 Neovascular Glaucoma. Peripheral anterior synechiae (PAS, *white arrows*). *EE*: scleral spur, *ESC* Sclera

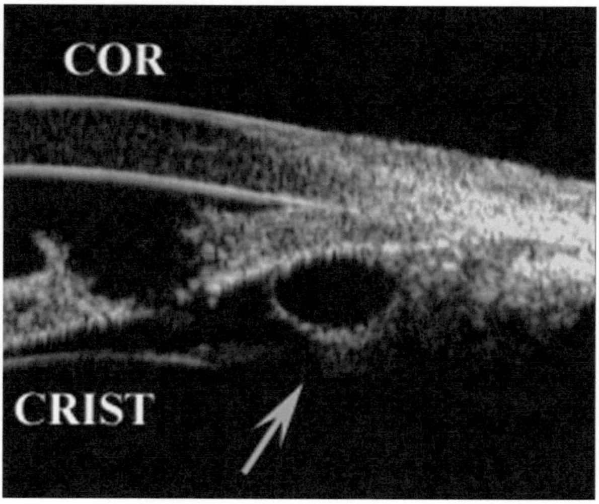

Fig. 4.11 Iris cysts pushing the peripheral iris forward and closing the angle. The iridotomy performed in this case did not resolve the angle closure. *COR* cornea, *CRIST* crystalline lens

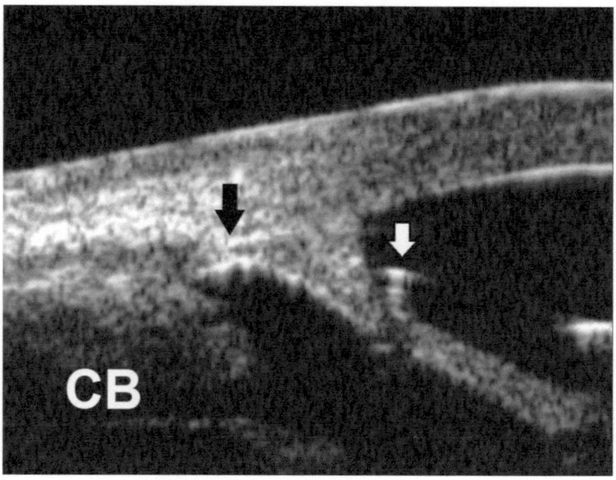

Fig. 4.12 Secondary angle-closure glaucoma caused by anterior chamber IOL (Z stepped haptics, *white arrow*). Peripheral anterior synechiae are blocking the outflow pathway (scleral spur: *black arrow*). *CB* ciliary body

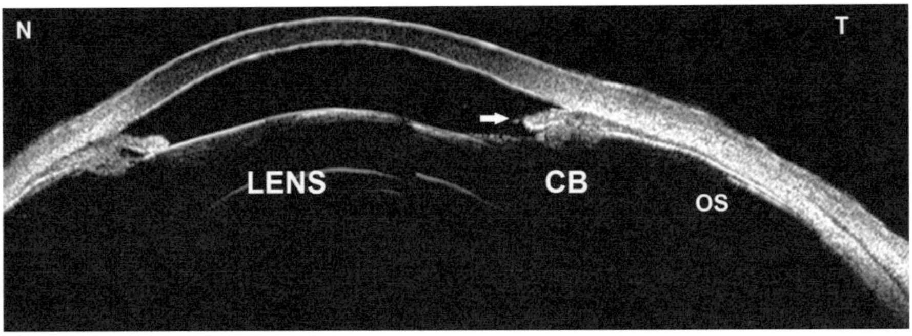

Fig. 4.13 UBM image in a patient with aniridia. Reconstruction from four consecutive radial scans (horizontal scans: 3–9 h). Partial absence of the iris (*arrow*). Crystalline lens (*LENS*) is displaced nasally. *CB* ciliary body, *OS* ora serrata, *T* temporal, *N* nasal

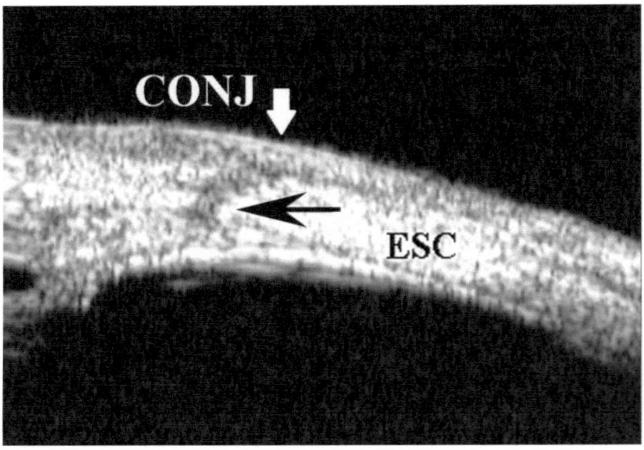

Fig. 4.14 UBM in Sturge-Weber Syndrome. Dilated intrascleral (*black arrow*) and conjunctival vessels (*white arrow*). *CONJ* conjunctiva, *ESC* sclera

4.6 Post-traumatic Glaucoma

After ocular trauma, UBM can be used to evaluate iris-angle abnormalities including angle recession, iridodialysis, and cyclodialysis (Figs. 4.15 and 4.16). Angle recession is characterized on UBM by a posterior displacement of the point of attachment of the iris to the sclera and a widening of the ciliary body face with no disruption of the interface between the sclera and ciliary body [26]. Cyclodialysis can be identified by detachment of the ciliary body from its normal location at the scleral spur [27]. UBM can also identify occult zonular damage in patients with anterior segment trauma [28]. The ability to diagnose zonular rupture preoperatively might reduce the chance of intraoperative complications.

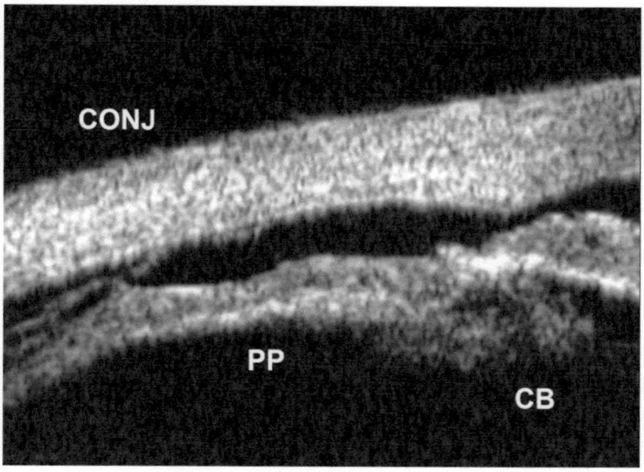

Fig. 4.15 Cyclodialysis. The ciliary body and iris root are disinserted from the scleral spur. The posterior pathway created by the detachment creates a choroidal effusion. *CB* ciliary body, *PP* ciliary body *pars plana*, *CONJ* conjunctiva

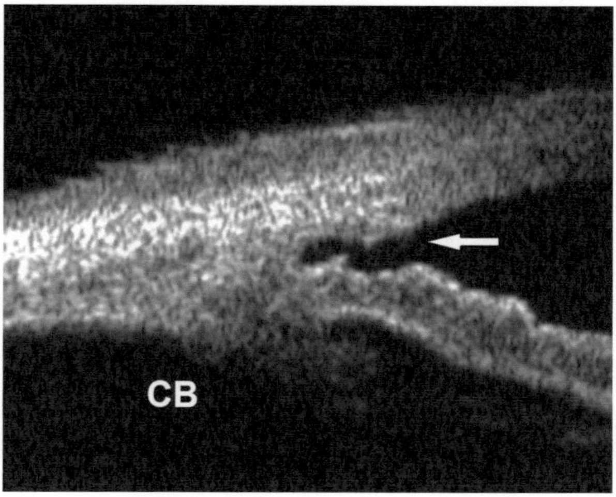

Fig. 4.16 Angle recession. The angle shows a tear into the ciliary body. See the widening of the ciliary body face and the posterior displacement of the iris (*arrow*). *CB* ciliary body

4.7 Pseudophakic and Lens-Induced Glaucoma

UBM can help to diagnose various types of lens-induced glaucomas such as phacomorphic glaucoma and glaucoma due to anterior subluxation of lens. It is helpful to know the circumference of intact zonules and the extent of zonular dialysis in pseudoexfoliation syndrome. In case of intraocular lens (IOL)-induced glaucoma, it can clearly delineate the position of the optic and haptic [29, 30] and is especially helpful in pseudophakic bullous keratopathy in determining the cause of glaucoma or in cases of secondary glaucoma related with posterior chamber phakic-IOL (Figs. 4.17 and 4.18a,b).

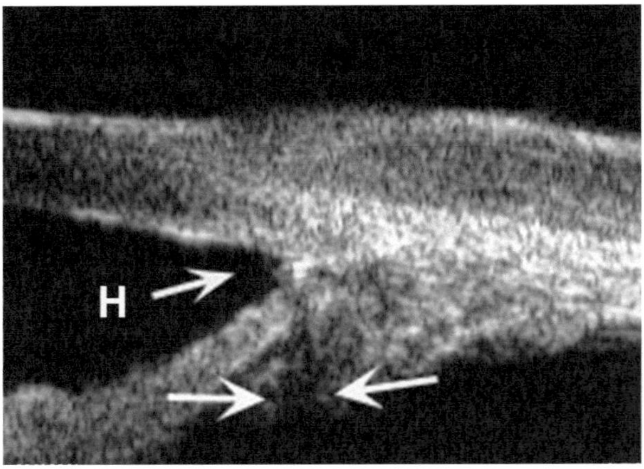

Fig. 4.17 Secondary glaucoma caused by anterior luxation of one haptic of a posterior chamber IOL. Corneal edema precludes the correct assessment of the anterior chamber. See the haptic in contact with the angle structures (*H and arrow* pointing the angle). The haptic of the IOL impedes the ultrasonic waves producing a characteristic acoustic shadow (*two arrows*)

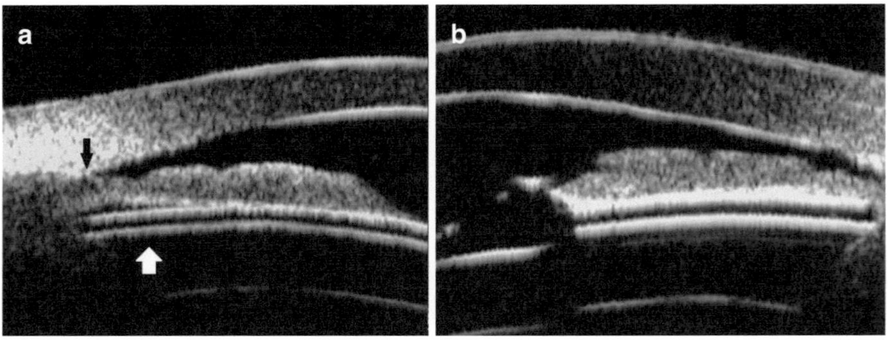

Fig. 4.18 (**a**, **b**) Secondary glaucoma caused by a PCP-IOL (PRL) caused by the excessive PRL size in relation to the patient's sulcus diameter. The iris has been pushed upwards by the PRL (*white arrow*: PRL haptic) and is in contact with the trabecular meshwork (*black arrow*). Note the decrease in the anterior chamber depth and the distance between the crystalline lens and the PRL

4.8 UBM in Glaucoma Surgery

4.8.1 Trabeculectomy

After trabeculectomy, UBM can show whether the sclerostomy aperture is patent or blocked internally (Fig. 4.19). Avitabile et al. [31] studied the correlation of bleb morphology on UBM and functional status with the effect of laser suture lysis. They found a statistically significant correlation between the UBM classification of function and the IOP control level. Both well-functioning and failed trabeculectomies could be identified by UBM. The UBM images of eyes with good IOP control are characterized by better visibility of the route under the scleral flap and a low reflectivity inside the bleb. Also in modified trabeculectomies, aimed to enhance the suprachoidal pathway, [32] UBM has allowed us to image the suprachoidal drainage (Figs. 4.20 and 4.21) [33]. Thus UBM can be a useful method to study and explain the mechanisms of filtering structures and, together with IOP control, to evaluate bleb function.

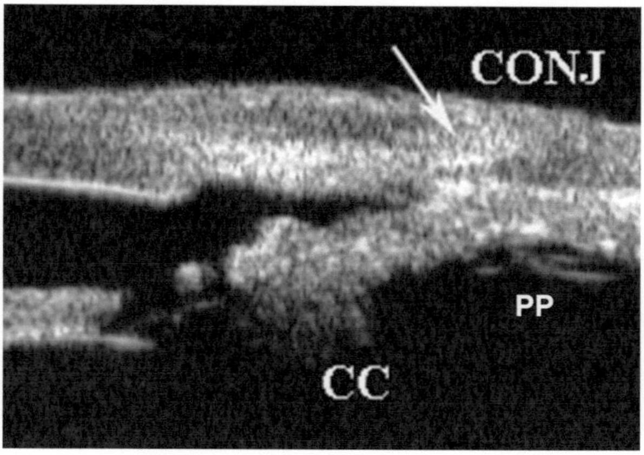

Fig. 4.19 Trabeculectomy. The trabeculectomy site can be easily studied, subconjunctival drainage can be observed through the scleral flap *(arrow)*. *CC* ciliary body, *PP* ciliary body *pars plana, CONJ* conjunctiva

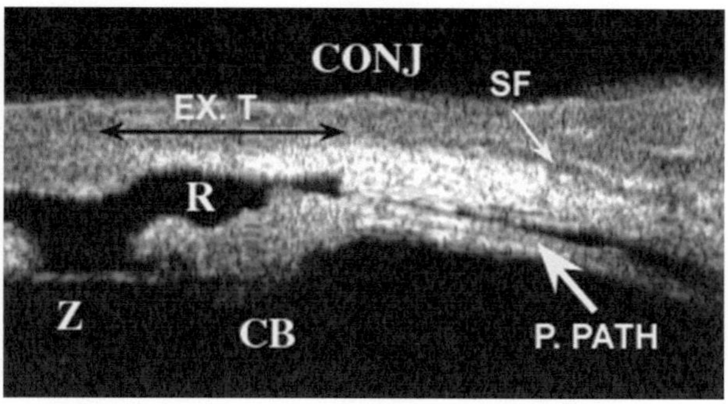

Fig. 4.20 Modified trabeculectomy. This surgery aims to create a suprachoroidal drainage pathway and/or the traditional subconjunctival drainage. In this case both coexisted. *Z* zonula, *CB* ciliary body, *P. Path* posterior drainage pathway, *SF* superficial or subconjunctival drainage pathway, *R* reservoir, *Ex T* excised scleral inner block size, *CONJ* conjunctiva

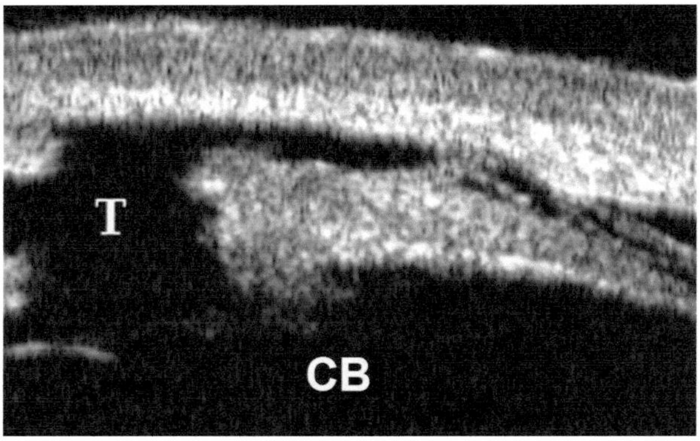

Fig. 4.21 Modified trabeculectomy. In this case no subconjunctival bleb can be seen, but the suprachoidal drainage is patent. *T* trabeculectomy site, *CB* ciliary body

4.8.2 Nonpenetrating Deep Sclerectomy

UBM may be used in eyes that have undergone nonpenetrating deep sclerectomy (NPDS) to evaluate the functional status of the surgery. It can evaluate the thickness and demonstrate a nonperforated continuous trabeculum and Descemet's membrane.

In patients undergoing deep sclerectomy, UBM examination after long-term follow-up shows the presence of an intrascleral space and a filtering bleb (Figs. 4.22 and 4.23a, b) [34]. The UBM allows the surgeon to detect three different signs related to the IOP-lowering mechanism of NPDS: filtering bleb, trans-scleral filtration and increased uveo-scleral filtration [35]. However a hipoecogenic band in the superficial area of the ciliary body is very common and should not be misinterpreted as a suprachoroidal aqueous humor drainage pathway. It is related to the difference in acoustic impedance between the sclera (hiperecogenic), the hipoecogenic ciliary body tissue close to the sclera, and the more ecogenic tissue of the inner portion of ciliary body the muscle (Figs. 4.1 and 4.24). Collagen implants used to augment deep sclerectomy can also be visualized (Figs. 4.25 and 4.26). Grading similar to the trabeculectomy bleb has also been used for NPDS blebs. Information provided by UBM is useful and assists in understanding the mechanisms of action of deep sclerectomy. After deep sclerectomy, the height and the length of the different collagen implants can be measured. It has been shown on UBM that these collagen implants dissolve slowly leaving an intrascleral lake [36]. Aptel et al. [37] identified the clinical and anatomic characteristics of filtering blebs after glaucoma surgery with a biodegradable collagen implant, Ologen, using UBM and Visante anterior segment optical coherence tomography. In this study, they found that lower IOP correlated with bleb height.

Wang et al. [38] studied causes of failure of NPDS with SKGeL implants. UBM showed that the filtering bleb disappeared in every failure. The scarring at conjunctiva and Tenon's capsule-superficial scleral flap interface was the most important cause of NPDS with SKGeL implant failure. Park et al. [39] studied UBM of the intrascleral lake after combined viscocanalostomy and cataract surgery. They found lower IOP without bleb formation. Postoperatively, the size of the lake and IOP decreased. The lake was undetected ultrasonographically in most of the cases 1 year postoperatively.

Other causes of failure as trabeculo-Descemet window block can be also imaged by UBM (Fig. 4.27a, b).

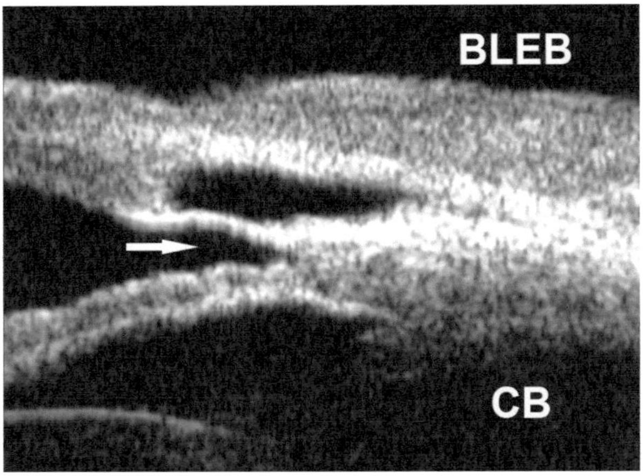

Fig. 4.22 Nonpenetrating deep sclerectomy. Nonperforated continuous trabeculum and Descemet's membrane (*arrow*). The reservoir/intrascleral lake and a subconjunctival bleb (*BLEB*) are patent. *CB* ciliary body

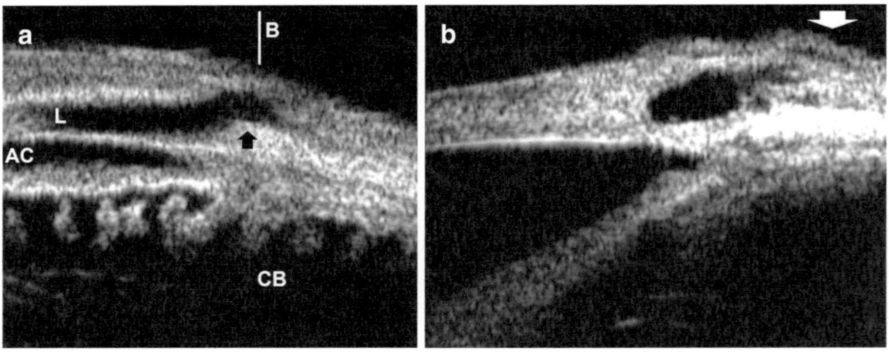

Fig. 4.23 (**a**) Nonpenetrating deep sclerectomy first week after surgery. Transversal scan. A tear in the superficial scleral flap (*black arrow*) facilitates the direct passage of the aqueous to the subconjunctival space leading to overfiltration. *White line* (*B*) indicates the location of the radial section (25 A). *CB* ciliary body, *AC* anterior chamber, *L* scleral lake. (**b**) Nonpenetrating deep sclerectomy first week after surgery. Radial scan. High conjunctival bleb (*arrow*)

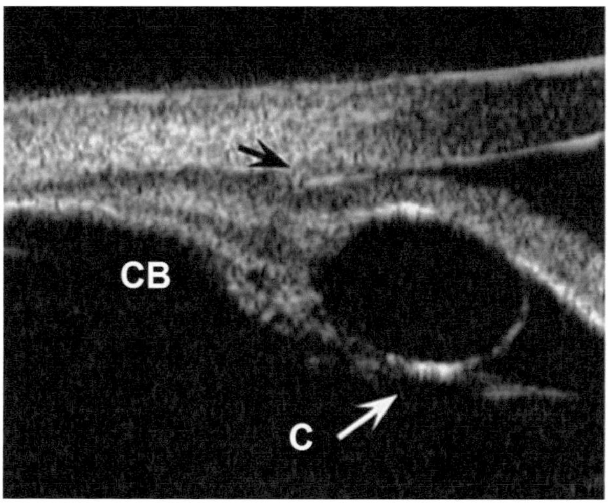

Fig. 4.24 Iris root-ciliary body cyst (iridociliary junction). The total lack of internal reflectivity indicates it is filled with fluid. In this case the hipoecogenic band in the ciliary body closer to the sclera is very patent. The angle is close by the cyst (*black arrow*: scleral spur). *CB* ciliary body, *C* cyst (*white arrow*)

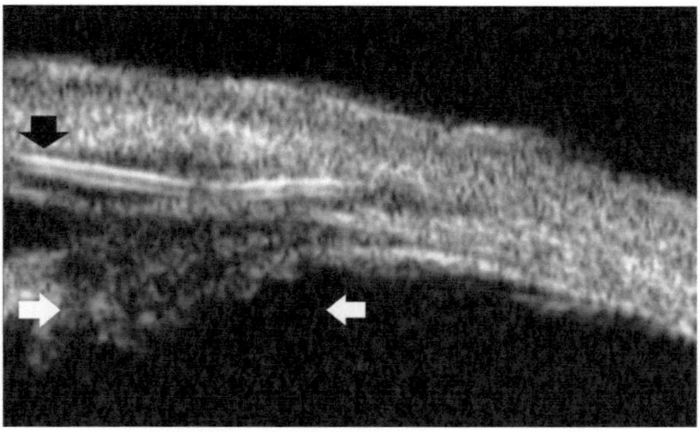

Fig. 4.25 Nonpenetrating deep sclerectomy. The implant can be seen (*black arrow*). The implant is highly reflective and produces a shadowing of the structures behind it (space between the *two white arrows*). The implant is surrounded with tissue and no free aqueous can the detected in the reservoir

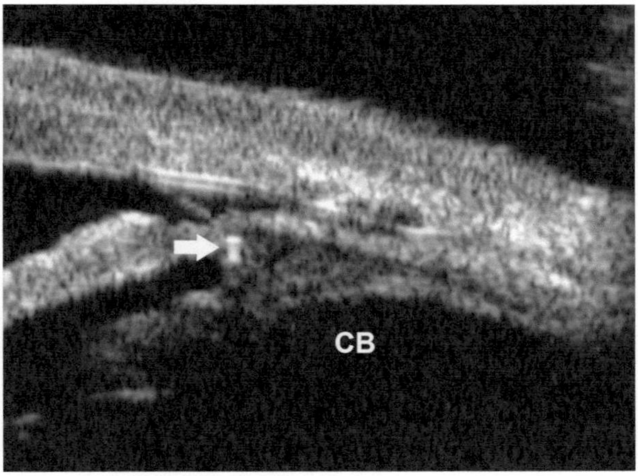

Fig. 4.26 Nonpenetrating deep sclerectomy. Twelve months after surgery. The implant is surrounded with tissue, but the areas of total lack of internal reflectivity indicate some are free aqueous. See the sulcus position of and IOP haptic (*arrow*). *CB*: ciliary body

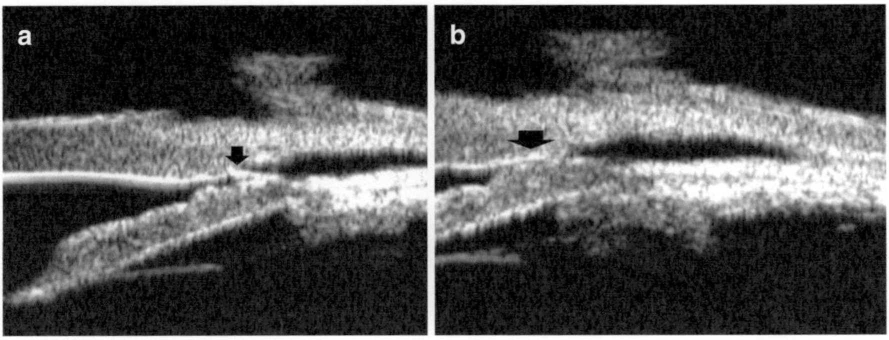

Fig. 4.27 (**a**) Nonpenetrating deep sclerectomy in a case of angle closure glaucoma (3 weeks after the surgery). The intrascleral lake is adequately formed and the Descemet's membrane can be imaged. But without an iridectomy the iris is very close to the membrane and will block the filtration. (**b**) Nonpenetrating deep sclerectomy in a case of angle closure glaucoma (6 weeks after the surgery). See the contact between the iris and the Descemet's membrane leading to the surgical failure

4.8.3 Aqueous Drainage Tubes

UBM can be used to determine the tube position, rule out causes of tube obstruction or tube-related complications and can be useful for surgical planning, for instance to find the best location for the tube insertion [22]. Carrillo et al. [40] reported two cases in which UBM was used to diagnose Ahmed valve obstruction by the iris. Occlusion of the end of the tube by iris tissue was demonstrated by UBM both in implants placed in the anterior chamber and the ciliary sulcus. An iridectomy over the tip of the tube restored filtration in each case. UBM has also been used to demonstrate peritubular filtration as a cause of ocular hypotony after glaucoma shunt device implant (Fig. 4.28) [41].

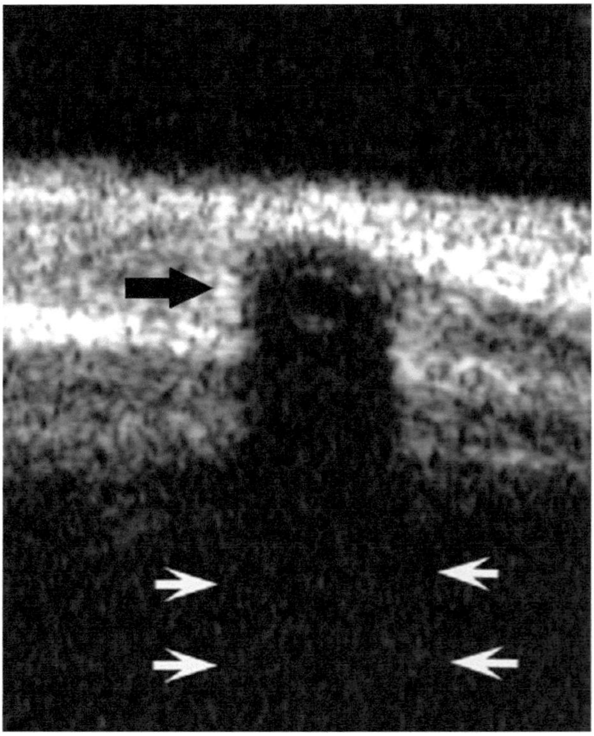

Fig. 4.28 Ahmed Drainage Device implant. Transversal scan. In this case there is no fluid around the tube (*black arrow*). See the acoustic shadow produce by the tube (*white arrows*)

4.8.4 Evaluation of Postoperative Complications After Trabeculectomy

After glaucoma filtering surgery, UBM can be used to detect and evaluate the extent of ciliochoroidal effusion and cyclodialysis. In ciliochoroidal effusion, UBM shows the ciliary body to be edematous and separated from the sclera by a collection of supraciliary fluid (Figs. 4.29 and 4.30). Many ciliochoroidal effusions that are too limited in extent to be detectable by indirect ophthalmoscopy and slit lamp biomicroscopy can be imaged by UBM. A study done by Sugimoto et al. [42] showed that the presence of suprachoroidal fluid is related to a low IOP after trabeculectomy, whereas the disappearance of suprachoroidal fluid increases IOP. Grigera et al. [43] studied the pathophysiology of flat anterior chamber without bleb leak. Ring-shaped effusions were detected on UBM even in cases in which conventional ultrasonography did not. UBM is a helpful tool in the diagnosis and management of flat anterior chamber and low IOP after trabeculectomy.

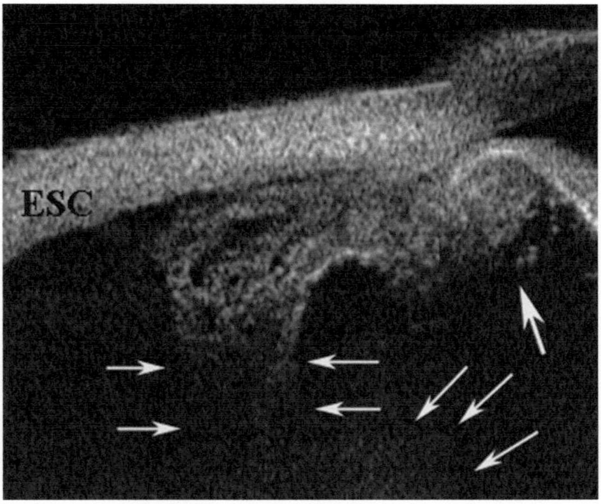

Fig. 4.29 Massive serous choroidal effusion after trabeculectomy (*small arrows*). Note the anterior displacement and rotation of the ciliary body (*big arrow*). *ESC* sclera

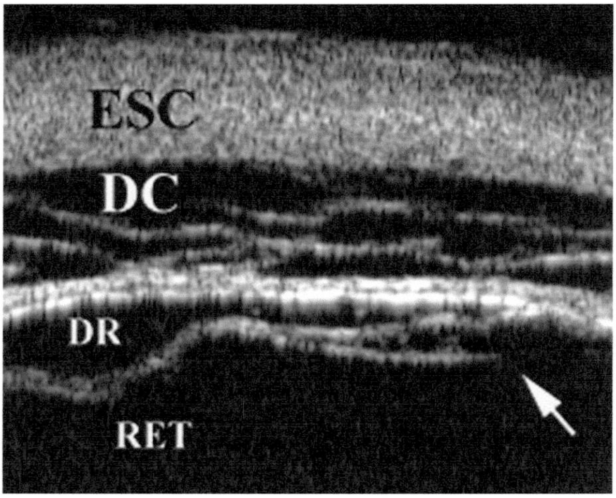

Fig. 4.30 Serous choroidal effusion (*DC*) and retinal detachment (*DR*). The *arrow points* to a retinal tear. *RET* retina, *ESC* sclera

4.9 Role of UBM in Other Surgeries

UBM has been used to to assess changes in the anterior chamber depth after both cataract and antiglaucomatous surgeries, synequiolysis or drainage implants.

More interestingly UBM images could very useful in the assessment of the effectiveness of the new minimally invasive glaucoma surgery. It can provide us with useful information about the mechanism of action of these implants, and its evaluation over time in relation to the causes of success or failure of the surgery.

4.9.1 Glaukos

UBM may be a useful imaging modality to identify iStent in the anterior or posterior chamber. The iStent (Glaukos Corporation, Laguna Hills, CA) is a 1-mm, titanium trabecular bypass stent implanted across the inner wall of Schlemm's canal under direct gonioscopy. In a study designed to determine the best modality to identify iStent placement when gonioscopic visualization is not possible on a human cadaver eye, UBM, anterior segment optical coherence tomography (AS-OCT), and B-scan ultrasonography were done to visualize and precisely locate two intentionally misplaced iStents. UBM could localize both intentionally misplaced stents, whereas AS-OCT could not visualize the iStent that was lodged in the sulcus. B-scan ultrasonography was unable to detect either of the stents. UBM may be useful to identify iStent in the anterior or posterior chamber, whereas AS-OCT is limited to detection of stents in the anterior chamber alone. B-scan ultrasonography is unable to identify iStent in either the anterior or posterior chamber (imaging modalities for localization of an iStent(®) [44]. However the titanium causes artifacts and image distortion so UBM is not able to provide us with information on the tilt and/or depth of the iStent in the scleral sulcus (Fig. 4.31).

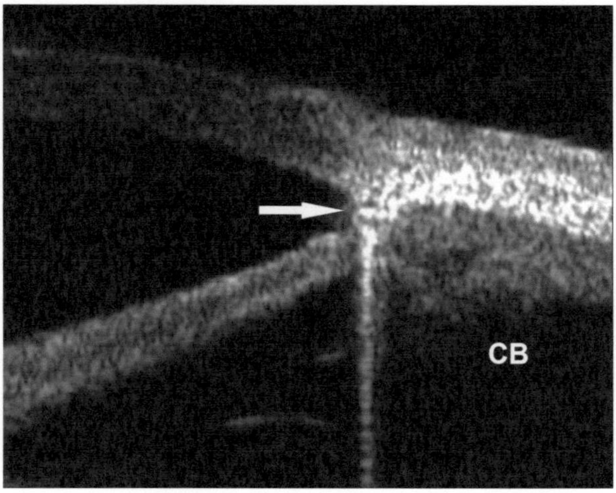

Fig. 4.31 Glaukos G1 implant (Glaukos Inc). UBM allows to locate the iStent in the angle (*arrow*), however due to artifacts and image distortion is not able to provide us with more information. *CB* ciliary body

4.10 Suprachoroidal Surgeries

4.10.1 Cypass

In a prospective study of patients with suprachoroidal glaucoma implant Cypass by our group, the presence of fluid in the suprachoroidal space was an indicator of good evolution in the postoperative period (Gonzalez-Pastor E et al. *UBM findings after suprachoroidal CyPass implant for glaucoma: 1 year follow up*. ARVO 2013). Two months after surgery, all patients presented suprachoroid fluid, while 12 months postoperatively, only eight patients (33 %) showed fluid in the suprachoroid space (Figs. 4.32 and 4.33). The decrease in suprachoroidal fluid coincided with an increase in IOP. The presence of fluid in the four quadrants was only found in five patients. In addition, it was possible to identify the presence of peritubular fluid in all patients 2 months after surgery but only in three patients was it observed at the end of the study. These results suggest tisular changes in the suprachoroidal space after surgery and possible processes of healing that would avoid the free flow of aqueous humor.

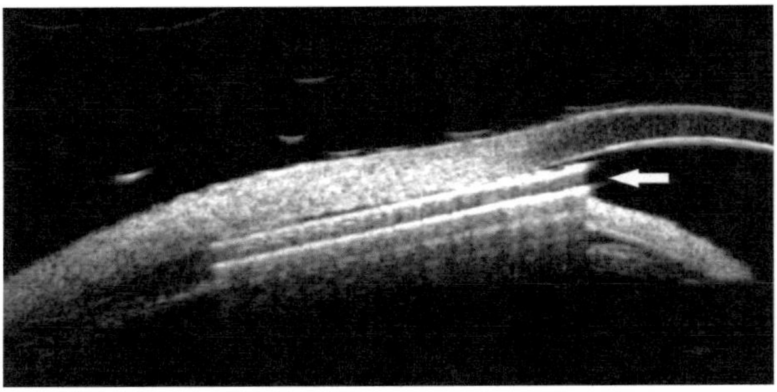

Fig. 4.32 CyPass suprachoidal implant (Transcend Medical). UBM allows to examine the position of the device (*arrow*) and the presence of fluid in the suprachoidal space. Image courtesy of Andrea Vásquez Roa (Clínica de Ojos Orillac-Calvo, Panama)

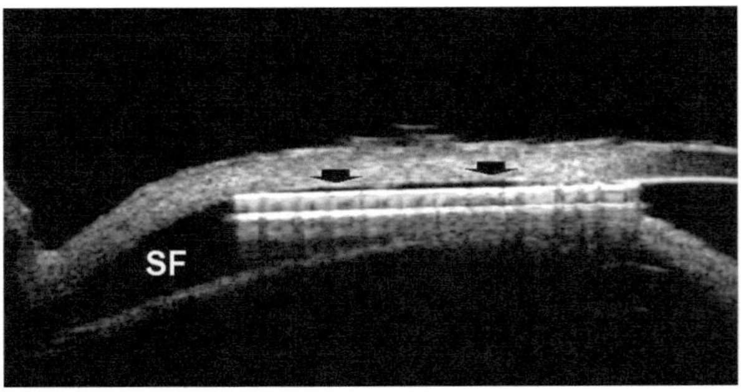

Fig. 4.33 CyPass suprachoidal implant (Transcend Medical). In this case there is more suprachoidal fluid (*SF*), note the fluid between the device and the sclera (*Arrow*). Image courtesy of Andrea Vásquez Roa (Clínica de Ojos Orillac-Calvo, Panama)

4.10.2 Gold Shunt

This implant decreases the IOP by means of drainage to the suprachoroidal space. UBM images show the presence of fluid in the suprachoroidal space as well as the correct position of the implant (Fig. 4.34). In the late postoperative period a decrease of the liquid can be found despite verifying the correct position of the implant.

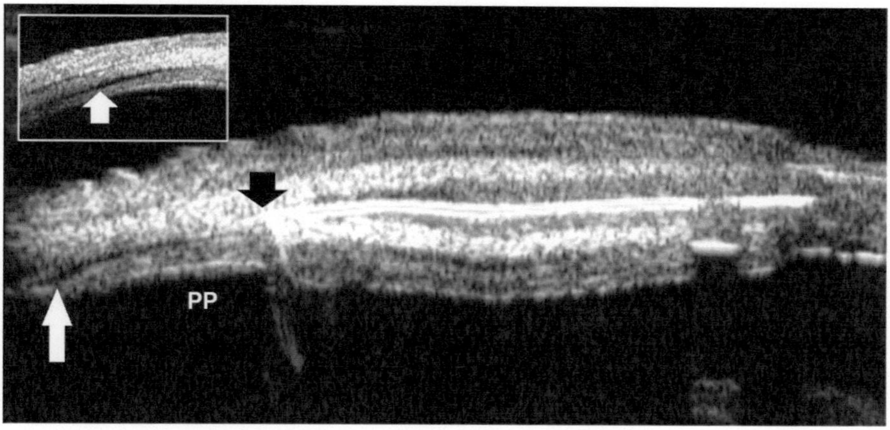

Fig. 4.34 Gold Glaucoma Shunt suprachoidal implant (SOLX). The device tail implanted in the suprachoidal space (*black arrow*). In this case fluid in the suprachoidal can be imaged (*white arrows*). The GGS is highly reflective and produces artifacts of the structures behind it, so no reliable information can be obtained behind the device. *PP* pars plana

References

1. Pavlin CJ, Harasiewicz K, Sherar MD, Foster FS (1991) Clinical use of ultrasound biomicroscopy. Ophthalmology 98(3):287–295
2. McWhae JA, Crichton AC (1996) The use of ultrasound biomicroscopy following trabeculectomy. Can J Ophthalmol 31(4):187–191
3. Liebmann JM (2001) Ultrasound biomicroscopy of the anterior segment. J Glaucoma 10(5 Suppl 1):S53–S55
4. Pavlin CJ, Sherar BA, Foster FS (1990) Subsurface ultrasound microscopic imaging of the intact eye. Ophthalmology 97:244–250
5. García Feijoó J, Benítez Del Castillo JM, Martín Carbajo M, García Sánchez J (1997) Orbital cup: a device to facilitate UBM examination of pars plana and peripheral retina. Arch Ophthalmol 115:1475–1476
6. Kapetansky FM (1997) A new water bath for ultrasonic biomicroscopy. Ophthalmic Surg Lasers 28:605–606
7. Esaki K, Ishikawa H, Leibmann JM et al (2000) A technique for performing ultrasound biomicroscopy in the sitting and prone positions. Ophthalmic Surg Lasers 31:166–169
8. Ishikawa H, Schuman JS (2004) Anterior segment imaging: ultrasound biomicroscopy. Ophthalmol Clin North Am 17:7–20
9. Potash SD, Tello C, Liebmann J, Ritch R (1994) Ultrasound biomicroscopy in pigment dispersion syndrome. Ophthalmology 101(2):332–339
10. Adam RS, Pavlin CJ, Ulanski LJ (2004) Ultrasound biomicroscopic analysis of iris profile changes with accommodation in pigmentary glaucoma and relationship to age. Am J Ophthalmol 138(4):652–654
11. Mora P, Sangermani C, Ghirardini S et al. Ultrasound biomicroscopy and iris pigment dispersion: a case-control study. Br J Ophthalmol 2010;94:428–32
12. Mendez-Hernandez C, Garcia-Feijoo J, Cuina-Sardina R et al (2003) Ultrasound biomicroscopy in pigmentary glaucoma. Arch Soc Esp Oftalmol 78:137–142
13. Pillunat LE, Bohm A, Fuisting B et al (2000) Ultrasound biomicroscopy in pigmentary glaucoma. Ophthalmologe 97:268–271
14. Diniz Filho A, Cronemberger S, Me'rula RV et al (2008) Plateau iris. Arq Bras Oftalmol 71:752–758
15. Pavlin CJ, Ritch R, Foster FS (1992) Ultrasound biomicroscopy in plateau iris syndrome. Am J Ophthalmol 113(4):390–395
16. Garudadri CS, Chelerkar V, Nutheti R (2002) An ultrasound biomicroscopic study of the anterior segment in Indian eyes with primary angle-closure glaucoma. J Glaucoma 11:502–507
17. Kumar RS, Tantisevi V, Wong MH et al (2009) Plateau iris in Asian subjects with primary angle closure glaucoma. Arch Ophthalmol 127:1269–1272
18. Parc C, Laloum J, Berge`s O (2010) Comparison of optical coherence tomography and ultrasound biomicroscopy for detection of plateau iris. J Fr Ophtalmol 33:266.e1–266.e3
19. Diniz Filho A, Cronemberger S, Ferreira DM et al (2010) Plateau iris configuration in eyes with narrow-angle: an ultrasound biomicroscopic study. Arq Bras Oftalmol 73:155–160
20. Diniz Filho A, Cronemberger S, Me'rula RV et al (2009) Comparative biometric study between plateau iris configuration and primary open angle glaucoma with narrow angle. Arq Bras Oftalmol 72:302–307
21. Ramani KK, Mani B, George RJ, Lingam V (2009) Follow-up of primary angle closure suspects after laser peripheral iri-dotomy using ultrasound biomicroscopy and A-scan biometry for a period of 2 years. J Glaucoma 18(7):521–527
22. García-Feijoó J, Sáenz-Francés F, Martínez de la Casa JM et al (2008) Angle-closure glaucoma after piggyback intraocular lens implantation. Eur J Ophthalmol 18(5):822–826
23. Okamoto F, Nakano S, Okamoto C et al (2004) Ultrasound biomicroscopic findings in aniridia. Am J Ophthalmol 137:858–862

24. Kranemann CF, Pavlin CJ, Trope GE (1998) Ultrasound biomicroscopy in Sturge-Weber-associated glaucoma. Am J Ophthalmol 125:119–121
25. Zhang M, Chen J, Liang L et al (2006) Ultrasound biomicroscopy of Chinese eyes with iridocorneal endothelial syndrome. Br J Ophthalmol 90:64–69
26. Berinstein DM, Gentile RC, Sidoti PA et al (1997) Ultrasound biomicroscopy in anterior ocular trauma. Ophthalmic Surg Lasers 28:201–207
27. Park M, Kondo T (1998) Ultrasound biomicroscopic findings in a case of cyclodialysis. Ophthalmologica 212:194–197
28. McWhae JA, Crichton AC, Rinke M (2003) Ultrasound biomicroscopy for the assessment of zonules after ocular trauma. Ophthalmology 110:1340–1343
29. Mendez-Hernandez C, Fernandez-Barrientos Y, Fernandez-Vidal AM, Martinez-de-la-Casa JM, Saenz-Frances F, Garcia-Feijoo J (2008) Secondary pigment dispersion syndrome after in-the-bag acrysof intraocular lens SN60AT implantation. Can J Ophthalmol 43(1):120–121
30. García-Feijoó J, Hernández Matamoros JL, Castillo-Gómez A, Méndez-Hernández C, Martínez de la Casa JM, Martín Orte T, García-Sánchez J (2004) Secondary glaucoma and severe endothelial damage after silicon posterior chamber phakic intraocular lens implantation. J Cataract Refract Surg 30:1786–1789
31. Avitabile T, Russo V, Uva MG et al (1998) Ultrasound-biomicroscopic evaluation of filtering blebs after laser suture lysis trabeculectomy. Ophthalmologica 212(Suppl 1):17–21
32. Lázaro García C, Benítez del Castillo JM, Castillo Gómez A, García Feijoó J, Macías Benítez JM, García Sánchez J (2002) Lens fluorophotometry following trabeculectomy in primary open angle glaucoma. Ophthalmology 109:76–79
33. García Feijoó J, García Sánchez J, Cuiña Sardiña R, Méndez Hernández C (2001) Biomicroscopía ultrasónica en el postoperatorio de la macrotrabeculectomía. In: Muñoz Negrete F, Rebolleda G (eds) Manejo postoperatorio de la cirugía filtrante y sus complicaciones. Rigorma Gráfica, Madrid
34. Khairy HA, Atta HR, Green FD et al (2005) Ultrasound biomicroscopy in deep sclerectomy. Eye 19:555–560
35. Marchini G, Marraffa M, Brunelli C et al (2001) Ultrasound biomicroscopy and intraocular-pressure-lowering mechanisms of deep sclerectomy with reticulated hyaluronic acid implant. J Cataract Refract Surg 24:507–517
36. Chiou AG, Mermoud A, Underdahl JP et al (1998) An ultrasound biomicroscopic study of eyes after deep sclerectomy with collagen implant. Ophthalmology 105:746–750
37. Aptel F, Dumas S, Denis P (2009) Ultrasound biomicroscopy and optical coherence tomography imaging of filtering blebs after deep sclerectomy with new collagen implant. Eur J Ophthalmol 19:223–230
38. Wang Y, Sun XH, Meng FR et al (2003) The failure causes of nonpenetrating trabecular surgery and reoperation. Zhonghua Yan Ke Za Zhi 39:87–90
39. Park M, Tanito M, Nishikawa M et al (2004) Ultrasound biomicroscopy of intrascleral lake after viscocanalostomy and cataract surgery. J Glaucoma 13:472–478
40. Carrillo MM, Trope GE, Pavlin C et al (2005) Use of ultrasound biomicroscopy to diagnose Ahmed valve obstruction by iris. Can J Ophthalmol 40:499–501
41. Garcia-Feijoo J, Cuina-Sardina R, Mendez-Hernandez C et al (2001) Peritubular filtration as cause of severe hypotony after Ahmed valve implantation for glaucoma. Am J Ophthalmol 132:571–572
42. Sugimoto K, Ito K, Esaki K et al (2002) Supraciliochoroidal fluid at an early stage after trabeculectomy. Jpn J Ophthalmol 46:548–552
43. Grigera D, Moreno C, Fava O et al (2002) Ultrasound biomicroscopy in eyes with anterior chamber flattening after trabeculectomy. Can J Ophthalmol 37:27–32
44. Ichhpujani P, Katz LJ, Gille R, Affel E (2010) Imaging modalities for location of an iStent. Ophthal Surg Lasers Imag: Off J Int Soc Imag Eye 41(6):660–663

Chapter 5
Retrobulbar Ocular Blood Flow Evaluation in Open-Angle Glaucoma

Antonio Martinez

This chapter aims to give an overview over:

1. To briefly review the underlying physical principles and the different CDI devices currently available in the market
2. To describe the following clinical protocol:
   (a) Preparation of the subject/patient
   (b) Evaluation procedure
   (c) Vessels studied
3. To evaluate the relationship between retrobulbar blood flow disturbances and glaucoma

5.1 Doppler Ultrasound

The color Doppler imaging (CDI) combines B-scan gray images from tissue structures with velocity information obtained from the Doppler shift of the moving blood cells. A Doppler ultrasound test uses reflected sound waves to evaluate blood as it flows through a blood vessel.

This method has been widely used in many different fields of medicine. In ophthalmology it is used to measure blood flow velocities in the retrobulbar vessels.

A. Martinez
Clinical Science, Science and Sports Research, Ames, Spain
e-mail: tontxu_1999@yahoo.com

A. Ferreras (ed.), *Glaucoma Imaging*, DOI 10.1007/978-3-319-18959-8_5

5.1.1 Basic Technology

The Doppler ultrasonography is based on a phenomenon, observed for sound waves and electromagnetic radiation, characterized by a change in the apparent frequency of a wave as a result of relative motion between the observer and the source (Fig. 5.1). The transducer sends and receives sound waves that are amplified through a microphone. The sound waves bounce off solid objects, including blood cells. The movement of blood cells causes a change in pitch of the reflected sound waves (called the Doppler effect).

The greater the blood flow velocity, the greater the Doppler shift. The Doppler shift (Δf) can be calculated as $\Delta f = 2.u.f_0/C$ (in which "u" is blood flow velocity, f_0 is the frequency of the sound source, and C is the sound velocity in the medium) in the situation where the transducer is parallel to the blood vessel. If this condition is not met, a Doppler angle (α) has to be considered by using a correction for the measurement angle in the following formula: $u = \Delta f.C/\ (2.f_0.\cos\ \alpha)$. When the transducer is aligned with a vessel ($\cos 0° = 1$), the largest Doppler shift will be obtained with the least possible effect of angle uncertainty. However, using very small angles may lead to technical difficulties because the vessel wall may totally reflect the sound waves. Therefore, in practice, angles between 30° and 60° are most commonly used. Angles exceeding 60° should be avoided because in this case even small errors in estimating the Doppler angle will result in very large correction errors.

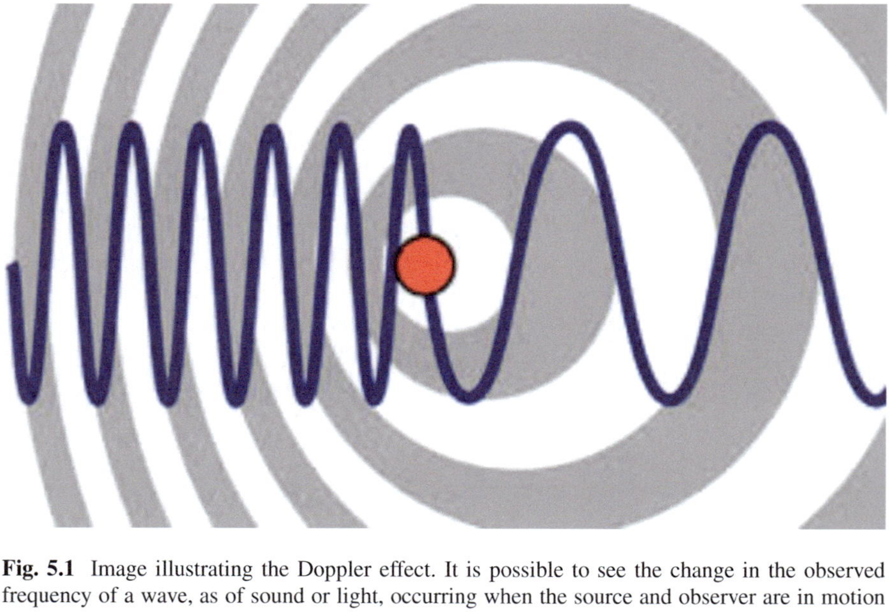

Fig. 5.1 Image illustrating the Doppler effect. It is possible to see the change in the observed frequency of a wave, as of sound or light, occurring when the source and observer are in motion relative to each other, with the frequency increasing when the source and observer approach each other and decreasing when they move apart. The motion of the source causes a real shift in frequency of the wave, while the motion of the observer produces only an apparent shift in frequency

5.1.2 Types of Doppler Ultrasound

There are four types of Doppler ultrasound:

- "Bedside" or continuous wave Doppler. This type uses the change in pitch of the sound waves to provide information about blood flow through a blood vessel.
- Duplex Doppler. Duplex Doppler ultrasound uses standard ultrasound methods to produce a picture of a blood vessel and the surrounding organs. In addition, a computer converts the Doppler sounds into a graph that provides information about the speed and direction of blood flow through the blood vessel being evaluated.
- Color Doppler. Color Doppler uses standard ultrasound methods to produce a picture of a blood vessel. In addition, a computer converts the Doppler sounds into colors that are overlaid on the image of the blood vessel and that represent the speed and direction of blood flow through the vessel.
- Power Doppler. Power Doppler is a newer ultrasound technique that is up to five times more sensitive in detecting blood flow than color Doppler. Power Doppler can obtain some images that are difficult or impossible to obtain using standard color Doppler. However, power Doppler is most commonly used to evaluate blood flow through vessels within solid organs.

The most commonly used in ophthalmology is the color Doppler imaging (Fig. 5.2). The CDI is a variation in the technology of pulse Doppler processing. The frequency shift information contained in the radiofrequency pulses returning to the transducer along one line is decoded at a given depth along this line, depending on the corresponding time delay. A mean value of the frequency shift is extracted for each point along this line. This is then done for multiple lines as defined as a color box [9, 20, 40, 49].

Unlike a conventional B scan, CDI uses a linear array transducer consisting of linearly arranged, sequentially excited piezoelectric elements. When choosing the probe frequency, we consider both the resolution and the depth of measurement: higher frequency improves resolution, but imposes limits on image depth due to attenuation.

The transducers for retrobulbar CDI have a frequency of about 7.5 MHz, but frequencies may range from 6 to 13 MHz. Table 5.1 summarizes the currently market available CDI devices and probes that have been used in the various studies on retrobulbar circulation.

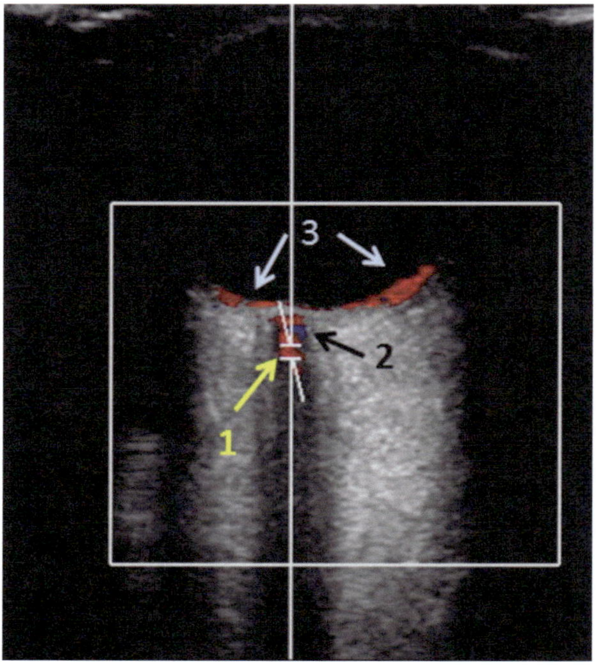

Fig. 5.2 Color Doppler imaging taken with a 7.5 MHz linear probe (Phillips HD11 XE). The arterial blood flow is represented in red and the venous blood flow in blue. The image shows the central retinal artery (*1*), the central retinal vein (*2*), and the short posterior ciliary arteries (*3*)

Table 5.1 Devices and probes, listed in alphabetical order, currently available in the market and that have been used in various studies on retrobulbar color Doppler imaging (CDI)

Manufacturer company	Device	Probe
Advanced Technology Laboratories	ATL Apogee 800 plus	7.5 MHz
	ATL HDI 3000	5–10 MHz
		7.5 MHz
	ATL ultramark 8	7.5 MHz
	ATL ultramark-9 HDI	5 MHz
		5–10 MHz
		7.5 MHz
Dynaview	TM II SSD-1700	6 MHz
General Electric Medical System	Logiq 400 MD	7.5 MHz
	Logic 500 Pro	6.0–9.0 MHz
	Logiq 700 MR	8.8 MHz
	Voluson	7.5 MHz
Quantum Medical	QUAD 1	7.5 MHz
	QAD 1	7.5 MHz
Hewlett Packard	Sonos 1000	5.5 MHz
Hitachi	AU-580 Asynchronous-Hitachi analyzer	7.5 MHz
Medasonic	Transpect TCD	2 MHz
Medison	Accuvix XQ	7.5 MHz
Multigon	Neurovision 500	4 MHz

Table 5.1 (continued)

Manufacturer company	Device	Probe
Philips	ATL-HDI 1500	7.5 MHz
	HDI 5000	5–10 MHz
	P700	7.5 MHz
	HD11 XE	5 MHz
		6 MHz
		7.5 MHz
		12 MHz
Siemens	Acuson	7.5 MHz
	Acuson 128 XP	5 MHz
		5.5 MHz
		7.5 MHz
		7 MHz
	Acuson 128XP/10	5 MHz
		7 MHz
	Albis AG	7.5 MHz
	Antares	7.5 MHz
	QAD 1	5/7.5 MHz
	QAD1/QAD 2000	7.5 MHz
	Quantum	UNK
	Quantum 2000	7.5 MHz
	Sonoline Elegra	6.5 MHz
		7.5 MHz
	Sonoline G40	6 MHz
		7.5 MHz
		13 MHz
	Sonoline Sienna	7.5 MHz
		7.5/12 MHz
		7.5 MHz
	Sonoline Versa	7.5 MHz
Toshiba	Aplio-80	11.5 MHz
	Aplio-300	6 MHz
		7.5 MHz
		12 MHz
	Aplio 500	6 MHz
		7.5 MHz
		12 MHz
	SSH-I40A	7.5 MHz
	SSA-270A	7.5 MHz
	SSA-340A	6/7.5 MHz
	SSA-380A	7 MHz
		7.5 MHz
Vingmed Sound	CFM 750	2 MHz
		3.25/7.5 MHz
		7.5 MHz

Adapted from Stalmans et al. [52]

5.2 Clinical Protocol

Comply with a clinical protocol facilitates the standardization of results and minimizes the potential negative impact of external influences on hemodynamic parameters.

5.2.1 *Preparation of the Study Subject and Examiner*

Before starting the CDI exam, both patient and examiner should take into consideration a series of recommendations. In brief, before starting the measurement, a resting period of at least 5–10 min should be scheduled. Stable hemodynamic conditions should be verified by repeated measurements of systemic blood pressure and pulse rate. Additionally, patients should be instructed to abstain from smoking and exercise for three hours and from drinking coffee or alcohol for 12 h.

Patient is placed in supine position and the head tilted forward at an angle of approximately 30° and legs uncrossed to avoid influence on venous return.

The patient is instructed to look straight while closing the eyes. If the patient has difficulty keeping eyes steady during the measurements, they may be asked to open the other eye in order to use this eye to guide their gaze to a fixation point above them.

The examiner should be kept in a comfortable and stable posture that minimizes the appearance of fatigue. Additionally, it must be kept a constant distance between the probe and the eye, and avoid any exerting pressure on the eye. It was proposed that it might be most easily accomplished when the examiner is seated behind the head of the patient, while the base of their hand rests on the patient's forehead and their finger is placed on the patient's cheek [52]. Nevertheless, the examiner being located beside the patient with the elbow resting on a pillow placed on the chest of the patient while the hand rests on the patient's cheek and his/her finger is placed on the temporal region of the patient is a perfectly valid option [21–27, 29, 31].

Moreover, supporting the cable of the probe by the examiner's shoulder and arm takes weight off the probe and further improves comfort and stability. The examiner's other hand operates the control panel of the CDI device.

5.2.2 *Evaluation Procedure*

Firstly, we use the B-scan mode to identify the back globe structures (Fig. 5.3).

The optic nerve is used as a landmark (Fig. 5.4). Then, color Doppler is applied to visualize the vessels (flow) (Fig. 5.5).

In order to obtain reliable and reproducible measurements using CDI, it is extremely important to have a thorough knowledge of the retrobulbar vascular anatomy. It proceeds to identify the blood vessel that we want to study, the sample volume is placed in the center of the vessel, the angle is set parallel to the vessel, and several seconds of Doppler waveform are recorded (Fig. 5.6).

On the other hand, it is essential to know the characteristics of the waves corresponding to different blood vessels and their specific locations that are conventionally chosen for measurement (Fig. 5.7).

According to the type of CDI device, it may be necessary to adapt the setting to the type of vessel that is being measured. For the smaller vessels [central retinal artery (CRA) and short posterior ciliary artery (SPCA)], "low flow" settings (to detect small Doppler frequency shifts) and a shallow measuring depth (e.g., 35–45 mm) may be used, whereas "high flow" settings and a higher measuring depth (e.g., 50–60 mm) may be more appropriate for the ophthalmic artery (OA) [52].

It is necessary to pay an especial attention to the measurement angle. As previously mentioned, the blood velocity (u) can be calculated as $u = \Delta f.C/(2.f_0.\cos\alpha)$. If the angle is small, an error in the angle correction will result in a very small error in the velocity measurement. However, if the angle exceeds 60°, the cos α will approach 0, and very small deviations in the angle will result in very large errors in velocity calculation. It is therefore crucial to perform the Doppler measurements at angles below 60°. In the OA and CRA, the angle can be determined relatively easily. In the SPCA, this is more difficult because of their smaller size and more tortuous course [53].

The CDI allows the measurement of blood flow velocities including peak systolic velocity (PSV) and end-diastolic velocity (EDV) in the retrobulbar vessels—that is, the ophthalmic artery, the central retinal artery, and the nasal and temporal short posterior ciliary arteries.

The operator identifies the PSV (highest velocity at systole) and the EDV (lowest velocity at diastole); from these points, both velocities are measured (Fig. 5.8).

Additionally, the resistivity (RI) [43] and pulsatility (PI) [8] indices can be calculated as follows:

$$\mathrm{RI} = \frac{\mathrm{PSV} - \mathrm{EDV}}{\mathrm{PSV}} \qquad \mathrm{PI} = \frac{\mathrm{PSV} - \mathrm{EDV}}{\text{Mean Velocity}\left(\mathrm{MV}\right)}$$

The advantage of these indices is that they are independent of Doppler angle, since changes in angle have a concomitant effect on PSV and EDV. The RI varies from 0 to 1, with higher values supposedly indicating higher vascular distal resistance. However, it is unclear whether the RI represents an adequate measure of retinal vascular resistance [41, 48].

Although the CDI has important advantages such as it is a noninvasive method, is not affected by poor ocular media, and requires no contrast or radiation, it has some limitations that should be mentioned in this section.

One important limitation of this technique is that no quantitative information of vessel diameter is obtained. Therefore, calculation of blood flow is not possible with this method. Nevertheless, if the blood perfusion pressure and blood viscosity remain constant, an increase in flow velocity is invariably associated with an increase in flow in terms of volume per time unit. Indeed, there is a general agreement that blood flow velocity assessed by color Doppler ultrasonography correlates with volume blood flow, provided there is no evidence of vascular stenosis or changes in perfusion pressure [50].

Additionally, as mentioned above, the validity of RI as a measure of vascular resistance is uncertain, and its value in the determination of resistivity distal from the measuring point is controversial [41, 48].

An important issue to take into consideration, especially when planning to conduct multicenter studies, is that the comparability between different instruments is problematic. One should realize that this also limits the comparability of the results from different studies.

Furthermore, CDI measurements are subjective, and adequate training is crucial for producing reliable and reproducible results. An important source of error is incorrect angle of incidence. It is crucial to perform the Doppler measurements at angles below 60°. Another potential source of error is increased intraocular pressure caused by excessive pressure applied to the eyelid [52].

An additional limitation of this technique is that the examination is time consuming: a thorough examination with repeated measurements of the four retrobulbar vessels can take up to 30–45 min.

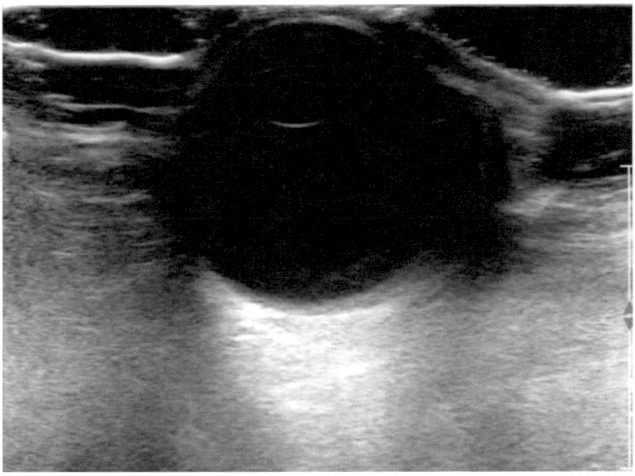

Fig. 5.3 Gray scale B-scan imaging of the eye taken with a 7.5 MHz linear probe (Phillips HD11 XE)

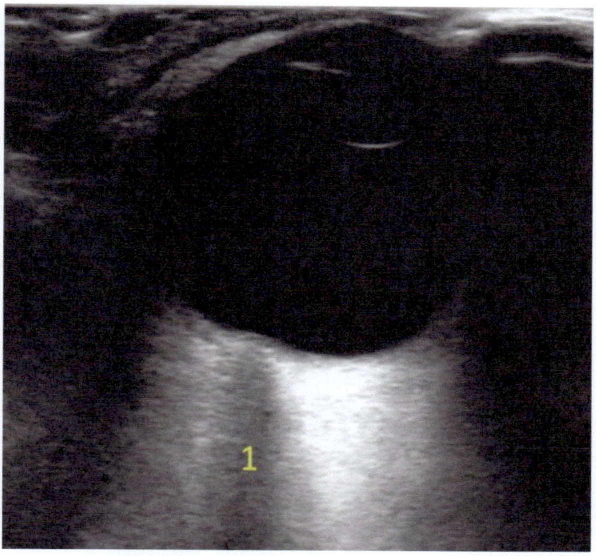

Fig. 5.4 Grayscale B-scan imaging of the eye showing the optic nerve shadow (*1*)

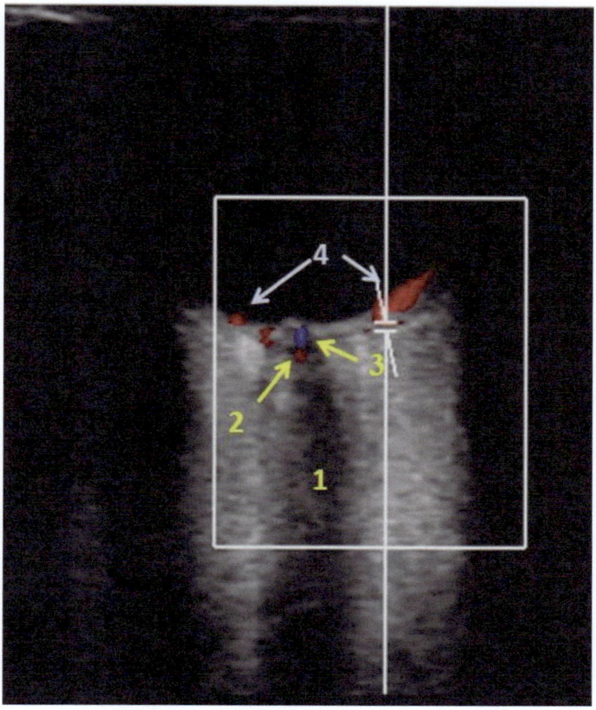

Fig. 5.5 Color Doppler imaging taken with a 7.5 MHz linear probe (Phillips HD11 XE). *Red* and *blue pixels* represent blood movement toward and away from the transducer, respectively. This image shows the optic nerve shadow (*1*), the central retinal artery (*2*), the central retinal vein (*3*), and the short posterior ciliary arteries (*4*)

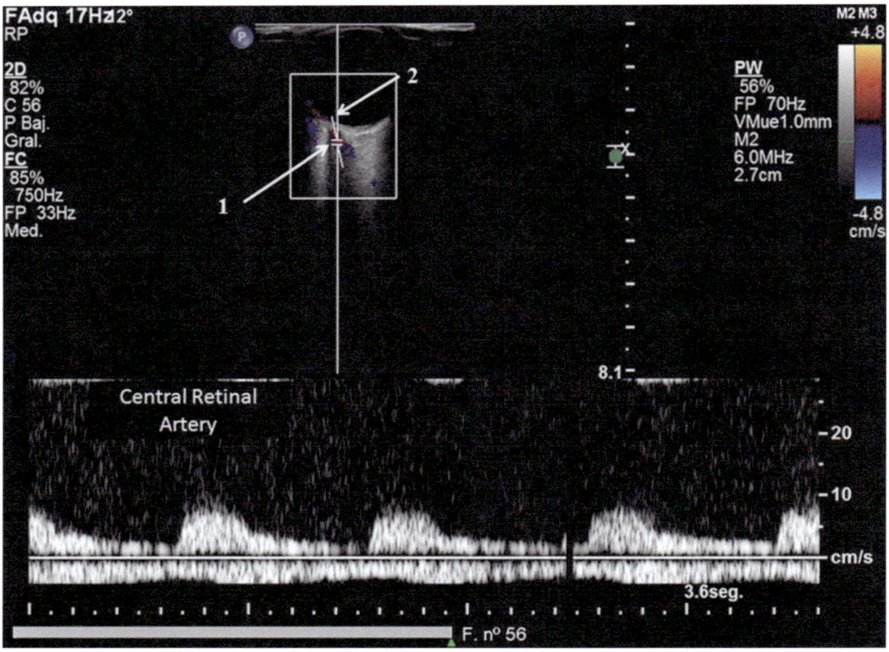

Fig. 5.6 Color Doppler imaging of the central retinal artery and vein taken with a 7.5 MHz linear probe (Phillips HD11 XE). Once identified the vessel to study the sample volume (*1*) is placed in the center of the vessel, the angle (*2*) is set parallel to the vessel, and several seconds of Doppler waveform are recorded

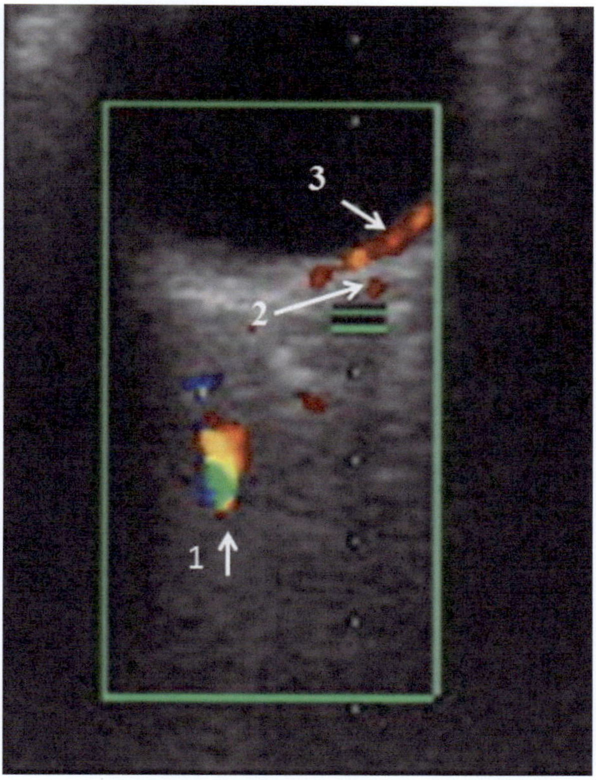

Fig. 5.7 Color Doppler imaging showing the different blood vessels and their specific locations that are conventionally chosen for measurement. This image shows the ophthalmic artery (*1*), central retinal artery (*2*), and short posterior ciliary arteries (*3*)

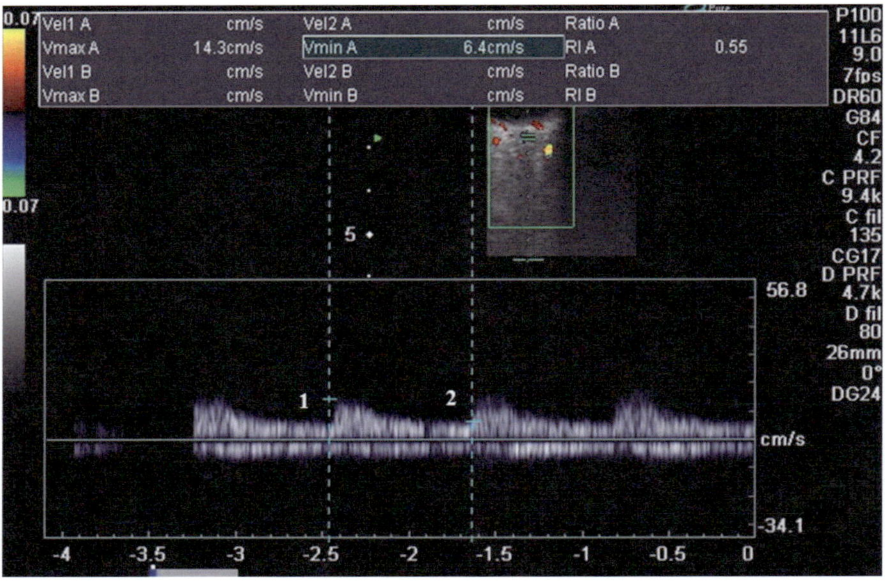

Fig. 5.8 Color Doppler imaging of the central retinal artery and vein taken with a 7.5 MHz linear probe (Toshiba Aplio 80). (*1*) Represents the peak systolic velocity (*PSV*) (the highest velocity at systole); (*2*) represents the end-diastolic velocity EDV) (the lowest velocity at diastole). Pourcelot's resistivity index (RI) can be calculated according to the following formula: $\mathrm{RI} = \frac{\mathrm{PSV} - \mathrm{EDV}}{\mathrm{PSV}}$

5.2.3 *Vessels Studied*

As previously mentioned, the CDI allows the measurement of the blood flow velocity in the retrobulbar vessels, more specifically in the CRA, the nasal PCA, the temporal PCA, and the OA. Unfortunately, individual short posterior ciliary vessels cannot be distinguished by CDI. Therefore, bundles of vessels, rather than individual ciliary vessels, are examined.

5.2.3.1 Central Retinal Artery

The CRA and central retinal vein (CRV) are measured 2–3 mm behind the surface of the optic disc (Fig. 5.9) and cannot be measured separately by CDI. Therefore, a double waveform is obtained with a distinct pulsatile arterial waveform above the zero line and a gentle sinusoidal venous variation below the zero line.

The Doppler of the CRA is that of a low resistance wave with a rounded peak systolic and continuous flow during diastole. Blood flow in the CRV produces a smoother Doppler waveform than in the CRA, and therefore, the terms maximal velocity and minimal velocity are used to describe the highest and lowest recorded velocities during the cardiac cycle.

In healthy subjects, the [mean (standard deviation) (SD)] PSV ranges from 6.6 (1.5) [16] to 20.5 (7.8) cm/s [17], the EDV ranges from 6.7 (1.0) [54] to 1.6 (0.4) cm/s [16], and the RI ranges from 0.85 (0.08) [11] to 0.44 (0.04) [13]. In healthy subjects, we found that the [mean (SD)] RI was 0.60 (0.02) in those patients younger than 70 years [mean age 65.1 (2.7) years] and 0.63 (0.03) in those patients of 70 years or older (mean age 75.3 (3.3) years).

On the other hand, in primary open-angle glaucoma (POAG) patients, the mean (SD) PSV ranges from 16.5 (6.2) [17] to 6.4 (2.1) cm/s [16], the EDV ranges from 5.4 (2.3) [17] to 1.4 (0.1) [56] cm/s, and the RI ranges from 0.89 (0.1) [11] to 0.46 (0.05) [13].

The reproducibility (class correlation coefficients) in the CRA in both healthy controls and glaucoma patients ranges from 0.53 to 0.80 for the PSV, 0.55 to 0.66 for the EDV, and 0.69 to 0.82 for the RI [48].

In addition, the coefficients of variation in healthy subjects range from 2.6 % [51] to 21 % [15] for the PSV, 4.2 % [51] to 25.8 % [45] for the EDV, and 1.8 % [51] to 9.4 % [45] for the RI.

In glaucoma patients, the coefficient of variation seems to be slightly higher ranging from 16.3 % [51] to 26.0 % [15] for the PSV, 13.2 % [51] to 30.0 % [36] for the EDV, and 4.0 % [36] to 7.5 % [51] for the RI.

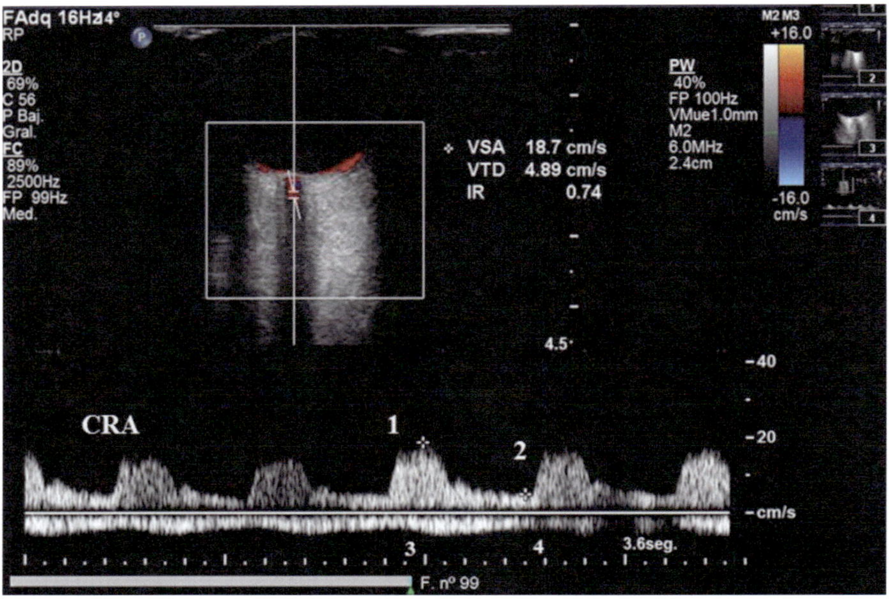

Fig. 5.9 Color Doppler imaging of the central retinal artery (*CRA*) and vein (*CRV*) taken with a 7.5 MHz linear probe (Phillips HD11 XE). The Doppler of the CRA is that of a low resistance wave with a rounded peak systolic and continuous flow during diastole. The peak systolic velocity (*1*) and the end-diastolic velocity (*2*) are measured. Blood flow in the CRV produces a smoother Doppler waveform than in the CRA, and therefore, the terms maximal velocity (*3*) and minimal velocity (*4*) are used to describe the highest and lowest recorded velocities during the cardiac cycle

5.2.3.2 Short Posterior Ciliary Artery

The nasal (NSPCA) and temporal (TSPCA) short posterior ciliary arteries are located on both sides of the optic nerve and should be measured at a position that is close to the optic nerve and as anterior as possible without receiving interference from the choroid (Fig. 5.10).

It is important to have in consideration the fact that individual short posterior ciliary vessels cannot be distinguished by CDI. Therefore, the obtained waveform represents the mass effect produced by a bundle of vessels, rather than from individual ciliary vessels. These arteries produce a more uniform arterial pulse without a venous wave (Fig. 5.10). The Doppler of the SPCA is that of a low resistance wave with a rounded peak systolic and continuous flow during diastole.

In healthy subjects, the [mean (standard deviation) (SD)] PSV ranges from 29.7 (9.5) [34] to 5.8 (1.0) cm/s [16], the EDV ranges from 7.6 (3.8) [34] to 1.4 (0.3) cm/s [46], and the RI ranges from 0.80 (0.1) [10] to 0.48 (0.04) [13].

In healthy subjects, our results found that the [mean (SD)] RI was 0.61 (0.02) in those patients younger than 70 years [mean age 65.1 (2.7) years] and 0.65 (0.03) in those patients of 70 years or older (mean age 75.3 (3.3) years).

Otherwise, in POAG patients, the mean (SD) PSV ranges from 15.0 (5.7) [17] to 5.4 (1.1) cm/s [16], the EDV ranges from 5.9 (1.3) [13] to 1.5 (0.1) [16], and the RI ranges from 0.78 (0.21) [17] to 0.53 (0.06) [13].

In POAG patients, we found that the [mean (SD)] RI was 0.65 (0.04) in those patients younger than 70 years [mean age 65.1 (2.7) years] and 0.68 (0.04) in those patients of 70 years or older (mean age 75.3 (3.3) years).

Measurement of the SPCA usually shows greater variability because the technical problems are greater. Coefficients of variation, in healthy subjects, range from 2.4 % [51] to 19.0 % [15] for the PSV, 2.7 % [51] to 38.8 % [3] for the EDV, and 1.6 % [51] to 24.0 % [15] for the RI.

On the other hand, in glaucoma patients, the coefficients of variation range from 15.8 % [51] to 26.0 % [15] for the PSV, from 22.4 % [51] to 64.0 % [15] for the EDV, and from 4.2 % [36] to 69.0 % [15] for the RI.

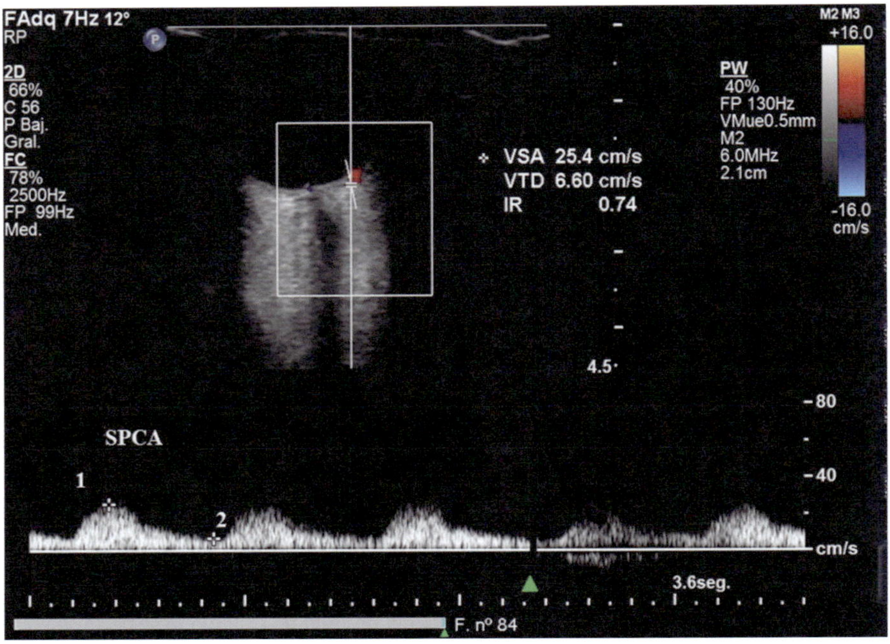

Fig. 5.10 Color Doppler imaging of the short posterior ciliary artery (SPCA) taken with a 7.5 MHz linear probe (Phillips HD11 XE). As the individual short posterior ciliary vessels cannot be distinguished by color Doppler imaging, the obtained waveform represents the mass effect produced by a bundle of vessels, rather than from individual ciliary vessels. As observed in the central retinal artery, the Doppler of the SPCA is that of a low resistance wave with a rounded peak systolic and continuous flow during diastole

5.2.3.3 Ophthalmic Artery

The ophthalmic artery (OA) is the first major branch of the internal carotid artery and divides into many branches in the orbital area. The ophthalmic artery is situated deeper in the orbit. Measurements of the OA are performed approximately 10–15 mm posterior to the globe, where the ecographic signals are stronger and by convention should be measured on the temporal side of the optic nerve, immediately after it crosses the optic nerve (Fig. 5.11).

When measuring the OA, "high flow" settings and a higher measuring depth (e.g., 50–60 mm) may be more appropriate. As in the CRA, the angle can be determined relatively easily in the OA.

The OA has a characteristic high resistance wave with a sharp systolic peak, one dicrotic depression, and reduced diastolic velocities (Fig. 5.12). The AO wave bears a certain resemblance with that of the common carotid artery or even with the external carotid artery rather than the internal carotid artery which it is a branch.

In healthy subjects, the [mean (standard deviation) (SD)] PSV ranges from 57.8 (14.0) [42] to 22.2 (5.3) cm/s [7], the EDV ranges from 14.1 (6.1) [34] to 3.7 (0.2) cm/s [60], and the RI ranges from 0.87 (0.01) [44, 60] to 0.66 (0.06) [32].

In healthy subjects, our results found that the [mean (SD)] RI was 0.70 (0.05) in those patients younger than 70 years [mean age 65.1 (2.7) years] and 0.73 (0.05) in those patients of 70 years or older (mean age 75.3 (3.3) years).

Moreover, in POAG patients, the mean (SD) PSV ranges from 44.6 (1.7) [1] to 27.3 (9.6) cm/s [17], the EDV ranges from 12.2 (1.5) [1] to 3.3 (2.6) cm/s [60], and the RI ranges from 0.90 (0.01) [56] to 0.67 (0.04) [1].

In POAG patients, we found that the [mean (SD)] RI in the OA ranged from 0.79 (0.07) [23] to 0.75 (0.09) [24].

The reproducibility (class correlation coefficients) in the OA in both healthy controls and glaucoma patients ranges from 0.66 to 0.98 for the PSV, 0.44 to 0.92 for the EDV, and 0.71 to 0.92 for the RI [33, 48].

Measurement of the OA usually shows lower variability than the SPCA. Coefficients of variation, in healthy subjects, range from 2.0 % [51] to 18.0 % [15] for the PSV, 3.6 % [51] to 25.5 % [3] for the EDV, and 1.1 % [51] to 9.0 % [15] for the RI.

On the other hand, in glaucoma patients, the coefficients of variation range from 5.0 % [15] to 10.1 % [51] for the PSV, from 4.0 % [15] to 24.9 % [51] for the EDV, and from 3.0 % [15] to 6.8 % [51] for the RI.

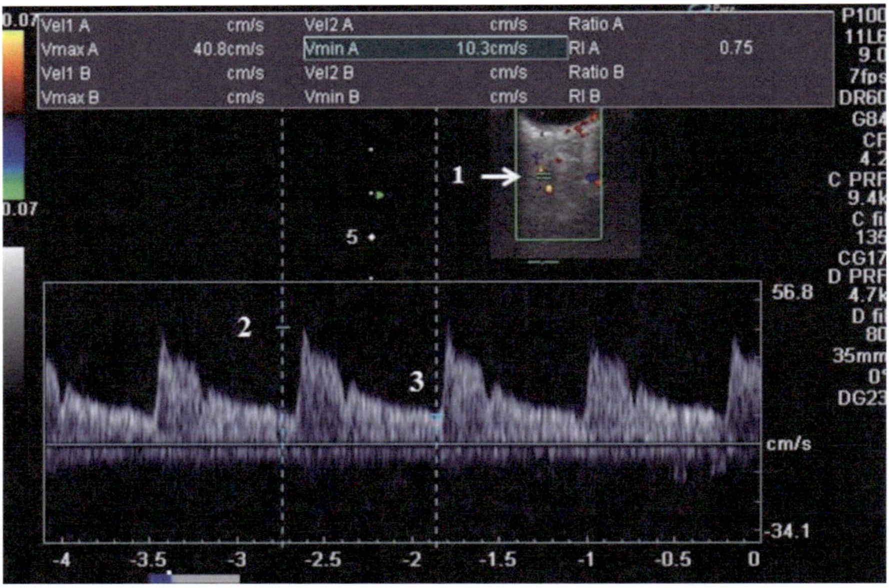

Fig. 5.11 Color Doppler imaging of the ophthalmic artery taken with a 7.5 MHz linear probe (Toshiba Aplio 80). Measurements of the OA are performed approximately 10 mm to 15 mm posterior to the globe immediately after it crosses the optic nerve (*1*). The peak systolic velocity (PSV) (the highest velocity at systole) (*2*) and the end-diastolic velocity (EDV) (the lowest velocity at diastole) (*3*) are measured by the examiner

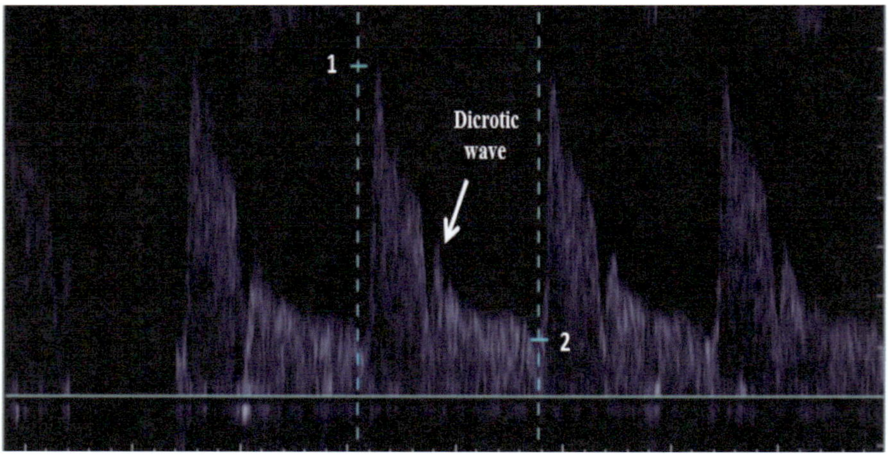

Fig. 5.12 Color Doppler imaging of the ophthalmic artery (OA) taken with a 7.5 MHz linear probe (Toshiba Aplio 80). The OA has a characteristic high resistance wave with a sharp systolic peak (*1*), one dicrotic depression, and reduced diastolic velocities (*2*)

5.3 Retrobulbar Blood Flow Disturbances in Glaucoma

Many different studies have evaluated the retrobulbar hemodynamic parameters in POAG patients [9, 11, 13, 22–26, 29, 31, 38, 39, 55], ocular hypertension [2, 35], angle-closure glaucoma (ACG) [5, 21, 37], pseudoexfoliative glaucoma (PXG) [6, 27, 28, 58, 59], and normal tension glaucoma (NTG) [14, 19, 57].

They have found, on average, reduced blood flow velocities and increased resistivity indices in the retrobulbar vessels of glaucoma patients.

Furthermore, within individuals, retrobulbar blood flow velocity reductions are greater in the eye with more advance damage.

Open-angle glaucoma seems to be associated with a decreased mean flow velocity and an increased mean resistivity index in the retrobulbar vessels. Reduced EDV and increased RI in the OA, reduced maximum and minimum velocities in the central retinal vein (CRV), and reduced PSV and EDV in the CRA and SPCA have been observed in eyes with POAG when compared with normal control eyes.

On the other hand, few studies investigated the ocular circulatory changes in angle-closure glaucoma patients.

Cheng et al. [5] suggested that as in POAG, the retrobulbar circulation was disturbed in the chronic angle-closure glaucoma. In the event of well-controlled IOP, retrobulbar hemodynamics were altered significantly more in chronic angle-closure glaucoma eyes with worse visual field than in those with better visual field.

Conversely, Marjanovic et al. [21] did not find blood flow disturbances in the retrobulbar vessels of the ACG patients.

On the other hand, Nong and Ninghua [37] investigated the hemodynamic changes of the ophthalmic and CRA in ACG patients and the effects of IOP on the retrobulbar hemodynamics. The results of this study suggested that compared with the normal subjects, the hypertension group of ACG showed significant reduction in the EDV and increases in pulsatility index and RI of CRA, whereas normal tension group of ACG also showed remarkable increase in RI of CRA. However, these authors concluded that the elevated IOP was a major cause of the vascular resistance increased in PACG, which will make the end-diastolic blood flow of CRA decreased.

In contrast to the study of Nong and Ninghua [37], Marjanovic et al [21] did not find either blood flow disturbances in the retrobulbar vessels of the ACG patients or any correlation between the IOP and the retrobulbar hemodynamic parameters.

A significant decreased for PSV and EDV and an increase for RI at the OA, SPCA, and CRA in exfoliation syndrome have been reported by previous studies [6, 58, 59].

Conversely, [28] showed that patients with pseudoexfoliation syndrome, compared with age-matched healthy subjects, had similar peak systolic, end-diastolic, and resistivity indices in all the arteries studied.

With regard to the comparison between pseudoexfoliative and primary open-angle glaucoma, literature data are still controversial. While Yüksel et al. [58] and Detorakis et al. [6] found that some retrobulbar hemodynamic parameters were more altered in PXG patients, [26] reported that color Doppler alterations were more pronounced in POAG than in PXG patients.

As regards the NTG patients, Harris et al. [14] reported that patients with NTG exhibited a low EDV and a high RI in the ophthalmic artery compared with controls.

Additionally, Kondo et al. [19] investigated the retrobulbar hemodynamics by means of color Doppler imaging in NTG patients with asymmetric visual field loss and asymmetric ocular perfusion pressure. The results of this study suggested that there are significant differences in blood velocities and in the RI in the retrobulbar vessels between the eyes with higher ocular perfusion pressure and a better mean deviation and those with higher ocular perfusion pressure and a worse mean deviation.

The influence of ocular blood flow disturbances on the progression of the glaucomatous damage has only been recognized more recently [4, 12, 18, 24, 31, 47, 60] (Table 5.2).

Galassi and coworkers [12] evaluated the effect of retrobulbar blood flow circulation on the progression of visual field damage in POAG patients. This study included 44 patients with POAG over a period of 7 years. The results of this study suggested that patients with low diastolic velocities and high resistivity indices in the ophthalmic artery had more progressive visual field.

Satilmis and collaborators [47] in a retrospective, observational, and case series study evaluate the correlation between progression rate of glaucomatous damage and retrobulbar blood flow. Based on the results of this study, independent of the extent of damage or IOP, the visual field deterioration significantly correlates with retrobulbar hemodynamic variables.

In addition, Martinez and Sanchez [24], in a prospective cohort study, assessed the value of color Doppler imaging of the ophthalmic artery and short posterior ciliary arteries in prognosis of disease progression in patients with primary open-angle glaucoma.

The results of this study suggested that poor blood flow in the retrobulbar vessels is closely link to deterioration in the visual field in patients with POAG and high IOP (Fig. 5.13).

Moreover, Martinez and Sanchez [31] in a prospective, randomized, evaluator-masked, parallel group study evaluated clinically relevant risk factors for progressive visual field loss in a cohort of patients with POAG. The results of this study suggested that lower diastolic blood pressure, systemic hypertension treatment, lower EDVs in the OA and SPCA, and higher RIs in the OA and SPCA were statistically significant predictors for progression of visual field damage in this group of patients with POAG over a 5-year period.

Additionally, Calvo et al. [4] suggested that an RI value higher than 0.75 in the ophthalmic artery was associated with the development of glaucoma.

Furthermore, Jimenez-Aragon et al. [18] reported statistically significant differences in the EDV and RI in the OA and CRA between glaucoma patients that progressed and those who remained stable.

Although these studies have shown promising and valuable results, further clinical studies, particularly multicenter clinical trials, including different types of glaucoma and different races, are needed to establish whether improved retrobulbar blood flow may prevent the progression of glaucomatous damage.

Table 5.2 Summary analysis of retrobulbar blood flow velocity studies and visual field progression

Study	Subjects	Time of follow-up	Doppler parameter	Visual field results
Galassi et al. [12]	44 POAG	7-years	RI OA $\geq$ 0.78	18/44 patients progressed RI OA $\geq$ 0.78 (14/18 progressed) RI OA $<$ 0.78 (4/18 progressed)
Satilmis et al. [47]	20 POAG	4.3 years	Reduced EDV CRA	Multiple $r = 0.63$ ($p = 0.0037$)
Martinez and Sanchez [24]	51 POAG	3 years	RI OA $>$ 0.72 RI SPCA $>$ 0.65	23/49 patients progressed RI OA $>$ 0.72 and RI SPCA $>$ 0.65 (21/23 progressed) RI OA $\leq$ 0.72 and RI SPCA $\leq$ 0.65 (2/23 progressed)
Zeitz et al. [60]	114 OAG	1 year	Reduced PSV CRA Reduced PSV SPCA Reduced EDV SPCA	12/114 patients progressed
Martinez and Sanchez [31]	215 eyes from 146 POAG	5 years	EDV OA $<$ 8.9 cm/s RI OA $\geq$ 0.74 EDV SPCA $<$ 4.6 cm/s RI SPCA $\geq$ 0.65	52/107 eyes progressed ($p < 0.001$) 67/105 eyes progressed ($p < 0.001$) 46/106 eyes progressed ($p = 0.007$) 48/122 eyes progressed ($p < 0.001$)
Calvo et al. [4]	262 glaucoma suspects	4 years	RI OA $\geq$ 0.75	36/262 progressed RI $<$ 0.75 (6/98 progressed) RI $\geq$ 0.75 (30/164 progressed)
Jimenez-Aragon et al. [18]	71 glaucoma suspects	5 years	Reduced EDV OA Reduced TAV OA Increased RI OA Reduced EDV CRA Reduced TAV CRA Increased RI CRA	12/71 progressed

Adapted from Martinez et al. [30]

Abbreviations: *POAG* primary open-angle glaucoma, *OAG* open-angle glaucoma, *OA* ophthalmic artery, *SPCA* short posterior ciliary artery, *CRA* central retinal artery, *PSV* peak systolic velocity, *EDV* end-diastolic velocity, *RI* resistivity index, *TAV* Time-average velocity

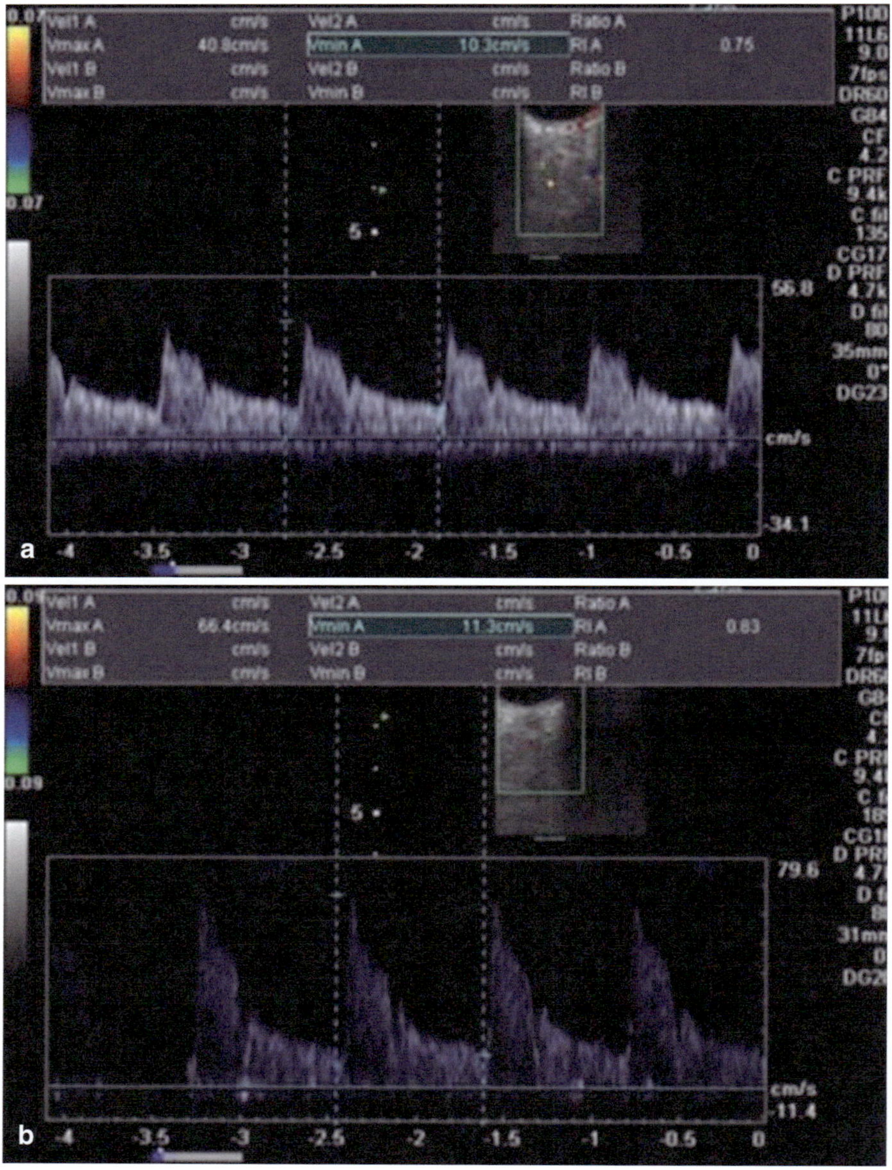

Fig. 5.13 Color Doppler imaging of the ophthalmic artery (OA) taken with a 7.5 MHz linear probe (Toshiba Aplio 80) from two patients with primary open-angle glaucoma. The resistivity index (0.75) of the stable patient (**a**) is much lower than that observed (0.83) in the patient that showed visual field progression (**b**)

References

1. Altan-Yaycioglu R, Türker G, Akdöl S, Acunaş G, Izgi B (2001) The effects of beta-blockers on ocular blood flow in patients with primary open angle glaucoma: a color Doppler imaging study. Eur J Ophthalmol 11(1):37–46
2. Akarsu C, Bilgili MY (2004) Color Doppler imaging in ocular hypertension and open-angle glaucoma. Graefes Arch Clin Exp Ophthalmol 242(2):125–129
3. Baxter GM, Williamson TH (1995) Color Doppler imaging of the eye: normal ranges, reproducibility, and observer variation. J Ultrasound Med 14(2):91–96
4. Calvo P, Ferreras A, Polo V, Güerri N, Seral P, Fuertes-Lazaro I, Pablo LE (2012) Predictive value of retrobulbar blood flow velocities in glaucoma suspects. Invest Ophthalmol Vis Sci 53(7):3875–3884
5. Cheng CY, Liu CJ, Chiou HJ, Chou JC, Hsu WM, Liu JH (2001) Color Doppler imaging study of retrobulbar hemodynamics in chronic angle-closure glaucoma. Ophthalmology 108(8): 1445–1451
6. Detorakis ET, Achtaropoulos AK, Drakonaki EE, Kozobolis VP (2007) Hemodynamic evaluation of the posterior ciliary circulation in exfoliation syndrome and exfoliation glaucoma. Graefes Arch Clin Exp Ophthalmol 245(4):516–521
7. Dimitrova G, Kato S, Tamaki Y, Yamashita H, Nagahara M, Sakurai M, Kitano S, Fukushima H (2001) Choroidal circulation in diabetic patients. Eye (Lond) 15(Pt 5):602–607
8. Evans DH, Barrie WW, Asher MJ, Bentley S, Bell PR (1980) The relationship between ultrasonic pulsatility index and proximal arterial stenosis in a canine model. Circ Res 46:470–475
9. Flammer J, Orgül S, Costa VP et al (2002) The impact of ocular blood flow in glaucoma. Prog Retin Eye Res 21:359–393
10. Fujioka S, Karashima K, Nishikawa N, Saito Y (2006) Correlation between higher blood flow velocity in the central retinal vein than in the central retinal artery and severity of nonproliferative diabetic retinopathy. Jpn J Ophthalmol 50(4):312–317
11. Galassi F, Nuzzaci G, Sodi A, Casi P, Vielmo A (1992) Color Doppler imaging in evaluation of optic nerve blood supply in normal and glaucomatous subjects. Int Ophthalmol 16(4–5): 273–276
12. Galassi F, Sodi A, Ucci F et al (2003) Ocular hemodynamics and glaucoma prognosis: a color Doppler imaging study. Arch Ophthalmol 121:1711–1715
13. Galassi F, Giambene B, Menchini U (2008) Ocular perfusion pressure and retrobulbar haemodynamics in pseudoexfoliative glaucoma. Graefes Arch Clin Exp Ophthalmol 246(3): 411–416
14. Harris A, Sergott RC, Spaeth GL, Katz JL, Shoemaker JA, Martin BJ (1994) Color Doppler analysis of ocular vessel blood velocity in normal-tension glaucoma. Am J Ophthalmol 118(5):642–649
15. Harris A, Williamson TH, Martin B, Shoemaker JA, Sergott RC, Spaeth GL, Katz JL (1995) Test/Retest reproducibility of color Doppler imaging assessment of blood flow velocity in orbital vessels. J Glaucoma 4(4):281–286
16. Hosking SL, Harris A, Chung HS, Jonescu-Cuypers CP, Kagemann L, Roff Hilton EJ, Garzozi H (2004) Ocular haemodynamic responses to induced hypercapnia and hyperoxia in glaucoma. Br J Ophthalmol 88(3):406–411
17. Januleviciene I, Sliesoraityte I, Siesky B, Harris A (2008) Diagnostic compatibility of structural and haemodynamic parameters in open-angle glaucoma patients. Acta Ophthalmol 86(5):552–557
18. Jimenez-Aragon F, Garcia-Martin E, Larrosa-Lopez R, Artigas-Martín JM, Seral-Moral P, Pablo LE (2013) Role of color Doppler imaging in early diagnosis and prediction of progression in glaucoma. Biomed Res Int 2013:871689. doi:10.1155/2013/871689, Epub 2013 Sep 17
19. Kondo Y, Niwa Y, Yamamoto T, Sawada A, Harris A, Kitazawa Y (2000) Retrobulbar hemodynamics in normal-tension glaucoma with asymmetric visual field change and asymmetric ocular perfusion pressure. Am J Ophthalmol 130(4):454–460

20. Lieb WE, Cohen SM, Merton DA et al (1991) Color Doppler imaging of the eye and orbit. Technique and normal vascular anatomy. Arch Ophthalmol 109:527–531
21. Marjanovic I, Milic N, Martinez A (2012) The impact of intraocular pressure reduction on retrobulbar hemodynamic parameters in patients with open-angle glaucoma. Eur J Ophthalmol 22(1):77–82
22. Marjanovic I, Milic N, Martinez A, Benitez-del-Castillo J (2012) Retrobulbar hemodynamic parameters in open-angle and angle-closure glaucoma patients. Eye (Lond) 26(4):523–528
23. Martinez A et al (1999) Dorzolamide effect on ocular blood flow. Invest Ophthalmol Vis Sci 40(6):1270–1275
24. Martínez A, Sánchez M (2005) Predictive value of colour Doppler imaging in a prospective study of visual field progression in primary open-angle glaucoma. Acta Ophthalmol Scand 83(6):716–722
25. Martínez A, Sánchez M (2006) A comparison of the effects of 0.005 % latanoprost and fixed combination dorzolamide/timolol on retrobulbar haemodynamics in previously untreated glaucoma patients. Curr Med Res Opin 22(1):67–73
26. Martinez A, Sanchez M (2008) Effects of dorzolamide 2 % added to timolol maleate 0.5 % on intraocular pressure, retrobulbar blood flow, and the progression of visual field damage in patients with primary open-angle glaucoma: a single-center, 4-year, open-label study. Clin Ther 30(6):1120–1134
27. Martinez A, Sanchez M (2008) Retrobulbar hemodynamic parameters in pseudoexfoliation syndrome and pseudoexfoliative glaucoma. Graefes Arch Clin Exp Ophthalmol 246(9): 1341–1349
28. Martinez A, Sanchez M (2008) Ocular haemodynamics in pseudoexfoliative and primary open-angle glaucoma. Eye 22(4):515–520
29. Martínez A, Sánchez-Salorio M (2009) A comparison of the long-term effects of dorzolamide 2 % and brinzolamide 1 %, each added to timolol 0.5 %, on retrobulbar hemodynamics and intraocular pressure in open-angle glaucoma patients. J Ocul Pharmacol Ther 25(3):239–248
30. Martinez A et al (2009) The impact of ischemia in glaucoma. In: Westerhouse AN (ed) Eye research developments: glaucoma, corneal transplantation, and bacterial Eye infections, 1st edn. Hauppauge, New York, pp 245–302, 11788–3619
31. Martínez A, Sanchez-Salorio M (2010) Predictors for visual field progression and the effects of treatment with dorzolamide 2 % or brinzolamide 1 % each added to timolol 0.5 % in primary open-angle glaucoma. Acta Ophthalmol 88(5):541–552
32. Martini E, Guiducci M, Campi L, Cavallini GM (2005) Ocular blood flow evaluation in injured and healthy fellow eyes. Eur J Ophthalmol 15(1):48–55
33. Matthiessen ET, Zeitz O, Richard G, Klemm M (2004) Reproducibility of blood flow velocity measurements using colour decoded Doppler imaging. Eye (Lond) 18(4):400–405
34. Modrzejewska M, Pieńkowska-Machoy E, Grzesiak W, Karczewicz D, Wilk G (2008) Predictive value of color Doppler imaging in an evaluation of retrobulbar blood flow perturbation in young type-1 diabetic patients with regard to dyslipidemia. Med Sci Monit 14(10): MT47–MT52
35. Nicolela MT, Wolman BE, Buckley AR, Drance SM (1996) Ocular hypertension and primary open-angle glaucoma: a comparative study of their retrobulbar blood flow velocity. J Glaucoma 5(5):308–310
36. Niwa Y, Yamamoto T, Kawakami H, Kitazawa Y (1998) Reproducibility of color Doppler imaging for orbital arteries in Japanese patients with normal-tension glaucoma. Jpn J Ophthalmol 42(5):389–392
37. Nong T, Ninghua F (1997) Color Doppler imaging in the study of retrobulbar hemodynamic changes of primary angle-closure glaucoma. Yan Ke Xue Bao 13(3):113–115
38. Plange N, Kaup M, Arend O, Remky A (2006) Asymmetric visual field loss and retrobulbar haemodynamics in primary open-angle glaucoma. Graefes Arch Clin Exp Ophthalmol 244(8):978–983
39. Plange N, Kaup M, Weber A, Arend KO, Remky A (2006) Retrobulbar haemodynamics and morphometric optic disc analysis in primary open-angle glaucoma. Br J Ophthalmol 90(12):1501–1504

40. PolaK JF (2004) Peripheral vascular sonography: a practical guide. 2nd Edn. Lippincott Williams & Wilkins, Philadelphia, PA 19106 USA; pp 23–25
41. Polska E, Kircher K, Ehrlich P et al (2001) RI in central retinal artery as assessed by CDI does not correspond to retinal vascular resistance. Am J Phisiol Heart Cir Physiol 280:H1442–H1447
42. Polska E, Polak K, Luksch A, Fuchsjager-Mayrl G, Petternel V, Findl O, Schmetterer L (2004) Twelve hour reproducibility of choroidal blood flow parameters in healthy subjects. Br J Ophthalmol 88(4):533–537
43. Pourcelot L (1974) Applications clinique de l'examen Doppler transcutané. INSRM 34:213–240
44. Rainer G, Kiss B, Dallinger S, Menapace R, Findl O, Schmetterer K, Georgopoulos M, Schmetterer L (1999) Effect of small incision cataract surgery on ocular blood flow in cataract patients. J Cataract Refract Surg 25(7):964–968
45. Rankin SJ, Walman BE, Buckley AR, Drance SM (1995) Color Doppler imaging and spectral analysis of the optic nerve vasculature in glaucoma. Am J Ophthalmol 119(6):685–693
46. Roff EJ, Harris A, Chung HS, Hosking SL, Morrison AM, Halter PJ, Kagemann L (1999) Comprehensive assessment of retinal, choroidal and retrobulbar haemodynamics during blood gas perturbation. Graefes Arch Clin Exp Ophthalmol 237(12):984–990
47. Satilmis M, Orgül S, Doubler B, Flammer J (2003) Rate of progression of glaucoma correlates with retrobulbar circulation and intraocular pressure. Am J Ophthalmol 135:664–669
48. Schmetterer L, Dallinger S, Findl O, Strenn K, Graselli U, Eichler HG, Wolzt M (1998) Noninvasive investigations of the normal ocular circulation in humans. Invest Ophthalmol Vis Sci 39(7):1210–1220
49. Schmetterer L, Garhofer G (2007) How can blood flow be measured? Surv Ophthalmol 52(Suppl):S134–S138
50. Sergott RC, Aburn NS, Trible JR, Costa VP, Lieb WE Jr, Flaharty PM (1994) Color Doppler imaging: methodology and preliminary results in glaucoma. Surv Ophthalmol 38(Suppl):S65–S70; discussion S70-1. Review. Erratum in: Surv Ophthalmol 1994;39(2):165
51. Stalmans I, Siesky B, Zeyen T, Fieuws S, Harris A (2009) Reproducibility of color Doppler imaging. Graefes Arch Clin Exp Ophthalmol 247(11):1531–1538
52. Stalmans I, Vandewalle E, Anderson DR, Costa VP, Frenkel RE, Garhofer G, Grunwald J, Gugleta K, Harris A, Hudson C, Januleviciene I, Kagemann L, Kergoat H, Lovasik JV, Lanzl I, Martinez A, Nguyen QD, Plange N, Reitsamer HA, Sehi M, Siesky B, Zeitz O, Orgül S, Schmetterer L (2011) Use of colour Doppler imaging in ocular blood flow research. Acta Ophthalmol 89(8):e609–e630
53. Taylor KJW, Holland S (1990) Doppler US, part I: basic principles, instrumentation, and pitfalls. Radiology 174:297–307
54. Toker E, Yenice O, Akpinar I, Aribal E, Kazokoglu H (2003) The influence of sex hormones on ocular blood flow in women. Acta Ophthalmol Scand 81(6):617–624
55. Trible JR, Costa VP, Sergott RC, Spaeth GL, Smith M, Wilson RP, Katz LJ, Moster MR, Schmidt CM (1993) The influence of primary open-angle glaucoma upon the retrobulbar circulation: baseline, postoperative and reproducibility analysis. Trans Am Ophthalmol Soc. 91:245–61; discussion 261–5
56. Wiermann A, Galambos P, Vafiadis J, Wagenfeld L, Richard G, Klemm M, Zeitz O (2007) Retrobulbar haemodynamics in normal and high tension glaucoma patients: the diagnostic importance of tinnitus, migraine and Raynaud-like symptoms. Klin Monbl Augenheilkd 224(5):396–400
57. Yamazaki Y, Hayamizu F (1995) Comparison of flow velocity of ophthalmic artery between primary open angle glaucoma and normal tension glaucoma. Br J Ophthalmol 79(8):732–734
58. Yüksel N, Karabaş VL, Arslan A, Demirci A, Cağlar Y (2001) Ocular hemodynamics in pseudoexfoliation syndrome and pseudoexfoliation glaucoma. Ophthalmology 108(6):1043–1049
59. Yüksel N, Karabaş VL, Demirci A, Arslan A, Altintaş O, Cağlar Y (2001) Comparison of blood flow velocities of the extraocular vessels in patients with pseudoexfoliation or primary open-angle glaucoma. Ophthalmologica 215(6):424–429
60. Zeitz O, Galambos P, Wagenfeld L, Wiermann A, Wlodarsch P, Praga R, Matthiessen ET, Richard G, Klemm M (2006) Glaucoma progression is associated with decreased blood flow velocities in the short posterior ciliary artery. Br J Ophthalmol 90(10):1245–1248

Chapter 6
Optic Nerve Head Assessment and Retinal Nerve Fiber Layer Evaluation

Antonio Ferreras

6.1 Introduction

Primary open-angle glaucoma is a progressive multifactorial optic neuropathy characterized by an acquired loss of retinal ganglion cells and their axons [1, 2]. The damage to the retinal nerve fiber layer (RNFL) is usually followed by changes in the optic nerve head (ONH) shape and specific visual field defects. Recognizing these changes is fundamental to the diagnosis and follow-up of glaucoma patients.

Glaucomatous damage to the ONH is observed as focal (notches) or diffuse neuroretinal rim narrowing with concentric enlargement of the optic cup or both [3]. While glaucoma produces different patterns of damage to the RNFL (e.g., wedge defect, diffuse loss) [4, 5], they are all associated with reduced RNFL thickness [6–11].

ONH evaluation can be performed by direct or indirect ophthalmoscopy, fundus photographs, and scanning laser devices (i.e., scanning laser ophthalmoscopy, optical coherence tomography, scanning laser polarimetry, etc.). Currently, there is a tendency to replace classical examinations of the RNFL and optic disc with the outcomes of objective technologies. Nevertheless, clinicians should base their first approach on simple examinations, which do not require expensive instruments and techniques that may not be available in all eye clinics.

Color fundus photographs or, even better, stereo-photographs, should be acquired to determine the baseline status of the optic disc, while monochromatic fundus photographs (RGB channel: blue color profile) should be used to evaluate the RNFL. These photographs should be repeated at follow-up visits to obtain a longitudinal series of photographs for detection of changes over time.

Commercially available fundus cameras are relatively easy to use, especially those that do not require pupil dilation (non-mydriatic fundus cameras). These

A. Ferreras
Department of Ophthalmology, Miguel Servet University Hospital,
University of Zaragoza, Zaragoza, Spain
e-mail: aferreras@msn.com

A. Ferreras (ed.), *Glaucoma Imaging*, DOI 10.1007/978-3-319-18959-8_6

cameras, however, usually require experienced operators to obtain stereo-photographs (photos are acquired from different angles) with good-quality images. Additionally, the quality of fundus photographs is influenced by the media opacity, retinal pigment epithelium status, and positioning and centering of the images. These limitations must be taken into account in clinical practice.

6.2 Normal Optic Disc Appearance

Typical healthy ONH morphology appears as a small or absent cup with a good color and size of the neuroretinal rim (Fig. 6.1). The high variability of normal human disc morphology, however, makes it difficult to detect optic disc damage.

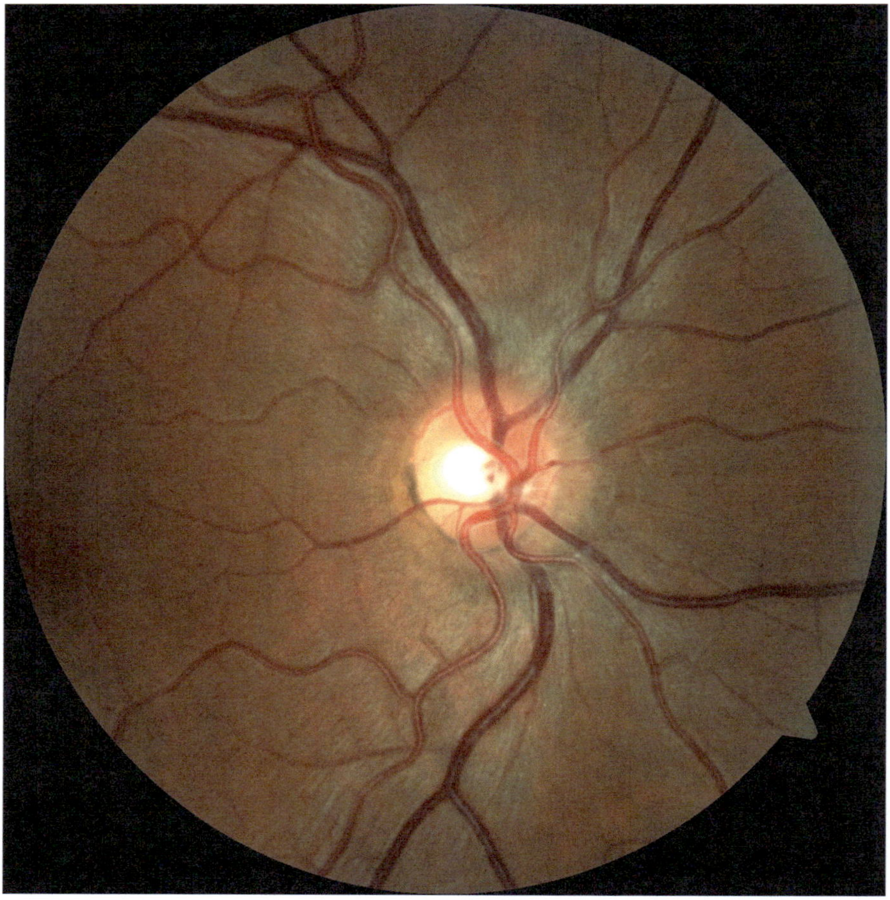

Fig. 6.1 Normal appearance of the optic nerve head

6.3 Classical Rules to Evaluate Optic Disc Morphology

Systematic studies of the optic disc are important to avoid missing details that may determine the difference between a healthy individual and an early glaucoma subject. Classically, five rules are applied for evaluating optic disc morphology:

1. Identify the scleral ring to establish the limits of the optic disc and calculate its size (Fig. 6.2).
2. Assess the neuroretinal rim limits (rim area; Fig. 6.3).
3. Determine the distribution of the RNFL bundles in the retina and evaluate the peripapillary RNFL integrity (Fig. 6.4).
4. Check for the presence and characteristics of peripapillary atrophy.
5. Look for optic disc hemorrhage.

Figure 6.5 illustrates these five steps for evaluating a potentially glaucomatous ONH.

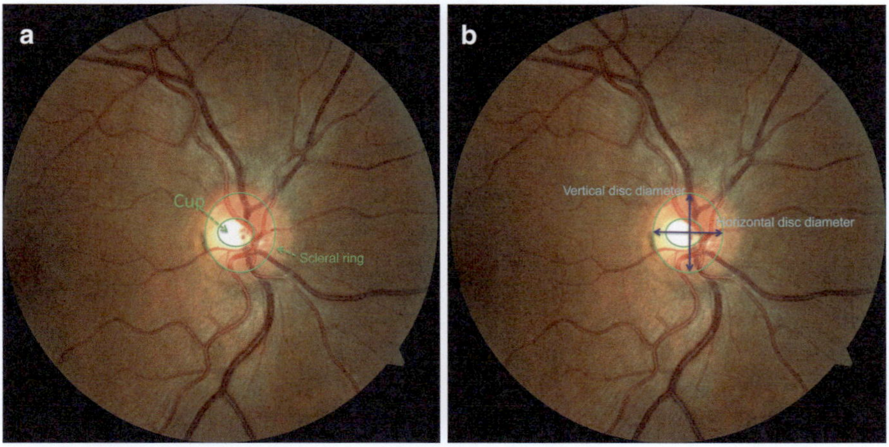

Fig. 6.2 (**a**) Scleral ring and optic disc limits in a healthy individual. (**b**) The vertical and horizontal disc diameters can be measured based on the length of the slit lamp beam

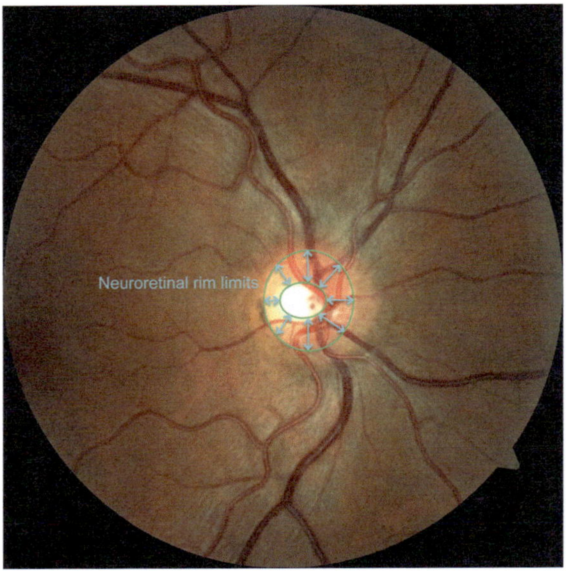

Fig. 6.3 The neuroretinal rim can be determined as the area between the scleral ring and the edge of the cup

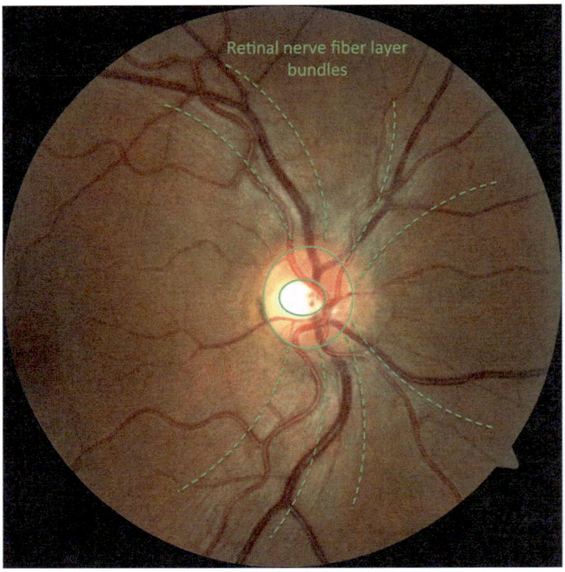

Fig. 6.4 The retinal nerve fiber layer bundles can be observed in high-quality color fundus photographs as striations on the surface of the retina leaving the margin of the optic disc and following an arcuate distribution

Fig. 6.5 Steps for assessing the optic nerve head morphology. (**a**) Color photograph of a glaucomatous optic disc. (**b**) Monochromatic fundus photograph of the same optic disc. (**c**) The dotted line corresponds to the margin of the optic nerve head (Elschnig's scleral ring). (**d**) The outer ring marks the limits of the optic disc while the inner ring shows the beginning of the cup. The area between the *two dotted lines* is the neuroretinal rim. This case shows inferior rim narrowing, suggesting that the ISNT rule is not respected. (**e**) Monochromatic fundus photograph with an inferior wedge defect (*yellow lines*) consistent with inferior rim narrowing. (**f**) The green area represents the alpha zone, *while the gray* area outside the alpha zone corresponds to the beta zone. The beta zone is more common in glaucoma. (**g**) The *green arrow points* to an optic disc hemorrhage, which is related to glaucoma progression. (**h**) Summary of the findings that can be observed in glaucomatous eyes

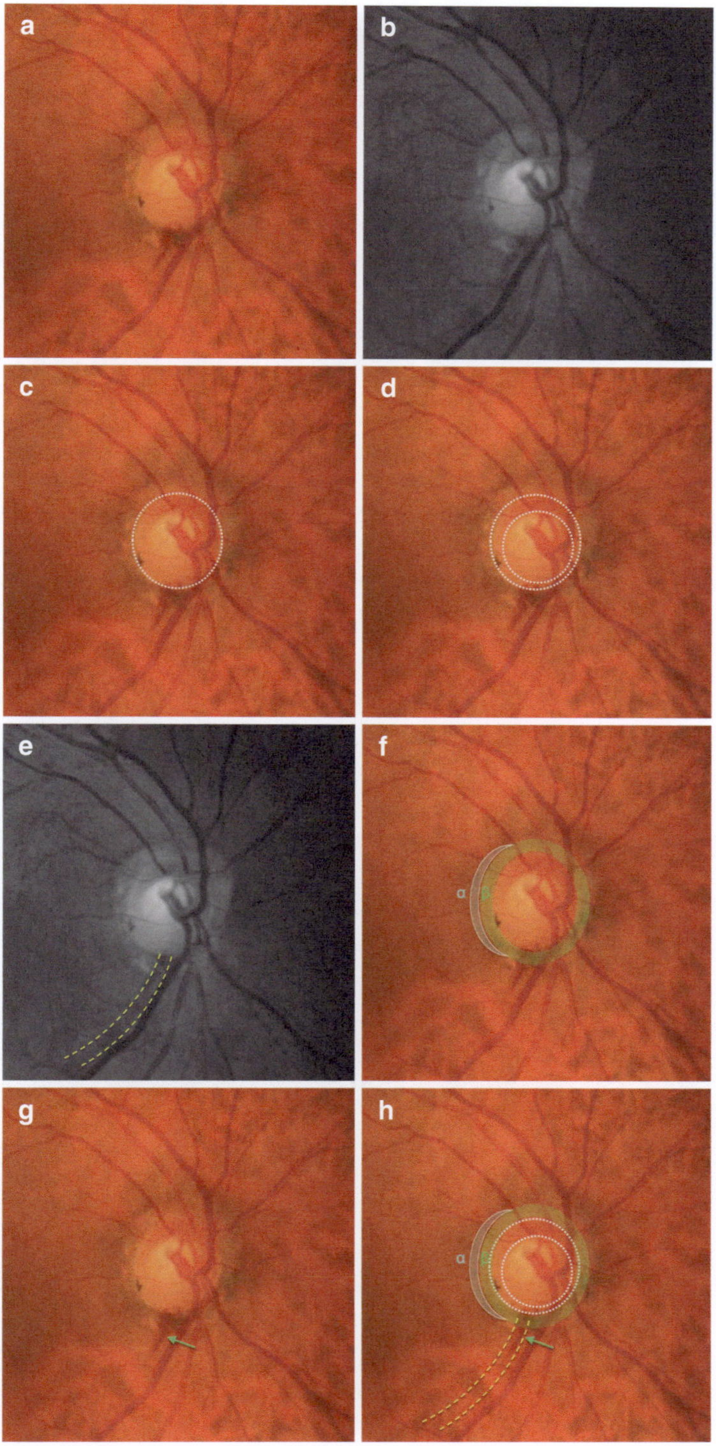
a
b
c
d
e
f
α
g
h
α

6.3.1 Identifying the Scleral Ring

The first step for evaluating ONH morphology is to identify the scleral ring limits and calculate the optic disc size, to determine if the optic disc is small, medium, or large (Fig. 6.5c).

The vertical and horizontal disc diameters can be measured with biomicroscopy. The end of the beam of the slit lamp must be placed at the edge of the vertical and horizontal scleral ring (Fig. 6.2b). The scale of the slit lamp will show the length of the beam, which corresponds to the disc diameter. This value should be corrected based on the power of the biomicroscopy lens to obtain a more accurate measurement. For a 60-diopter biconvex lens, the correction factor would be ×1, for a 78-diopter lens it would be ×1.1, and for a 90-diopter lens it would be ×1.3. Mean optic disc size generally ranges from 1.6–1.7 to 2.2–2.4 mm [2]. Nevertheless, there is no general agreement regarding the limits defining small, average, and large optic discs.

The vertical cup-to-disc ratio is highly dependent on the optic disc size [12, 13]. Large optic discs have physiologically increased cupping that may be confused with glaucoma, and conversely, small glaucomatous discs may not show any perceptible cupping or neuroretinal rim atrophy. Thus, clinicians should take into account that large discs in healthy eyes may have large cups, while small discs in eyes with glaucoma may have small cups (Fig. 6.6).

Calculating the border of the ONH is particularly difficult in highly myopic eyes, in discs with large chorioretinal atrophy areas, and in atypical optic discs. In these cases, changes in the direction of the blood vessels (blood vessel bending) may help to identify the contour of the optic disc.

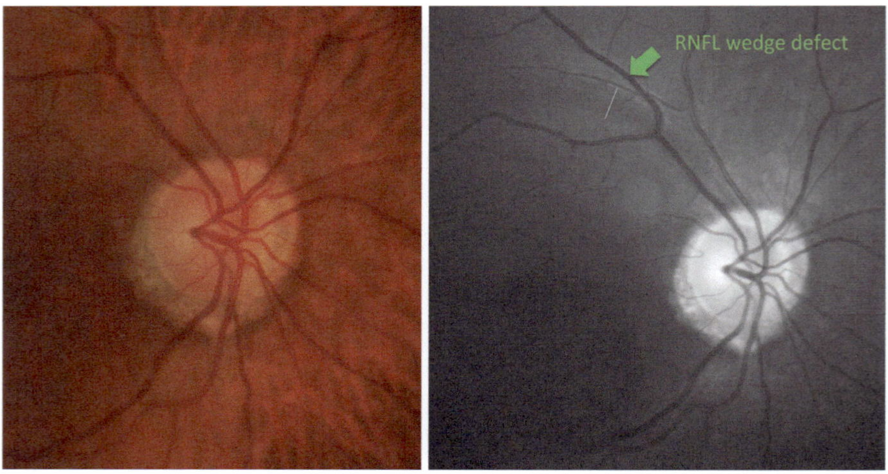

Fig. 6.6 The color fundus photograph (*left image*) shows a small optic disc with an apparently small optic disc cup. Nevertheless, on the monochromatic fundus photograph (*right image*), a small RNFL wedge defect (*white line near the green arrow*) is starting to be identifiable. This is a sign of early glaucomatous damage

6.3.2 Assessing Neuroretinal Rim Limits

The typical distribution of the RNFL bundles in the neuroretinal rim of the optic disc is usually thicker in the inferior pole, followed by the superior pole, the nasal area, and then the temporal area, which is the thinnest part of the rim (inferior ≥ superior ≥ nasal ≥ temporal). This characteristic distribution is known as the ISNT (inferior-superior-nasal-temporal) rule (Fig. 6.7) [14–16]. In glaucoma patients, however, the ISNT rule is frequently broken (Figs. 6.8 and 6.9), leading to localized rim narrowing, known as notching.

In addition to the RNFL distribution in the optic disc, it is important to observe the color of the rim area. The color of a healthy neuroretinal rim varies between orange and pink, while a white-yellowish rim suggests neuro-ophthalmologic disease other than glaucoma. In general, a pale neuroretinal rim is related to non-glaucomatous optic neuropathy (Fig. 6.10).

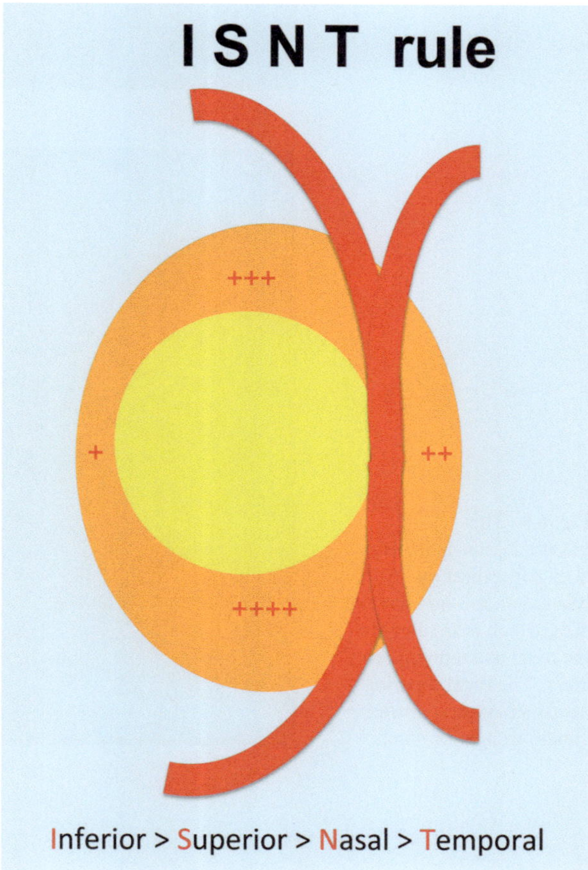

Fig. 6.7 In healthy eyes, the inferior sector of the neuroretinal rim tends to be greater than the superior, nasal, and temporal sectors (Inferior > Superior > Nasal > Temporal). This distribution is known as the ISNT rule

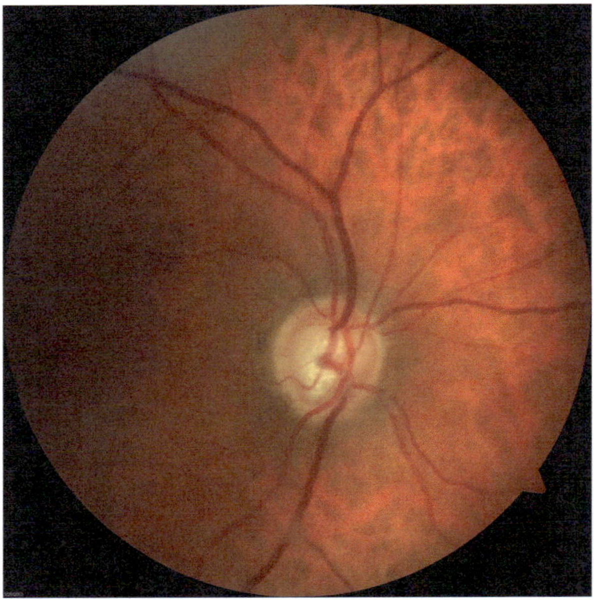

Fig. 6.8 The ISNT rule is broken in this glaucomatous eye, in which there is inferior neuroretinal rim narrowing (inferior notch) with enlargement of the optic disc cup. The superior rim area is larger than the inferior rim area

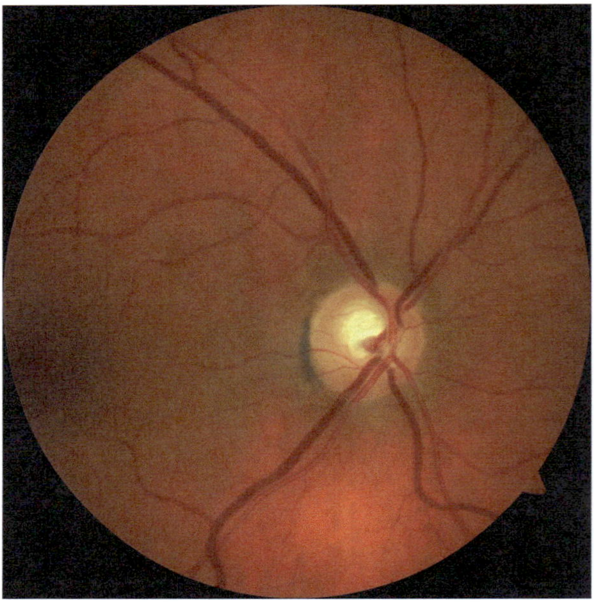

Fig. 6.9 This glaucomatous optic disc does not respect the ISNT rule due to the superior rim area, which is smaller than the nasal and temporal rim areas. The focal superior neuroretinal rim narrowing creates a superior notch

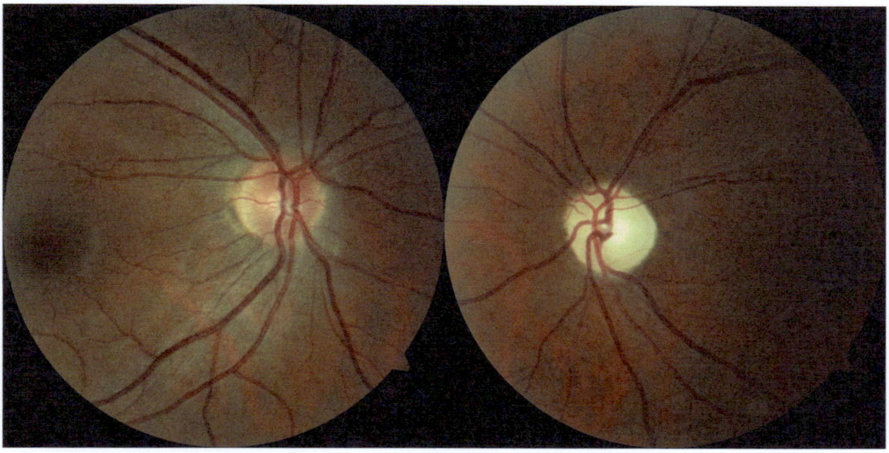

Fig. 6.10 These retinographies correspond to a 34-year-old male with chronic relapsing inflammatory optic neuropathy in the left eye. The different color of the neuroretinal rim is evident between the healthy eye (*right eye on the left side*) and the affected eye (*left eye, on the right side*). A pale neuroretinal rim increases the likelihood of non-glaucomatous optic neuropathy

6.3.3 *Determining the RNFL Bundle Distribution in the Retina*

The RNFL bundles in the retina are more easily observed with monochromatic fundus photographs (short wavelength light, such as blue light) than with color photographs (Fig. 6.11). The low penetration of blue light in the retina usually requires dilated pupils and transparent ocular media to obtain high-quality images. To evaluate the RNFL, a series of digital fundus photographs of each eye should be acquired: one photograph must be centered on the optic disc, another on the macula, and the other two on each arcuate zone (temporal superior and temporal inferior).

The RNFL corresponds to the axons of the ganglion cells. In healthy individuals, the normal RNFL has fine and bright striations following an arcuate distribution on the inner retina (Fig. 6.12). The RNFL is most easily visible in the inferior temporal part of the fundus, and then in the superior temporal region, the nasal superior region, and the nasal inferior region [17–19]. In particular, the RNFL is easiest to identify around the optic disc. In contrast, the RNFL is least visible in the peripheral retina (Fig. 6.13).

The visibility of the RNFL decreases with age, in part due to the physiologic loss of ganglion cells (3000–5000 per year) of the mean total of 1.4 million cells present at birth [20–22]. In addition, age-related opalescence or opacification of the lens makes it difficult to assess the RNFL status.

Two different patterns of reduction of the RNFL are observed in glaucoma patients: [4]

1. Localized RNFL defects or wedge defects (Figs. 6.14, 6.15, 6.16, 6.17, and 6.18) are darker focal areas with reduced or lost visibility of the normal striation pattern. These areas must be wider than a first-order branch vein, beginning at the disc margin and arching from the ONH to the periphery.

   Wedge defects can be observed in mild to moderate glaucoma patients, but they can also be detected in patients with normal standard automated perimetry scores as a sign of early glaucomatous damage. The age-related RNFL loss is diffuse and therefore focal losses cannot be attributed to patient age. Nevertheless, wedge defects are not pathognomonic for glaucoma and can be observed in other types of neuropathies.

   Wedge defects must be differentiated from slit-like RNFL defects, which are darker focal areas with reduced visibility of the normal striation pattern, but are smaller than a first-order branch vein, and do not extend to the border of the optic disc (Fig. 6.19). Slit-like RNFL defects can be observed in healthy individuals and do not indicate glaucoma.
2. Diffuse loses are a generalized rarefaction of the normal RNFL striation pattern, which seems to blur into a uniform or slightly granular light-gray area (Fig. 6.20). The retinal vessels normally course through the RNFL, but in eyes with diffuse RNFL loss, they are covered only by the inner limiting membrane. Thus, the retinal vessels appear more visible and sharper (Fig. 6.21). This pattern, however, is also not pathognomonic for glaucoma. Diffuse loss is usually related to more advanced glaucomatous disease than wedge defects. Frequently, a detailed inspection of the images is necessary to identify this pattern.

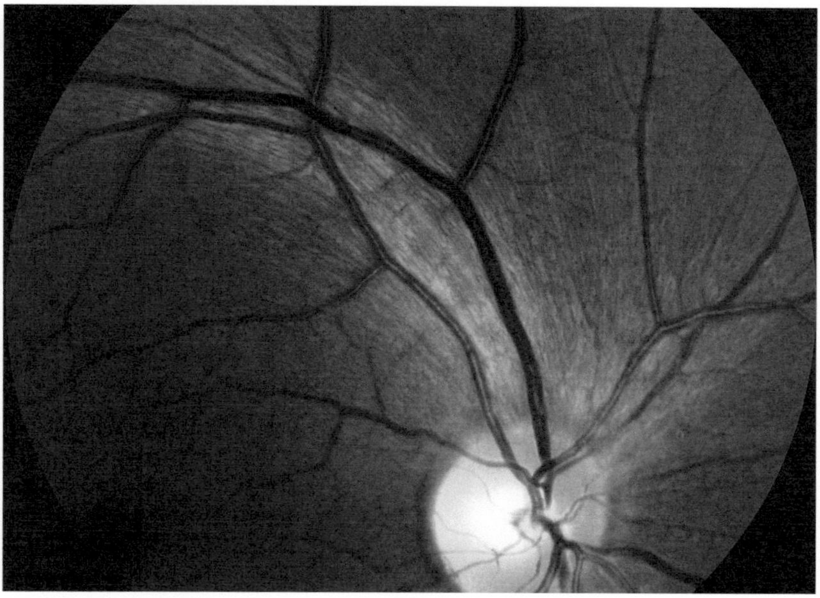

Fig. 6.11 Monochromatic fundus photograph showing the bright striation pattern of the RNFL bundles

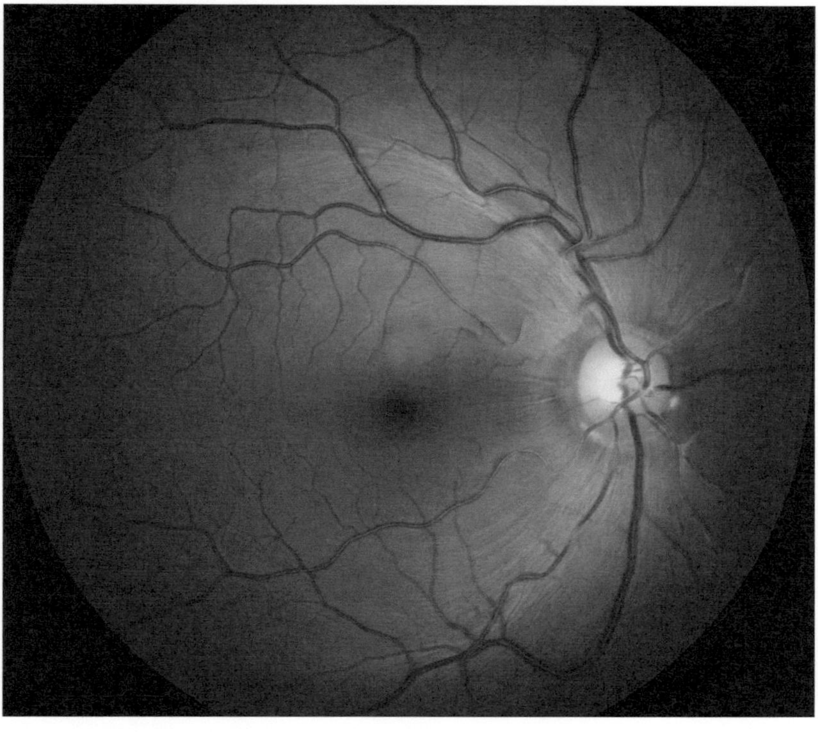

Fig. 6.12 The bundles of the RNFL follow an arcuate distribution under the inner limiting membrane

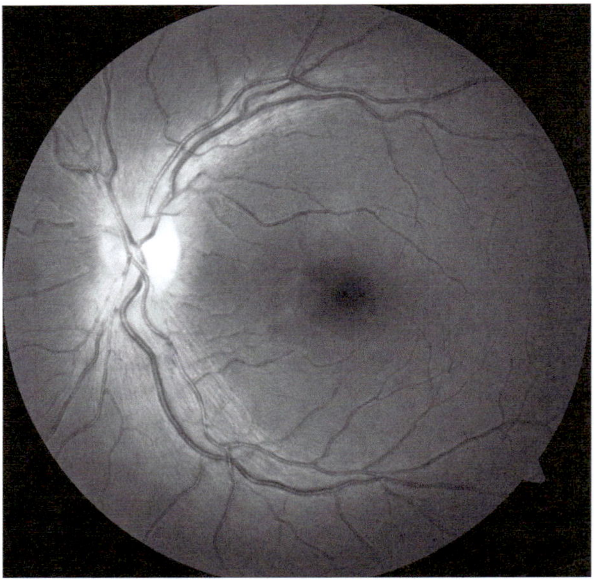

Fig. 6.13 In healthy individuals, the RNFL is more visible around the optic disc, while it is less detectable in the peripheral retina

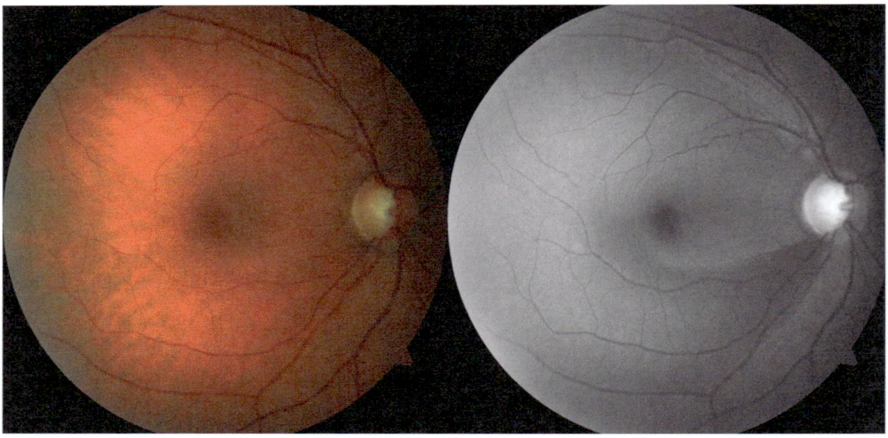

Fig. 6.14 Wedge defects can be identified in color photographs (*left image*), but are more visible in monochromatic fundus photographs (*right image*). This is an image from a patient with primary open-angle glaucoma. The inferior wedge defect appears as a darker area with loss of the normal striation pattern, near the notch in the optic disc

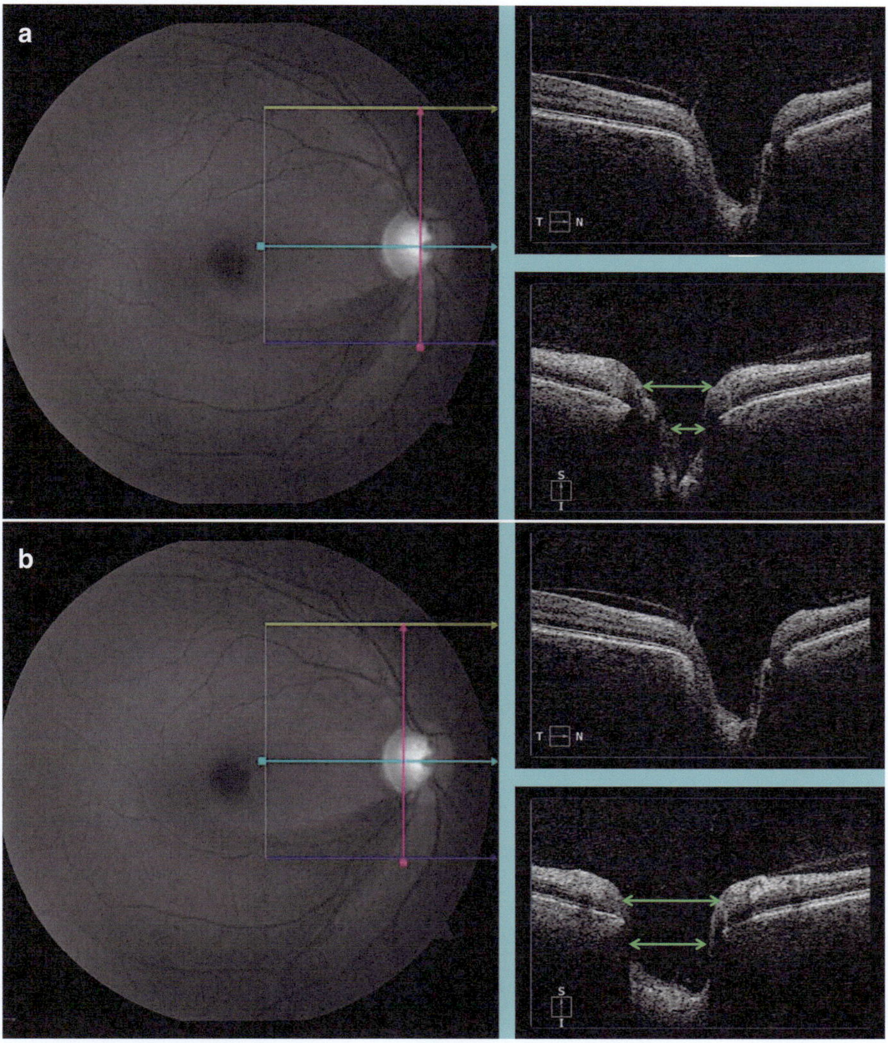

Fig. 6.15 Combined report of a fundus photograph and optical coherence tomography of the case shown in Fig. 6.14. When the vertical scan (*pink line*) is located outside the notch (**a**) the optic disc cup (*green lines*) is smaller than when the vertical scan is on the notch (**b**)

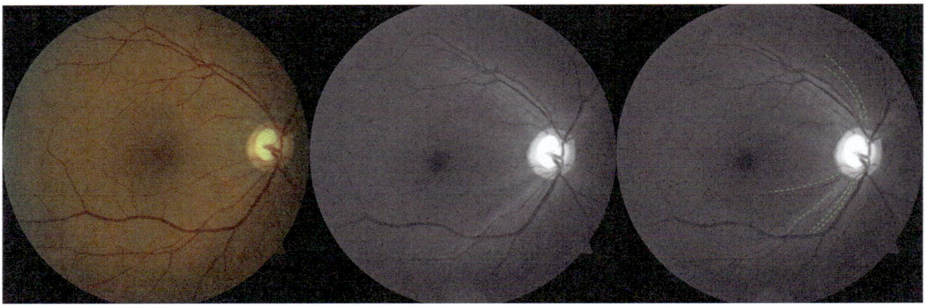

Fig. 6.16 The wedge defects can hardly be identified in the color retinography (*left picture*). In the monochromatic fundus photograph (*middle picture*), a wide inferior wedge defect is evident as well as other small inferior and superior wedge defects (*highlighted with green lines in the right picture*)

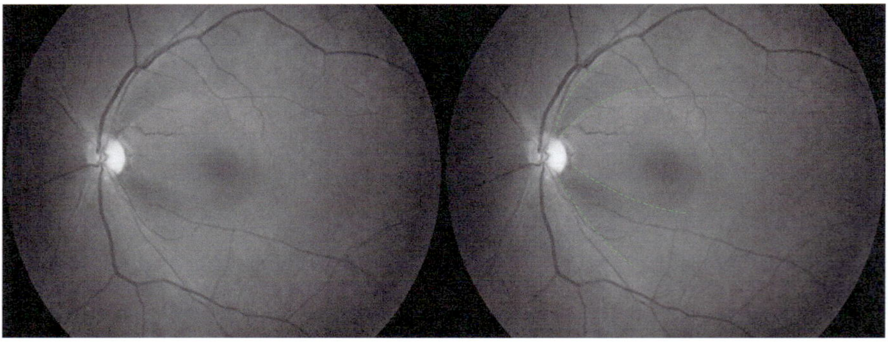

Fig. 6.17 This monochromatic retinography shows two wedge defects in the RNFL. The *green lines* in the *right picture mark* the limits of both defects

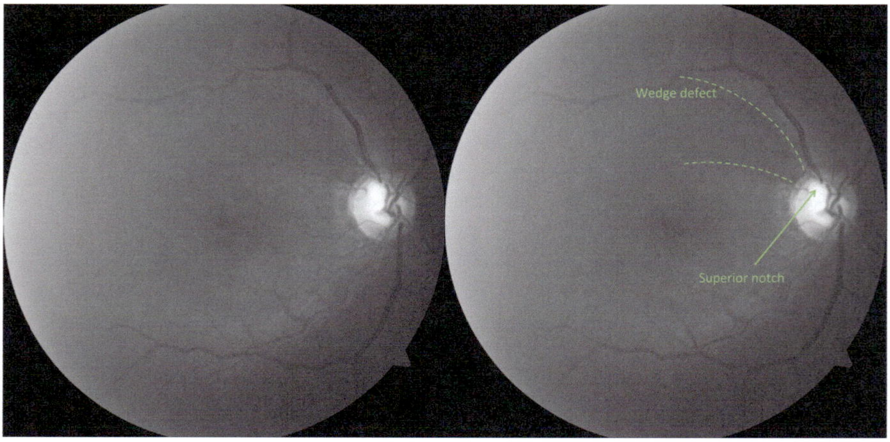

Fig. 6.18 A monochromatic fundus photograph of a 67-year-old glaucomatous female with a cataract. Besides the poor visibility of the RNFL striations, a superior wedge defect can be observed close to a superior notch (*left image*). The green lines and green arrow indicate these defects (*right picture*)

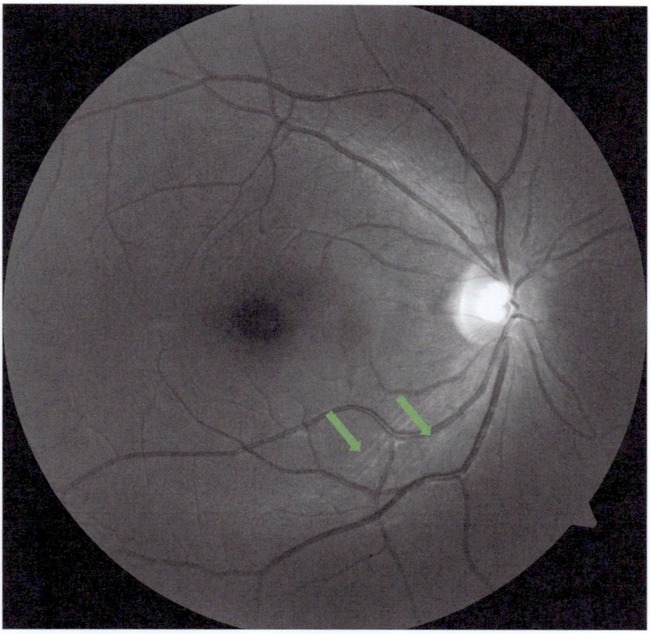

Fig. 6.19 Slit-like defects must be differentiated from wedge defects. Slit-like defects are not indicative of glaucomatous damage and can be observed in healthy individuals. These defects are small dark areas in the normal striation pattern that do not reach the optic disc border (*green arrows*)

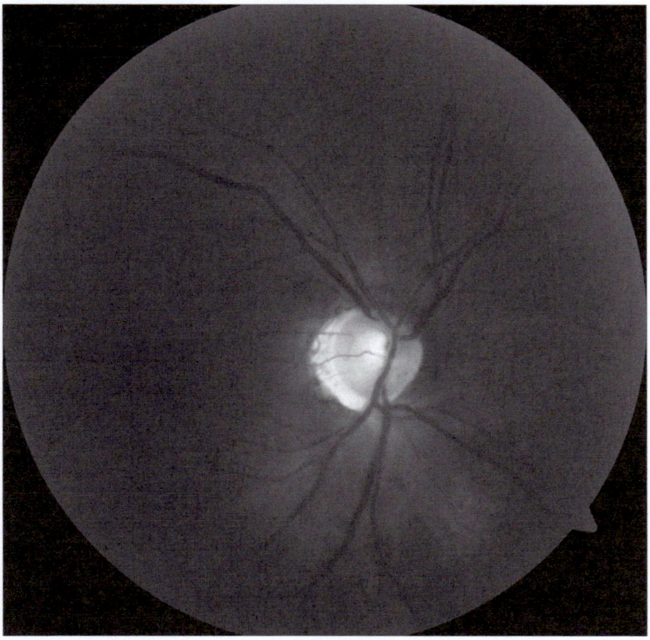

Fig. 6.20 Monochromatic retinography of a patient with advanced glaucoma. There is a generalized loss of the normal bright striations of the RNFL, leading to a dark and uniform appearance of the fundus. This pattern is known as diffuse loss

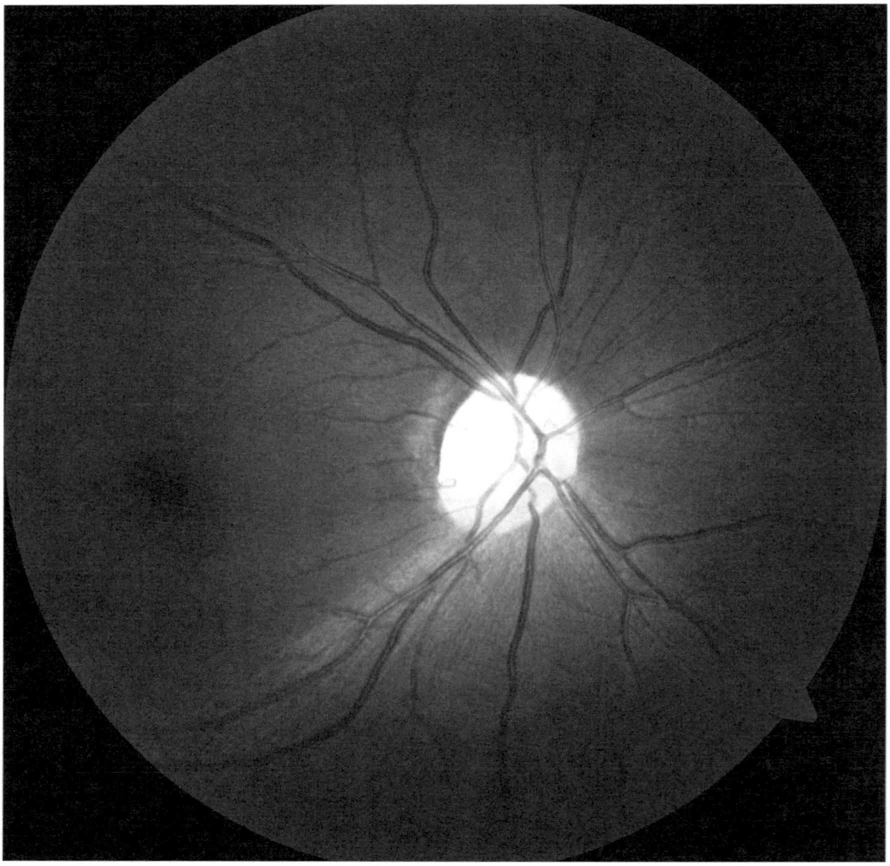

Fig. 6.21 This case illustrates the difference between the normal bright striations of the RNFL, clearly visible in the inferior retina, and a diffuse loss in the superior retina. The retinal vessels appear sharper in the superior area due to the lack of the RNFL covering and surrounding them under the inner limiting membrane

6.3.4 Evaluating Peripapillary Atrophy

Peripapillary atrophy has been associated with glaucoma since the early twentieth century [23]. Clinically, peripapillary atrophy is classified into alpha zone (α-zone) and the beta zone (β-zone) [24]. The alpha zone is defined as an area of irregular hypopigmentation and hyperpigmentation located in the periphery of the peripapillary atrophy. The beta zone is an area of visible sclera and the large choroidal vessels situated between the peripapillary scleral ring and the alpha zone (Fig. 6.22) [25]. The alpha zone corresponds histologically to irregularities in the retinal pigment epithelium (cells of uneven size and melanin content), while the beta zone, which is closer to the ONH, is a region with almost complete loss of photoreceptors and closure of the choriocapillaris (lack or atrophy of the retinal pigment epithelium) [26–29].

Based on histology, a new classification of peripapillary atrophy was recently suggested [30]. In addition to the alpha and beta zones, the new classification includes gamma and delta zones. The gamma zone is the distance between the end of Bruch's membrane and the outer margin of the optic nerve (covered by pia mater). The gamma zone represents the peripapillary sclera without the overlying choroid, Bruch's membrane, and deep retinal layers. The delta zone is defined as the central part of the gamma zone in which blood vessels of at least 50 μm in diameter are not detected over a length of at least 300 μm. The gamma and delta zones are not related to glaucoma, but rather to axial globe elongation.

The alpha zone is present in normal eyes, and can also be observed in glaucomatous eyes. The association between the beta zone and glaucoma is widely known [24, 25, 31]. The beta zone is more prevalent and extensive in glaucoma patients compared with healthy subjects [25]. Moreover, the location of the beta zone correlates with the location of the glaucomatous optic disc damage and visual field defects [24]. The width of the beta zone inversely correlates with the neuroretinal rim width in the corresponding area (i.e., the larger the beta zone, the thinner the neuroretinal rim). The beta zone is an important risk factor for visual field deficit progression in glaucoma patients [31–33]. Nevertheless, it seems that there is no association between the size of the beta zone and conversion from ocular hypertension to glaucoma [34].

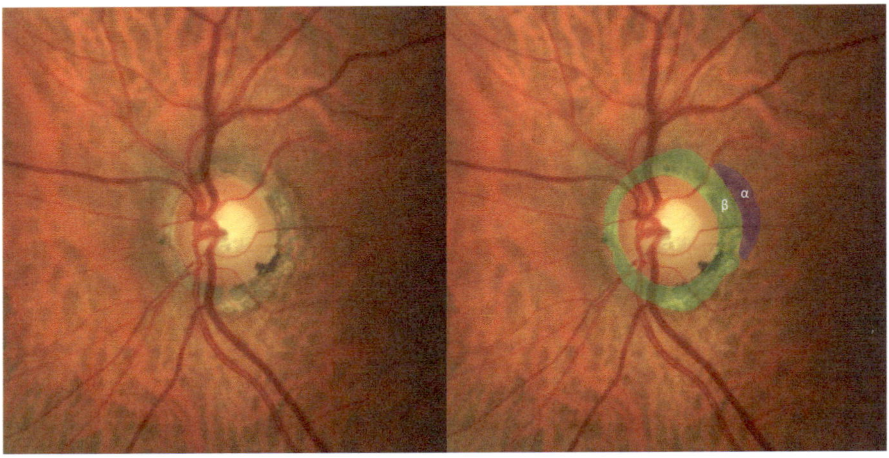

Fig. 6.22 The green ring on the right side corresponds to the beta zone of this glaucomatous optic disc. The alpha zone is located in the periphery of the beta zone (*purple ring*) and is not related to glaucoma

6.3.5 Checking for the Presence of Optic Disc Hemorrhage

Detecting disc hemorrhage requires careful optic disc examination. Many times, the hemorrhages are small and may go unnoticed. Splinter-shaped or flame-shaped hemorrhages at the margin of the ONH are usually a hallmark of glaucoma. Although optic disc hemorrhage is rarely found in healthy individuals, it is not pathognomonic of glaucomatous optic neuropathy. Optic disc hemorrhage is more frequently located at the inferotemporal or superotemporal sectors. Flame-shaped hemorrhages are usually associated with RNFL wedge defects, notches, and visual field defects in the corresponding area (Fig. 6.23).

Normal-tension glaucoma patients have a higher incidence of disc hemorrhage than high-tension glaucoma subjects (1.9–5 fold in prevalence vs. 1.3–2.8 fold in incidence) [35–41]. Some studies, however, suggest that the development of optic disc hemorrhage is not consistently related to intraocular pressure [35, 36, 42–44]. In primary open-angle glaucoma, disc hemorrhage could be larger and longer in eyes with normal-baseline intraocular pressure than in eyes with high-baseline intraocular pressure. Thus, disc hemorrhage could be more easily detected in cases with normal-baseline intraocular pressure, suggesting that findings of previous studies were partially biased to a higher prevalence and incidence of disc hemorrhage in normal-tension glaucoma eyes due to this topographic characteristic [44].

Flame-shaped hemorrhages are indicative of glaucoma progression [42, 45–52]. Nonetheless, a recent study suggested that disc hemorrhage is an ongoing sign of structural progression rather than a discrete event that leads to subsequent progression [53].

A series of fundus photographs can be helpful for following glaucoma suspects over time (Figs. 6.24 and 6.25). A comparison of images obtained through the years may reveal changes due to glaucoma progression.

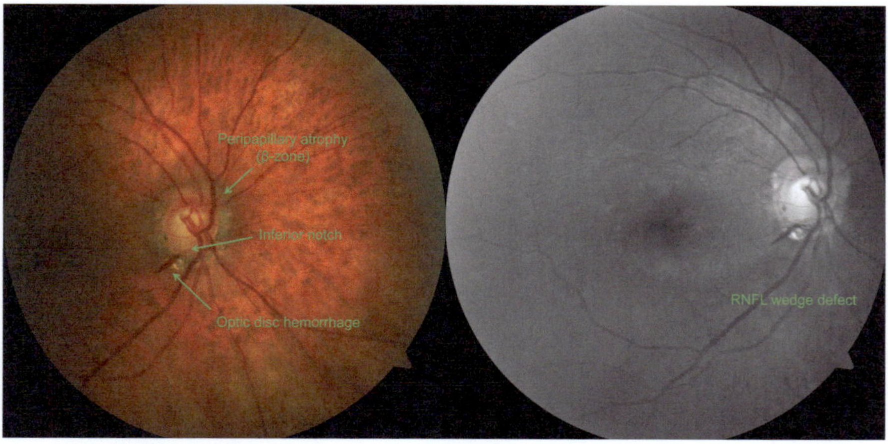

Fig. 6.23 In the color retinography (*left picture*) a flamed-shape hemorrhage can be identified at the inferior pole of the optic disc. The hemorrhage is located close to a notch in the neuroretinal rim and a RNFL wedge defect, clearly visible in the monochromatic fundus photograph (*right picture*)

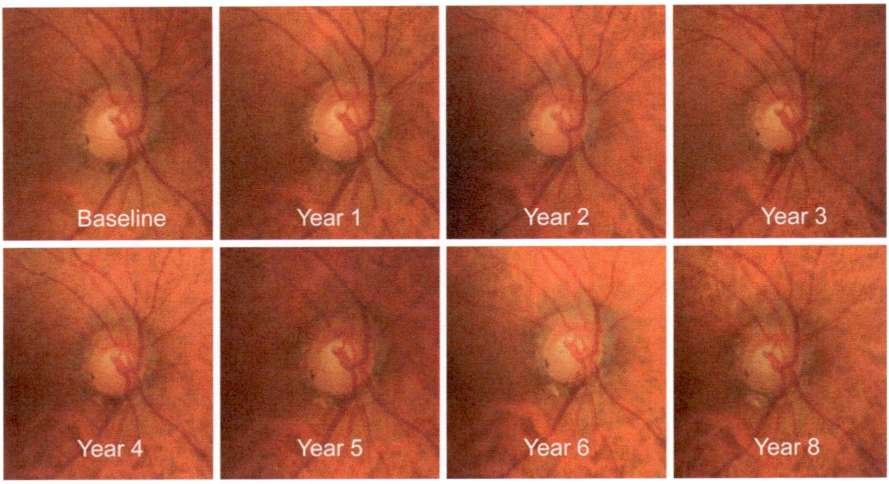

Fig. 6.24 A series of retinographies can be used to monitor changes in the optic disc over time. This is the same case shown in Figs. 6.5 and 6.23. A small optic disc hemorrhage was present at baseline. The hemorrhage changed in the follow-up period while the neuroretinal rim narrowing progressed, the peripapillary atrophy became more evident, and the direction of the vessels was modified

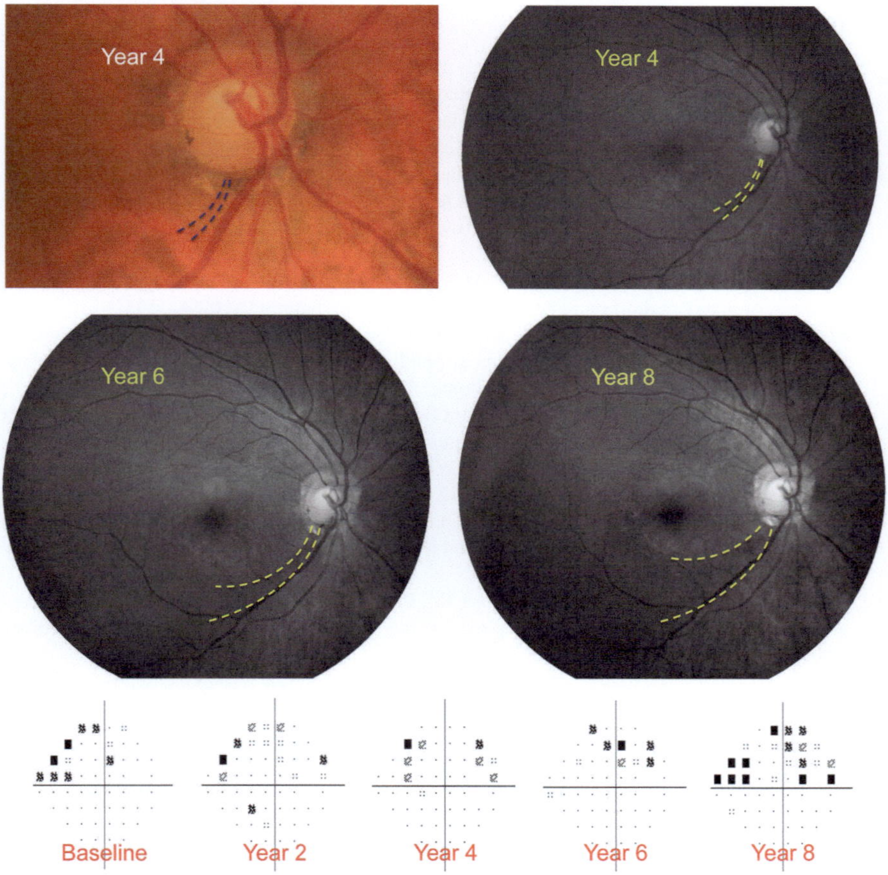

Fig. 6.25 The changes in the optic disc observed in the retinography of the glaucoma patient shown in Figs. 6.23 and 6.24 corresponded with progression of the RNFL defect and the visual field defect in standard automated perimetry (*bottom pictures*). Clinicians should check for agreement between the fundus photographs findings and other tests: clinical assessment, visual field, and imaging technologies

References

1. Quigley HA (1999) Neuronal death in glaucoma. Prog Retin Eye Res 18:39–57
2. American Academy of Ophthalmology Glaucoma Panel (2005) Preferred practice pattern. Primary open-angle glaucoma. American Academy of Ophthalmology, San Francisco, p 3
3. Tuulonen A, Airaksinen PJ (1991) Initial glaucomatous optic disk and retinal nerve fiber layer abnormalities and their progression. Am J Ophthalmol 111:485–490
4. Jonas JB, Dichtl A (1996) Evaluation of the retinal nerve fiber layer. Surv Ophthalmol 40: 369–378
5. Quigley HA, Miller NR, George T (1980) Clinical evaluation of nerve fiber layer atrophy as an indicator of glaucomatous optic nerve damage. Arch Ophthalmol 98:1564–1571
6. Medeiros FA, Zangwill LM, Bowd C et al (2004) Comparison of the GDx VCC scanning laser polarimeter, HRT II confocal scanning laser ophthalmoscope, and Stratus OCT optical coherence tomograph for the detection of glaucoma. Arch Ophthalmol 122:827–837
7. Nouri-Mahdavi K, Hoffman D, Tannenbaum DP et al (2004) Identifying early glaucoma with optical coherence tomography. Am J Ophthalmol 137:228–235
8. Budenz DL, Michael A, Chang RT et al (2005) Sensitivity and specificity of the Stratus OCT for perimetric glaucoma. Ophthalmology 112:3–9
9. Jeoung JW, Park KH, Kim TW et al (2005) Diagnostic ability of optical coherence tomography with a normative database to detect localized retinal nerve fiber layer defects. Ophthalmology 112:2157–2163
10. Ferreras A, Pablo LE, Pajarín AB, Larrosa JM, Polo V, Honrubia FM (2008) Logistic regression analysis for early glaucoma diagnosis using optical coherence tomography. Archives Ophthalmol 126:465–470
11. Sharma A, Oakley JD, Schiffman JC, Budenz DL, Anderson DR (2011) Comparison of automated analysis of Cirrus HD OCT spectral-domain optical coherence tomography with stereo photographs of the optic disc. Ophthalmology 118(7):1348–1357
12. Garway-Heath D, Ruben ST, Viswanathan A, Hitchings RA (1998) Vertical cup/disc ratio in relation to optic disc size: its value in the assessment of the glaucoma suspect. Br J Ophthalmol 82:1118–1124
13. Ferreras A, Pajarín AB, Polo V et al (2007) Diagnostic ability of Heidelberg retina tomograph 3 classifications: glaucoma probability score versus Moorfields regression analysis. Ophthalmology 114:1981–1987
14. Jonas JB et al (1998) Neuroretinal rim width ratios in morphological glaucoma diagnosis. Br J Ophthalmol 82:1366–1371
15. Jonas JB, Gusek GC, Naumann GOH (1988) Optic disc, cup and neuroretinal rim size, configuration and correlation in normal eyes. Invest Ophthalmol Vis Sci 29:1151–1158
16. Harizman N, Oliveira C, Chiang A et al (2006) The ISNT rule and differentiation of normal from glaucomatous eyes. Arch Ophthalmol 124:1579–1583
17. Jonas JB, Nguyen NX, Naumann GOH (1989) The retinal nerve fiber layer in normal eyes. Ophthalmology 96:627–632
18. Fitzgibbon T, Taylor SF (1996) Retinotopy of the human retinal nerve fibre layer and optic nerve head. J Comp Neurol 375:238–251
19. FitzGibbon T (1997) The human fetal retinal nerve fiber layer and optic nerve head: a DiI and DiA tracing study. Vis Neurosci 14:433–447
20. Dolman CL, McCormick AQ, Drance SM (1980) Aging of the optic nerve. Arch Ophthalmol 98:2053–2058
21. Balazsi AG, Rootman J, Drance SM et al (1984) The effect of age on the nerve fiber population of the human optic nerve. Am J Ophthalmol 97:760–766
22. Johnson BM, Miao M, Sadun AA (1987) Age-related decline of human optic nerve axon populations. Age 10:5–7
23. Airaksinen PJ, Tuulonen A, Werner EB (1996) Clinical evaluation of the optic disc and retinal nerve fiber layer. In: Ritch R, Shields MB, Krupin T (eds) The glaucomas, vol 1. Mosby, St. Louis, pp 617–657

24. Jonas JB, Nguyen XN, Gusek GC, Naumann GO (1989) Parapapillary chorioretinal atrophy in normal and glaucoma eyes. I. Morphometric data. Invest Ophthalmol Vis Sci 30:908–918
25. Jonas JB (2005) Clinical implications of peripapillary atrophy in glaucoma. Curr Opin Ophthalmol 16:84–88
26. Jonas JB, Königsreuther KA, Naumann GO (1992) Optic disc histomorphometry in normal eyes and eyes with secondary angle-closure glaucoma. II. Parapapillary region. Graefes Arch Clin Exp Ophthalmol 230:134–139
27. Kubota T, Jonas JB, Naumann GO (1993) Direct clinico-histological correlation of parapapillary chorioretinal atrophy. Br J Ophthalmol 77:103–106
28. Curcio CA, Saunders PL, Younger PW, Malek G (2000) Peripapillary chorioretinal atrophy: Bruch's membrane changes and photoreceptor loss. Ophthalmology 107:334–343
29. Spaide RF (2009) Age-related choroidal atrophy. Am J Ophthalmol 147:801–810
30. Jonas JB, Jonas SB, Jonas RA et al (2012) Parapapillary atrophy: histological gamma zone and delta zone. Plos One 7, e47237
31. Uchida H, Ugurlu S, Caprioli J (1998) Increasing peripapillary atrophy is associated with progressive glaucoma. Ophthalmology 105:1541–1545
32. Teng CC, De Moraes CG, Prata TS et al (2010) Beta-zone parapapillary atrophy and the velocity of glaucoma progression. Ophthalmology 117:909–915
33. Lee EJ, Kim TW, Weinreb RN et al (2011) Beta-zone parapapillary atrophy and the rate of retinal nerve fiber layer thinning in glaucoma. Invest Ophthalmol Vis Sci 52:4422–4427
34. Savatovsky E, Mwanza JC, Budenz DL et al (2015) ; Ocular Hypertension Treatment Study. Longitudinal changes in peripapillary atrophy in the Ocular Hypertension Treatment Study: a case-control assessment. Ophthalmology 122:79–86
35. Kitazawa Y, Shirato S, Yamamoto T (1986) Optic disc hemorrhage in low-tension glaucoma. Ophthalmology 93:853–857
36. Hendrickx KH, van den Enden A, Rasker MT, Hoyng PF (1994) Cumulative incidence of patients with disc hemorrhages in glaucoma and the effect of therapy. Ophthalmology 101:1165–1172
37. Jonas JB, Xu L (1994) Optic disk hemorrhages in glaucoma. Am J Ophthalmol 118:1–8
38. Healey PR, Mitchell P, Smith W, Wang JJ (1998) Optic disc hemorrhages in a population with and without signs of glaucoma. Ophthalmology 105:216–223
39. Jonas JB, Budde WM (2000) Optic nerve head appearance in juvenile onset chronic high-pressure glaucoma and normal-pressure glaucoma. Ophthalmology 107:704–711
40. Miyake T, Sawada A, Yamamoto T, Miyake K, Sugiyama K, Kitazawa Y (2006) Incidence of disc hemorrhages in open-angle glaucoma before and after trabeculectomy. J Glaucoma 15:164–171
41. Suh MH, Park KH (2011) Period prevalence and incidence of optic disc haemorrhage in normal tension glaucoma and primary open-angle glaucoma. Clin Exp Ophthalmol 39:513–519
42. Siegner SW, Netland PA (1996) Optic disc hemorrhages and progression of glaucoma. Ophthalmology 103:1014–1024
43. Tezel G, Siegmund KD, Trinkaus K, Wax MB, Kass MA, Kolker AE (2001) Clinical factors associated with progression of glaucomatous optic disc damage in treated patients. Arch Ophthalmol 119:813–818
44. Kim YK, Park KH, Yoo BW, Kim HC (2014) Topographic characteristics of optic disc hemorrhage in primary open-angle glaucoma. Invest Ophthalmol Vis Sci 55:169–176
45. Airaksinen PJ, Mustonen E, Alanku HI (1981) Optic disc haemorrhages precede retinal nerve fibre layer defects in ocular hypertension. Acta Ophthalmol (Copenh) 59:627–641
46. Ahn JK, Park KH (2002) Morphometric change analysis of the optic nerve head in unilateral disk hemorrhage cases. Am J Ophthalmol 134:920–922
47. Kim SH, Park KH (2006) The relationship between recurrent optic disc hemorrhage and glaucoma progression. Ophthalmology 113:598–602
48. Leske MC, Heijl A, Hyman L, Bengtsson B, Dong L, Yang Z, EMGT Group (2007) Predictors of long-term progression in the early manifest glaucoma trial. Ophthalmology 114:1965–1972
49. Prata TS, De Moraes CG, Teng CC, Tello C, Ritch R, Liebmann JM (2010) Factors affecting rates of visual field progression in glaucoma patients with optic disc hemorrhage. Ophthalmology 117:24–29

50. Medeiros FA, Alencar LM, Sample PA, Zangwill LM, Susanna R Jr, Weinreb RN (2010) The relationship between intraocular pressure reduction and rates of progressive visual field loss in eyes with optic disc hemorrhage. Ophthalmology 117:2061–2066
51. Hayamizu F, Yamazaki Y, Nakagami T, Mizuki K (2013) Optic disc size and progression of visual field damage in patients with normal-tension glaucoma. Clin Ophthalmol 7:807–813
52. Kim JM, Kyung H, Azarbod P, Lee JM, Caprioli J (2014) Disc haemorrhage is associated with the fast component, but not the slow component, of visual field decay rate in glaucoma. Br J Ophthalmol 98:1555–1559
53. Chung E, Demetriades AM, Christos PJ, Radcliffe NM (2015) Structural glaucomatous progression before and after occurrence of an optic disc haemorrhage. Br J Ophthalmol 99:21–25

Chapter 7
Confocal Scanning Laser Ophthalmoscopy

Michele Iester

7.1 Heidelberg Retina Tomograph

The Heidelberg retina tomograph (HRT) is a confocal laser scanning system designed to acquire and analyse three-dimensional images of the posterior segment of the eye [1, 2]. It is the oldest glaucoma imaging device on the marketing. The major clinical applications of the instrument are the quantitative analysis of the optic nerve head (ONH) in glaucoma at baseline or during a follow-up.

In a confocal laser scanning system, a focused laser beam scans the fundus, and the amount of light reflected from each scanned point is measured (Fig. 7.1a). A diaphragm sits in front of the light detector, the confocal pinhole, so that light originating mainly from the corresponding focal plane reaches the detector and contributes to the image. Light reflected from outside the focal plane is masked. The image is an optical section through a three-dimensional object. Sequential optical sections are acquired at different depths to produce a layered three-dimensional image. This imaging process is called scanning laser tomography (SLT).

The HRT acquires a series of up to 64 optical sections in depth at 1/16 mm intervals (Fig. 7.1b). The number of images acquired may vary from 1 mm to 4 mm, depending on the thickness of the tissue of interest. The image field is 15 by 15°, with a density of 384 by 384 pixels.

At each location in the image stack, the reflected light intensity varies through the depth of the scan series. It is assumed that this intensity variation has a maximum at the tissue surface. The surface topography is derived from an estimation of the intensity maximum at each pixel in the image, resulting in a matrix of 384×384 surface height measurements. The topography is presented as a colour-coded map,

M. Iester, MD, PhD
Associate Professor, Laboratorio clinico anatomo-funzionale per la diagnosi e il trattamento del glaucoma e della malattie neurooftalmologiche, Clinica Oculistica, DiNOGMI, University of Genoa, Genoa, Italy
e-mail: iester@unige.it

A. Ferreras (ed.), *Glaucoma Imaging*, DOI 10.1007/978-3-319-18959-8_7

with darker colours representing more superficial structures and lighter colours representing deeper structures.

In an examination of the ONH with the HRT, three image stacks are acquired automatically. During the acquisition process, the software determines, and automatically sets, the required scan depth and image brightness. Following this, 3 topography images, and a mean, are computed. The repeatability of height measurements at each pixel is calculated. This is used to assess the significance of detected changes in follow-up measurements.

In order to derive 3-dimensional ONH structures, the ONH margin is drawn manually by placing a contour line at the inner margin of Elschnig's ring (Fig. 7.1c), and the software calculates stereometric parameters within this line. The stereometric parameter values are computed for the whole ONH and for 6 predefined sectors.

The average reproducibility at each of the 384 × 384 local surface height measurements is around 20 μm for healthy and glaucomatous eyes with acuity of 6/12 or better and cylindrical refractive error <1 dioptre. Reproducibility is worse in eyes with larger degrees of cylindrical refractive error [3, 4].

Clinical evaluation of the ONH is mainly based on HRT parameter and their formulas such as the Moorfields regression analysis (MRA) and the various linear discriminant functions. Most of these analyses have reference plane-dependent values incorporated into their formulation.

The reference plane is an arbitrary plane set below and parallel to the retinal surface within an HRT topographic image. Within the scleral ring, space that is above the plane is defined as 'neuroretinal rim' and space that is below the plane is defined as the 'cup'. Figure 7.1d demonstrates the position of the reference plane relative to the optic nerve head.

The stereometric parameter values (such as rim area and volume) are dependent on the position of the reference plane, while other parameters such as cup shape measure (CSM) are reference plane independent.

The standard reference plane is located 50 um below the contour line at the temporal disc margin, between −10° and −4°, and it is parallel to the retina surface; in this way if the optic disc is tilted, also the reference plane will have the same inclination. This location was selected on the basis of the mean surface inclination angle of the optic nerve head and because it coincides with the papillomacular bundle [5]. It was assumed that the papillomacular bundle would maintain a relatively stable thickness because central visual acuity is not impacted upon until the later stages of the glaucomatous process. However, this has not been supported by OCT-derived retinal thickness measurements, which show reduced papillomacular bundle thickness in glaucomatous subjects despite maintenance of a good visual acuity [6]. There may, therefore, be some change in the reference plane height as disease progresses [7, 8].

The first step in the analysis is to draw the contour line around the outer edge of the ONH rim. The disc margin was delimited by a contour line placed around the margin of the peripapillary scleral ring. Once the contour line is drawn, the computer can analyse the ONH and calculate all the HRT parameters. Small changes in the contour line position do not change the diagnostic capacity of the HRT [9]; however, the user can also use the linear profile that shows a small depression where there is the Elschnig's ring just before the outer edge of the rim (Fig. 7.1e).

The main 12 variables measured by the Heidelberg retina tomograph include disc area, cup to disc ratio, cup shape, height variation contour, rim area, rim volume, maximum and mean cup depth, cup area, cup volume, RNFL cross-sectional area and mean RNFL thickness. The parameters can be global, when the ONH is considered all together, or sectorial when the ONH is divided into six sectors (Fig. 7.1fg).

All the methods inside the device are purely statistical description and have nothing to do with disease status.

No commercially available imaging device is able to discriminate perfectly between normal and glaucomatous eyes – there is an overlap in measurements between the two. When an eye with glaucoma will be classified as 'borderline' or 'outside normal limits', the final decision as to whether an eye is glaucomatous or not is a clinical judgement, based on all available clinical data. Inside the system there are different database to use to compare patients' data with healthy population (Fig. 7.2).

Efforts should be made during image acquisition to ensure that the variability of the images is the lowest it can be (a low standard deviation) (Fig. 7.1hi), and the clinician should check to ensure that serial images are on focus (Fig. 7.1jk), well aligned to avoid movement and fixation loss (Fig. 7.1lm) and not overexposed (Fig. 7.1n). Obviously misaligned images should be removed and the analysis repeated to obtain a good image (Fig. 7.1o).

During acquisition it is possible to detect floaters (Fig. 7.1pq), peripapillary haemorrhages (Fig. 7.1r), scleral ring (Fig. 7.1s) and peripapillary atrophy (Fig. 7.1t).

When a printout is read, the following parameters must be checked:

- Quality (Figs. 7.3a and 7.1h)
- Disc size (Fig. 7.3b)
- Configuration of the cup (Fig. 7.3c)
- CSM which is the slope of the cup
- RNFL (Fig. 7.3d–g)

Then all the algorithm inside the system should be considered.

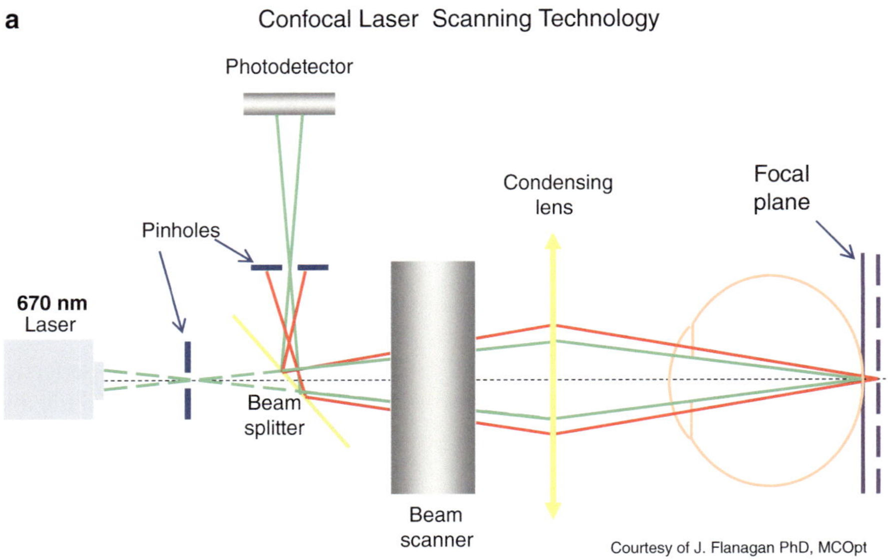

Fig. 7.1 (**a**) In a laser scanning system, a laser is used as a light source. The laser beam is focused to one point of the examined object. The light reflected from that point goes the same way back through the optics and is separated from the incident laser beam and deflected to a detector. This allows the instrument to measure the reflected light only at one individual point of the object. In order to produce a two-dimensional image, the illuminating laser beam is deflected periodically in two dimensions perpendicular to the optical axis using scanning mirrors. Therefore, the object is scanned point by point sequentially in two dimensions. A confocal laser scanning system has a high optical resolution not only perpendicular but also parallel to the optical axis, that means into depth. A two-dimensional image acquired at the focal plane therefore carries only information of the object layer located at or near the focal plane. It can be considered as an optical section of the three-dimensional object at the focal plane (Courtesy of J. Flanagan PhD, MCOpt). (**b**) HRT acquisition and signal processing. (**c**) How to draw the contour line. Place about 6–8 points to draw the contour line. Too many points result in an irregular shape and the contour line is difficult to modify. (**d**) The reference plane. Schematic of a cross section through the ONH and parapapillary retina. The reference plane (*dashed line*) is parallel to the retinal surface. The standard reference plane is set 50 μ below the contour line height at the temporal disc margin (Burk et al. [5]). (**e**) Look for the scleral ring. The scleral ring might appear as a depressed pale band on the topography image, a high reflective zone on the reflectance image. The contour line should be placed at the inner edge of the scleral ring. On the interactive height profile, the band can be identified as a 'valley'. (**f**) Global and sectorial parameters automatically calculated by the system. (**g**) Global and sectorial parameters automatically calculated by the system and the printout. (**h**) Standard deviation as a parameter of image quality. (**i**) Image quality. In order to detect glaucomatous progression, image quality is essential. Reproducibility of serial images is critical in detecting progressive structural change. The HRT is proven reproducible and has automatic quality control (standard deviation measure) to provide exact comparison of data and accurate follow-up of patients over time. (**j**) Focused and unfocused image. (**k**) Image acquisition with an uncorrected astigmatism. (**l**) Fixation loss during acquisition: see the double vessels. (**m**) Movement of the eye during acquisition. (**n**) Wrong focus; see the overexposure image. (**o**) Good image for the analysis. (**p**) Presence of floaters. (**q**) Presence of floaters in the TCA map (see below). (**r**) Presence of haemorrhages. (**s**) Scleral ring. (**t**) Peripapillary atrophy

b

c

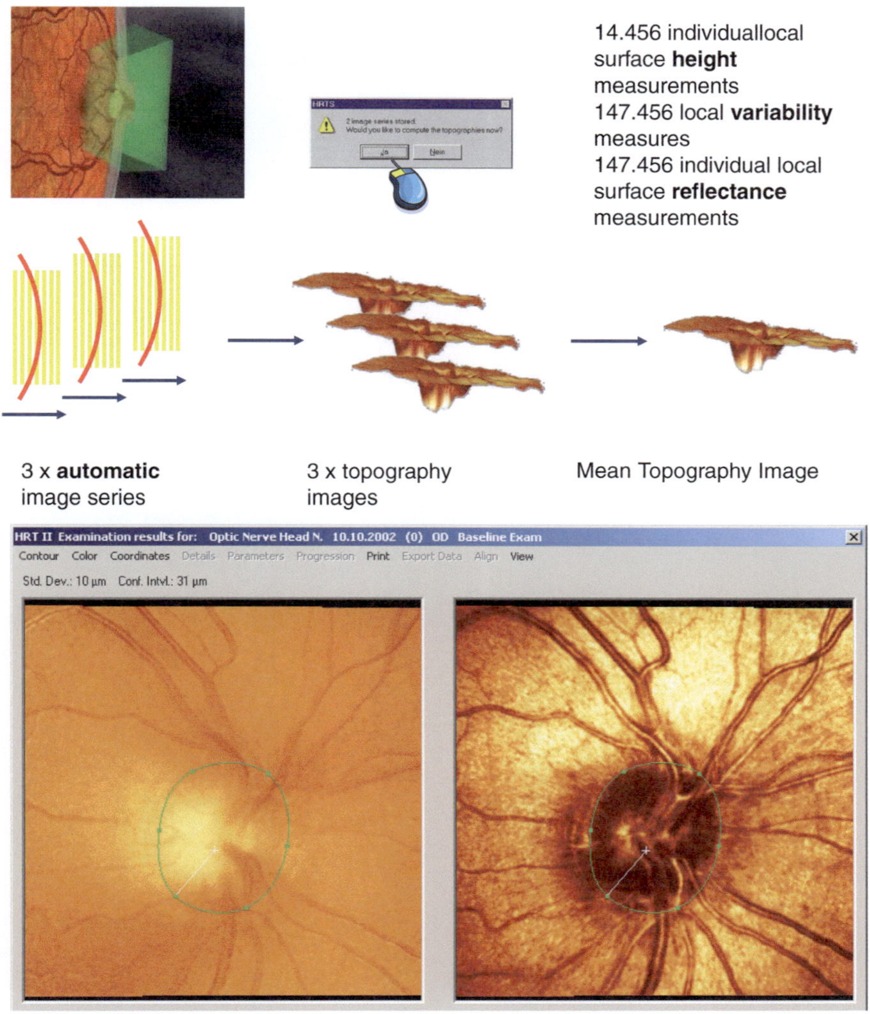

Fig. 7.1 (continued)

d

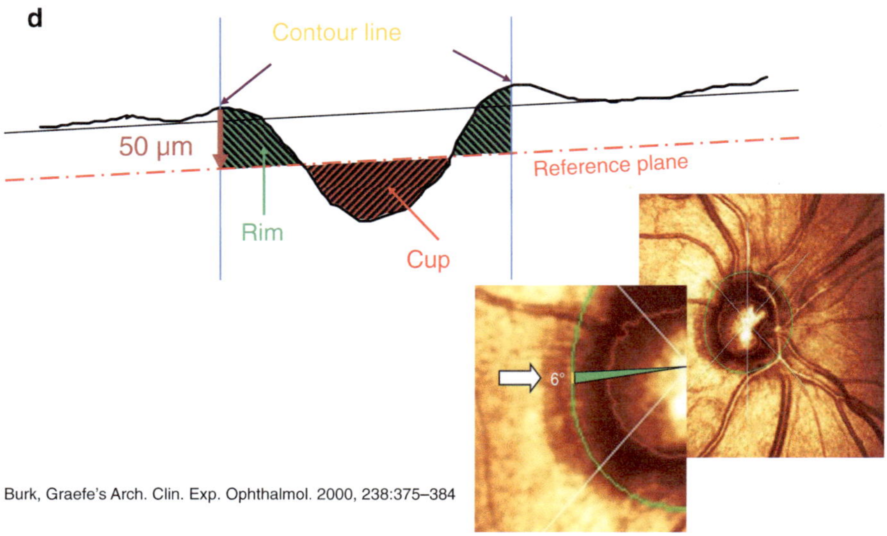

e

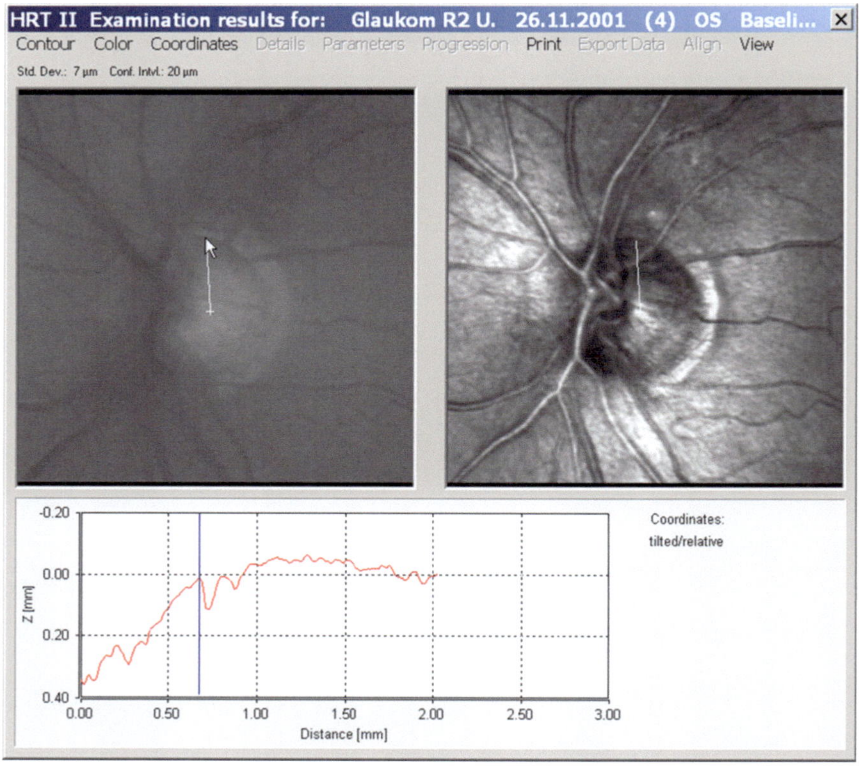

Fig. 7.1 (continued)

f

Parameters	global	normal range	p-value	temporal	tmp/sup	tmp/inf	nasal	nsl/sup	nsl/inf
disc area [mm²]	2.03	1.63 - 2.43	-	0.47	0.26	0.28	0.48	0.28	0.25
cup area [mm²]	0.33	0.11 - 0.68	> 0.5	0.25	0.03	0.05	0.00	0.00	0.00
rim area [mm²]	1.70	1.31 - 1.96	> 0.5	0.23	0.23	0.24	0.48	0.28	0.25
cup/disc area ratio [ ]	0.16	0.07 - 0.30	> 0.5	0.52	0.12	0.17	0.00	0.00	0.00
rim/disc area ratio [ ]	0.84	0.70 - 0.93	> 0.5	0.48	0.88	0.83	1.00	1.00	1.00
cup volume [mm³]	0.02	-0.01 - 0.18	> 0.5	0.02	0.00	0.00	0.00	0.00	0.00
rim volume [mm³]	0.40	0.30 - 0.61	> 0.5	0.02	0.04	0.05	0.12	0.08	0.08
mean cup depth [mm]	0.13	0.10 - 0.27	> 0.5	0.16	0.13	0.16	0.06	0.06	0.06
maximum cup depth [mm]	0.32	0.32 - 0.76	> 0.5	0.33	0.29	0.33	0.16	0.18	0.17
height variation contour [mm]	0.31	0.31 - 0.49	0.34	0.13	0.18	0.17	0.13	0.03	0.08
cup shape measure [ ]	-0.13	-0.28 - -0.15	0.24	-0.02	-0.07	-0.02	-0.15	-0.18	-0.15
mean RNFL thickness [mm]	0.23	0.20 - 0.32	> 0.5	0.09	0.27	0.28	0.24	0.34	0.32
RNFL cross sectional area [mm²]	1.19	0.99 - 1.66	> 0.5	0.11	0.17	0.19	0.29	0.23	0.21
linear cup/disc ratio [ ]	0.40	0.27 - 0.55	> 0.5	-	-	-	-	-	-
maximum contour elevation [mm]	-0.06	-0.21 - -0.04	0.42	-	-	-	-	-	-
maximum contour depression [mm]	0.25	0.17 - 0.39	> 0.5	-	-	-	-	-	-
CLM temporal-superior [mm]	0.18	0.14 - 0.27	> 0.5	-	-	-	-	-	-
CLM temporal-inferior [mm]	0.19	0.13 - 0.29	> 0.5	-	-	-	-	-	-
average variability (SD) [µm]	11	-	-	-	-	-	-	-	-
reference height [µm]	299	-	-	-	-	-	-	-	-
FSM discriminant function value [ ]	1.48	-	-	-	-	-	-	-	-
RB discriminant function value [ ]	1.15	-	-	-	-	-	-	-	-
modified ISNT rule fulfilled	yes	-	-	-	-	-	-	-	-

g

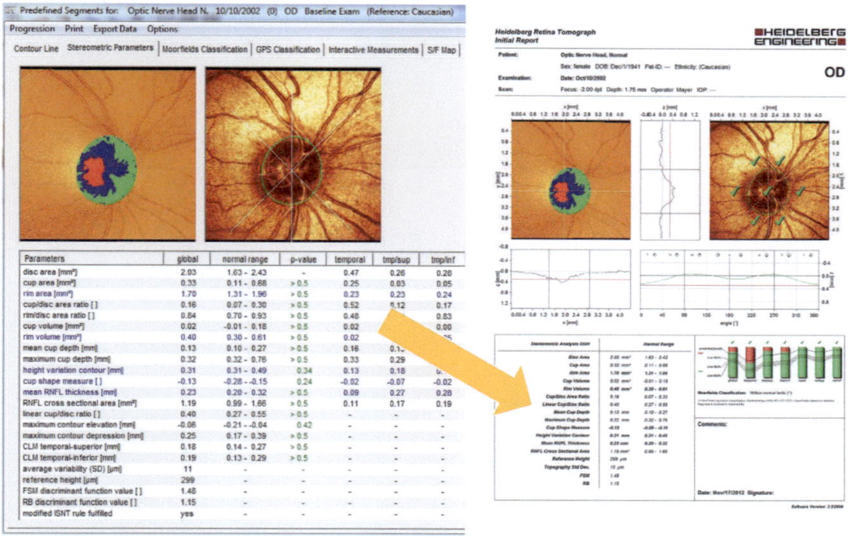

h

< 10 µm Excellent

10–20 µm Very Good

20–30 µm Good

30–40 µm Acceptable

40–50 µm Try to improve

> 50 µm Poor quality documentation only

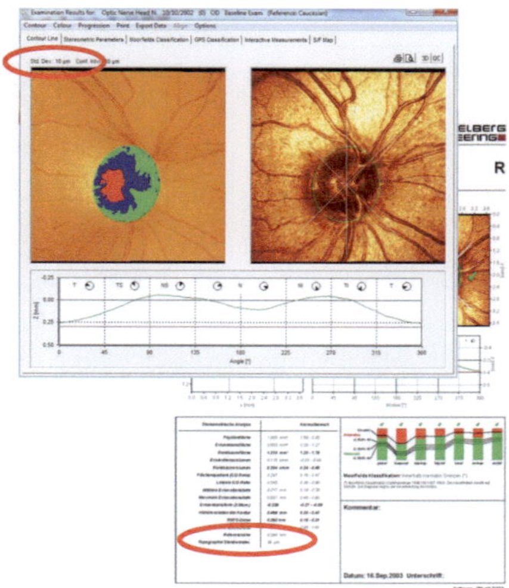

Fig. 7.1 (continued)

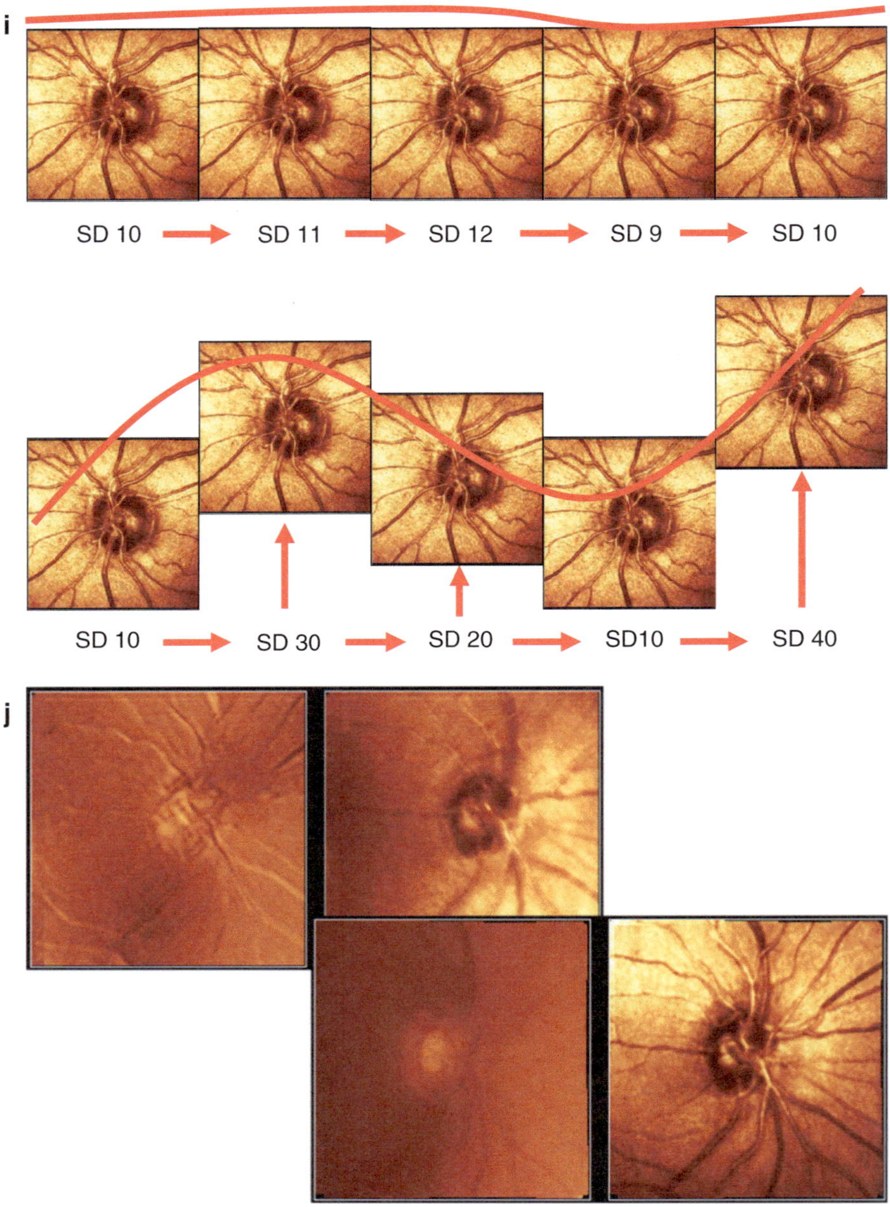

Fig. 7.1 (continued)

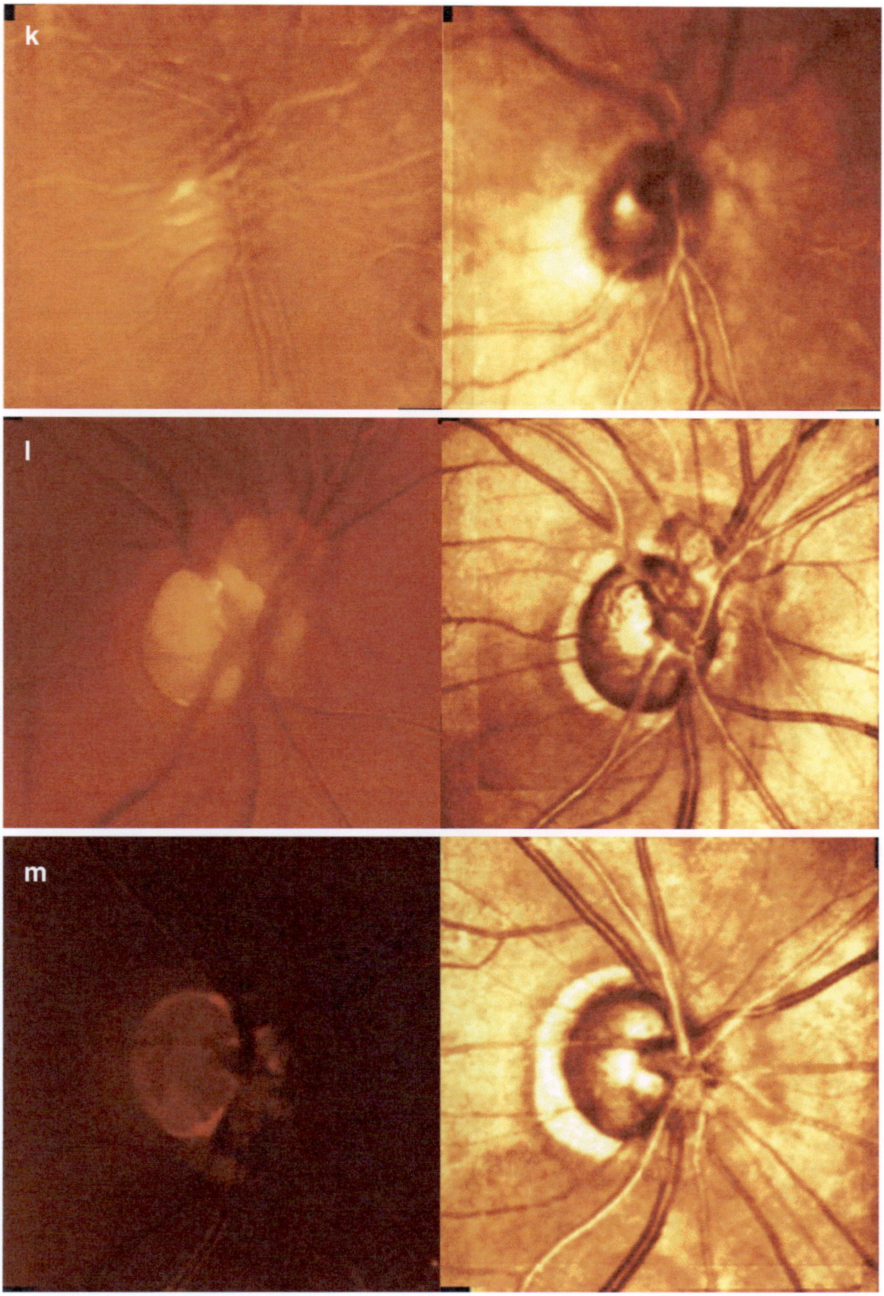

Fig. 7.1 (continued)

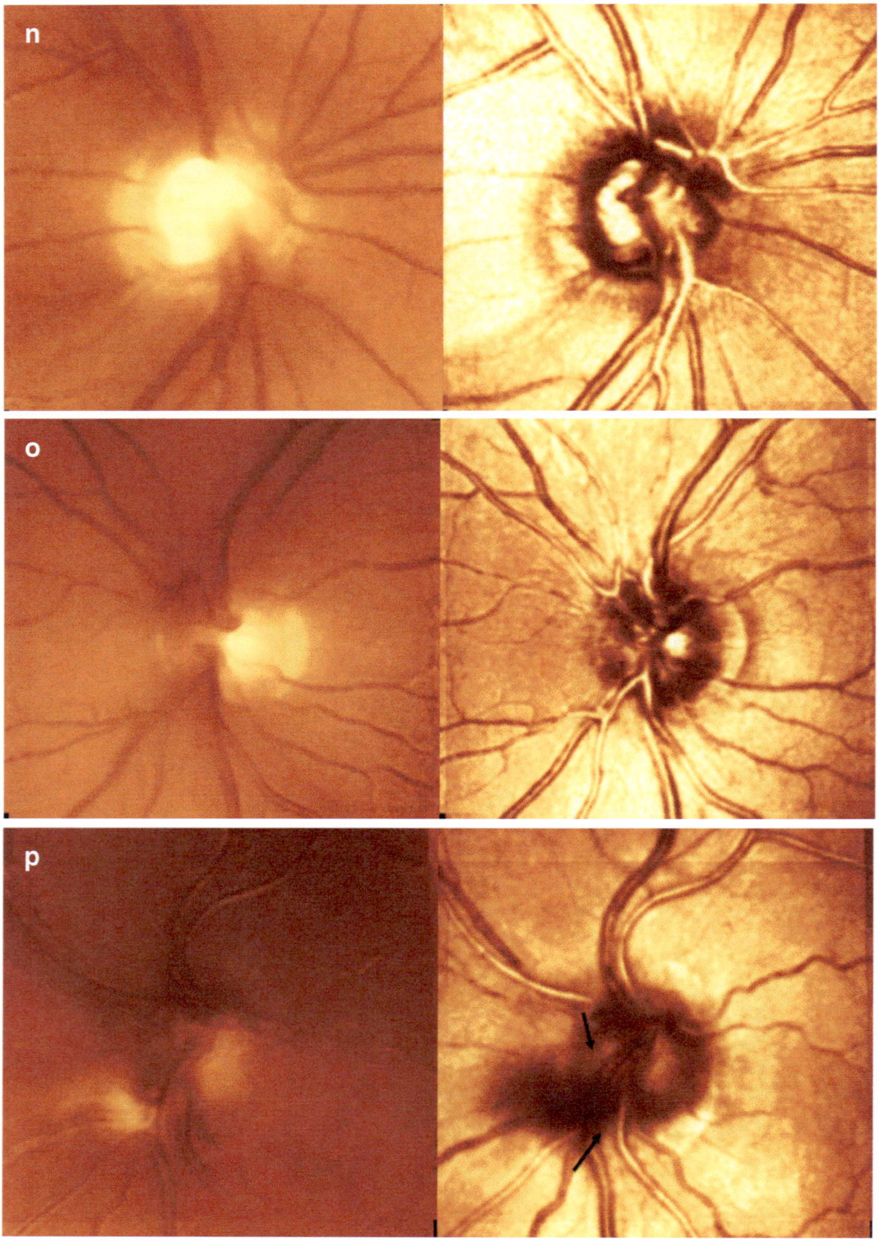

Fig. 7.1 (continued)

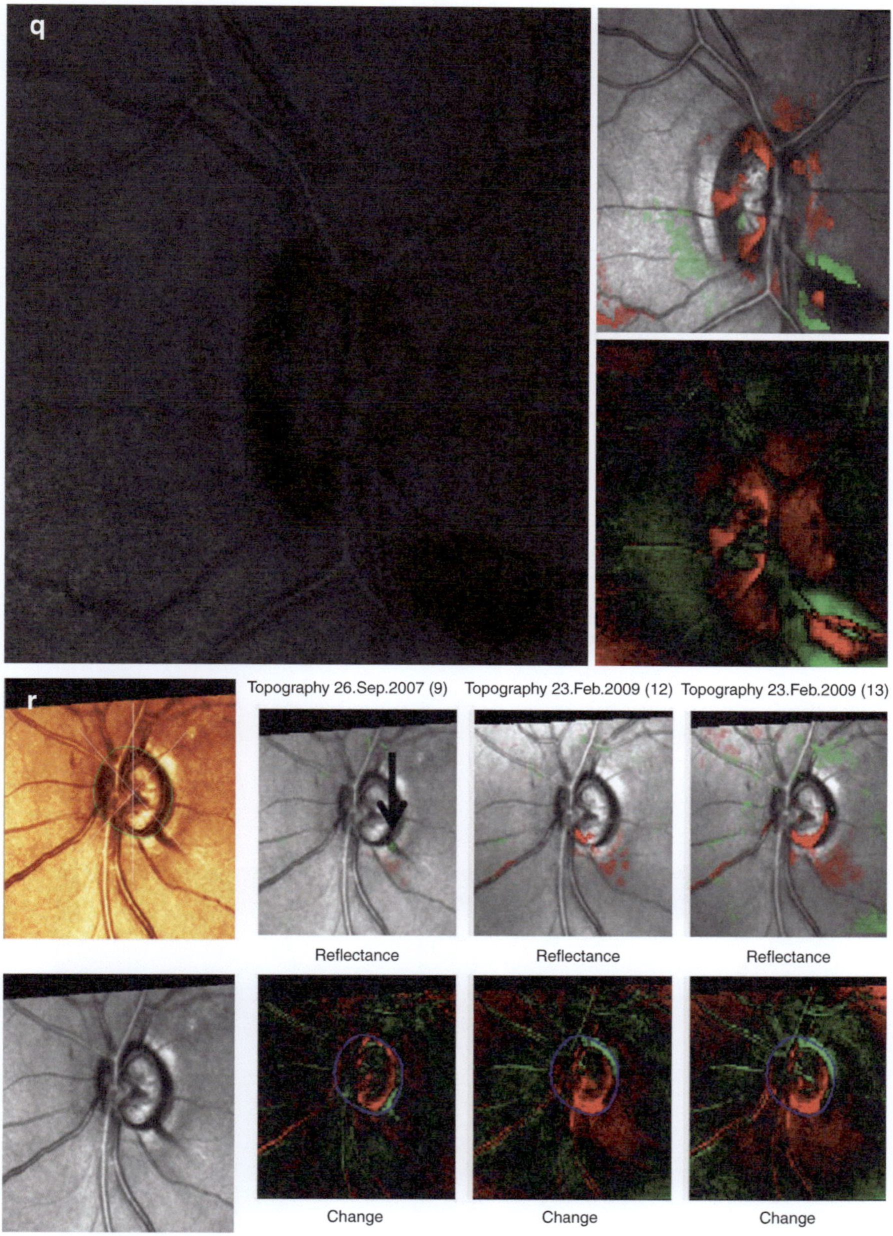

Fig. 7.1 (continued)

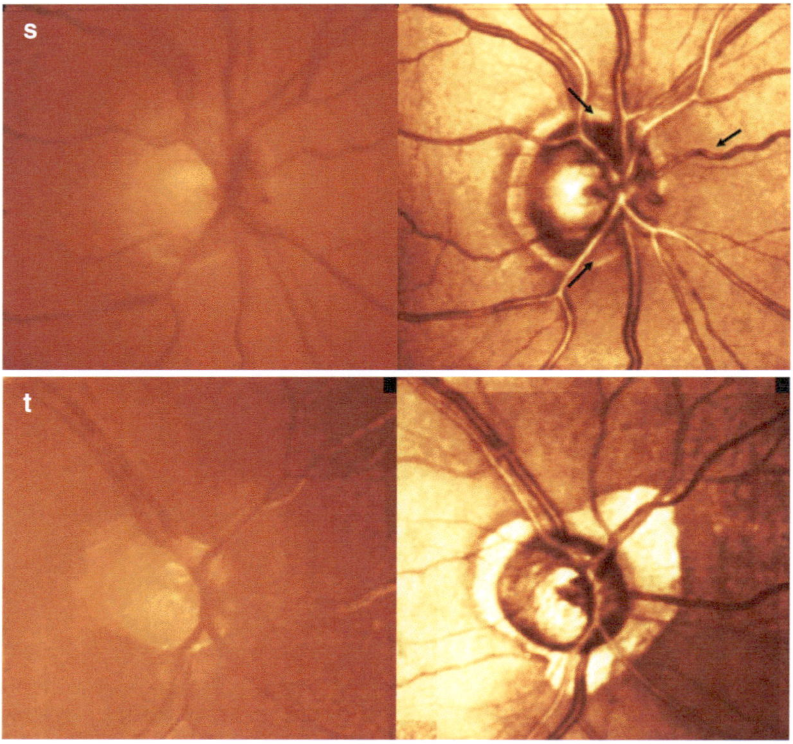

Fig. 7.1 (continued)

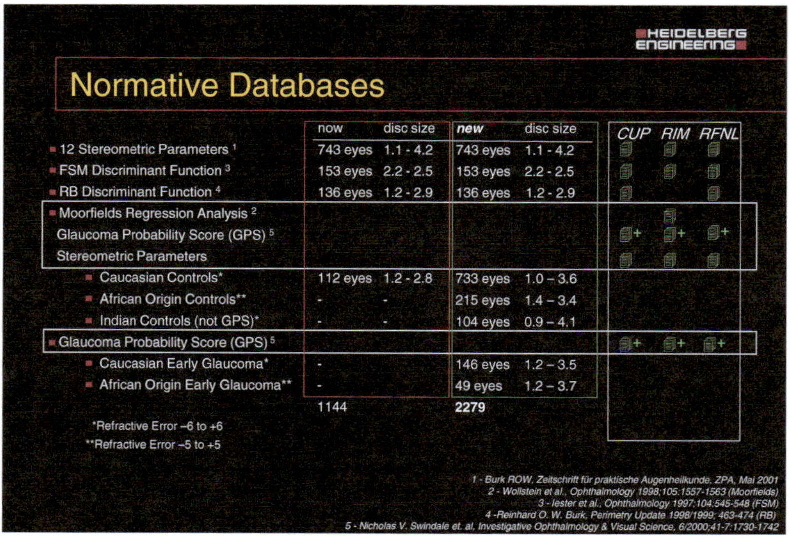

Fig. 7.2 Normative Databases

7.2 Moorfields Regression Analysis (MRA)

This is a method based on a logarithmic transformation which is made to normalise the distribution, and the normal limits are derived from the prediction intervals of a regression analysis of log neuroretinal rim area against ONH area and age, because of the known relationship between neuroretinal rim area and ONH size [10] and subject age [11]. Furthermore, in glaucoma, although neuroretinal rim narrowing is said to occur preferentially at the poles of the ONH, it may occur anywhere in the ONH; thus, the classification algorithm is based on an analysis of all ONH segments predefined in the software, with the most abnormal segment giving rise to the overall ONH classification.

In the software analysis, the neuroretinal rim and cup areas, in relation to the prediction intervals, for the whole disc and each predefined segment are displayed as a series of bars (Fig. 7.3i). The classification for each ONH segment is also displayed on the reflectivity image. A red cross denotes ‘outside normal limits’, a yellow exclamation mark denotes ‘borderline’ and a green tick denotes ‘within normal limits’ (Fig. 7.3r).

The lower three lines represent the lower 95.0, 99.0 and 99.9 % prediction intervals. These intervals are calculated for the ONH as a whole and for each of the six predefined sectors. An ONH is classified as ‘within normal limits’ if the global and segmental neuroretinal rim areas are all greater than (above) the 95 % prediction interval. If the rim area of any segment lies between the 95 and 99.9 % prediction intervals, then the ONH is classified as ‘borderline’. If the rim area of any segment lies below the 99.9 % prediction interval, then the ONH is classified as ‘outside normal limits’.

However, because glaucoma is associated with narrowing of the neuroretinal rim, the great majority of eyes with glaucoma will be classified as ‘borderline’ or ‘outside normal limits’. The final decision as to whether an eye is glaucomatous or not is a clinical judgement, based on all available clinical data (Fig. 7.3r, s).

Clinically some correlations between MRA results and visual fields have been found, and the system can offer a good and easy to read print-out (see below; Fig. 7.5a–c).

The OHTS Ancillary Study found that the MRA superior temporal region had the highest positive predictive value for glaucoma. A patient with an abnormal MRA at this location was likely to be six times more at risk of glaucoma compared to any other risk factors. And 40 % of eyes flagged as ‘outside normal limits’ at the baseline examination went on to develop glaucoma [12].

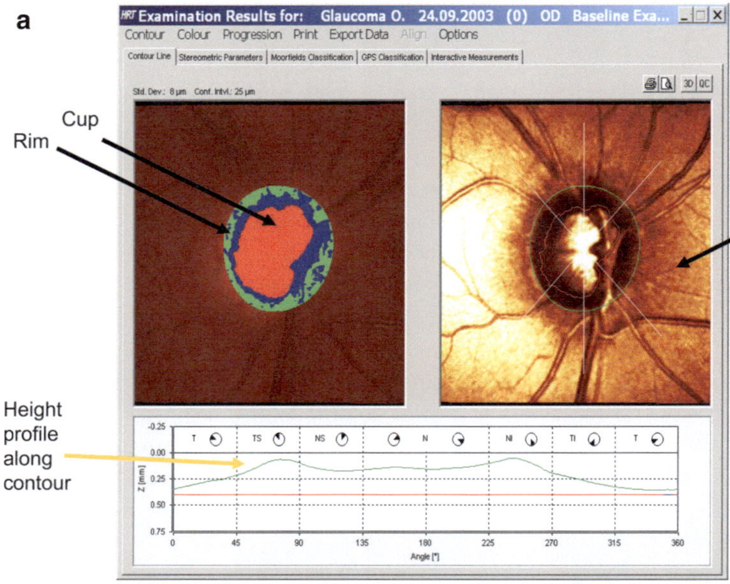

b

Parameters	global	normal range	p-value	temporal	tmp/sup	tmp/inf	nasal	nsl/sup	nsl/inf
disc area [mm²]	2.61	1.63 - 2.43	-	0.65	0.33	0.34	0.66	0.32	0.31
cup area [mm²]	1.22	0.11 - 0.68	0.01	0.39	0.15	0.21	0.20	0.16	0.12
rim area [mm²]	1.39	1.31 - 1.96	0.01	0.26	0.18	0.13	0.47	0.16	0.19
cup/disc area ratio [ ]	0.47	0.07 - 0.30	0.04	0.60	0.45	0.61	0.30	0.50	0.39
rim/disc area ratio [ ]	0.53	0.70 - 0.93	> 0.5	0.40	0.55	0.39	0.70	0.50	0.61
cup volume [mm³]	0.52	-0.01 - 0.18	< 0.001	0.13	0.08	0.10	0.07	0.07	0.07
rim volume [mm³]	0.27	0.30 - 0.61	0.04	0.02	0.04	0.02	0.10	0.03	0.05
mean cup depth [mm]	0.40	0.10 - 0.27	0.03	0.36	0.52	0.52	0.28	0.42	0.50
maximum cup depth [mm]	0.95	0.32 - 0.76	0.12	0.86	0.99	0.89	0.89	0.95	0.98
height variation contour [mm]	0.30	0.31 - 0.49	0.21	0.14	0.15	0.13	0.06	0.07	0.14
cup shape measure [ ]	-0.13	-0.28 - -0.15	0.35	-0.11	0.05	0.09	-0.27	-0.10	-0.05

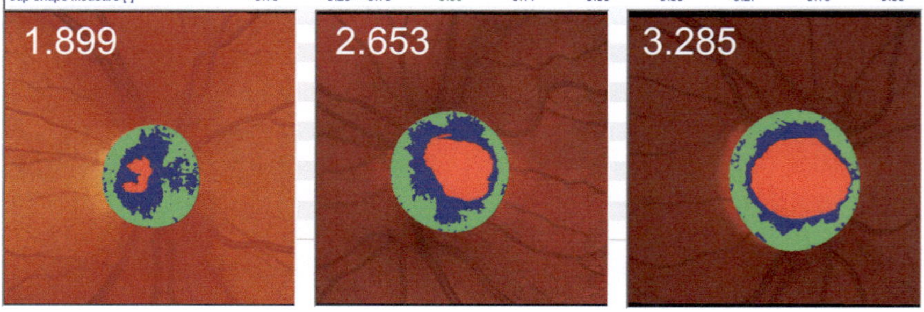

Fig. 7.3 (**a**) Qualitative overview. (**b**) Disc size is important because you need to assess the disc size relative to the normative values of the other parameters. For example, a cup shape measure of –0.2 is OK on a normal size disc but on a large disc, –0.1 is normal. (**c**) Configuration of cup. Vertical orientation of the cup would be a risk factor. (**d**) Height profile along contour line. (**e**) Cross check looking at RNFL profile. The retinal surface height variation graph should be above the red reference plane. Typically you see the RNFL double hump configuration. The retinal surface height should not dip below the reference plane. If it does, it generally means the contour line is drawn too narrow. (**f**) Normal RNFL profile. (**g**) Abnormal RNFL profile. (**h**) Reflectivity and RNFL loss. (**i**) Moorfields regression analysis (MRA). (**j**) Moorfields regression analysis (MRA). (**k**) Discriminant analysis formulas: FSM and RB. (**l**) Stereometric parameters and discriminant functions. (**m**) Glaucoma probability score (GPS): parameters used. (**n**) Glaucoma probability score (GPS). (**o**) Rim configuration. Does the disc follow the ISNT rule? (**p**) Rim configuration example. (q) OU report. How to read. (**r**) OU report. example. (**s**) OU report example. (**t**) OU report GPS

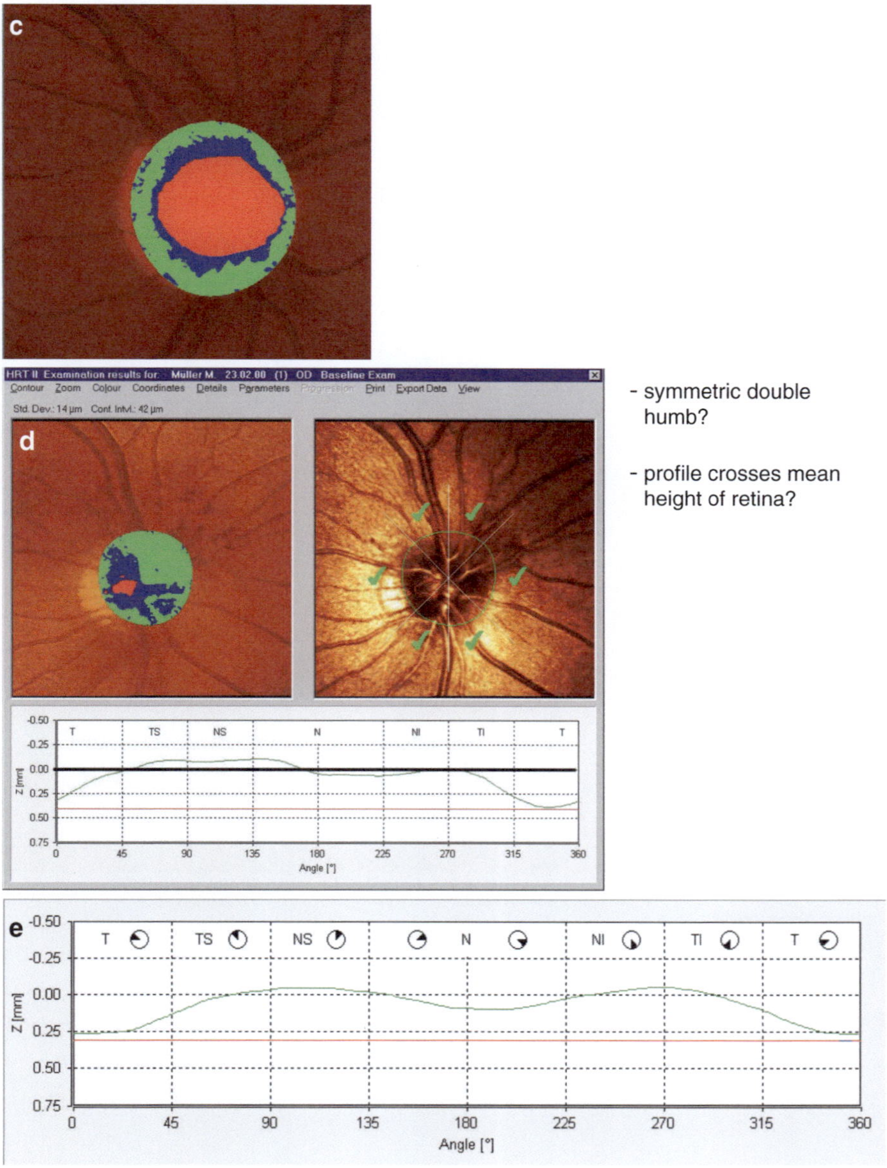

Fig. 7.3 (continued)

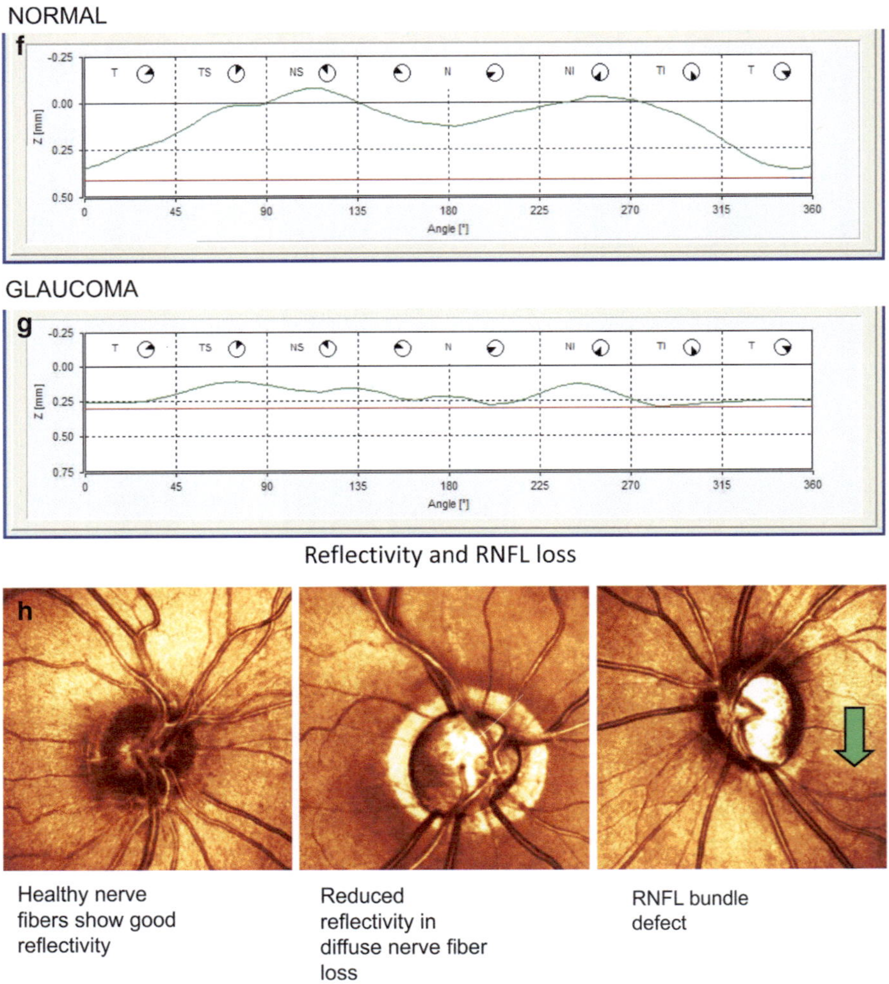

Fig. 7.3 (continued)

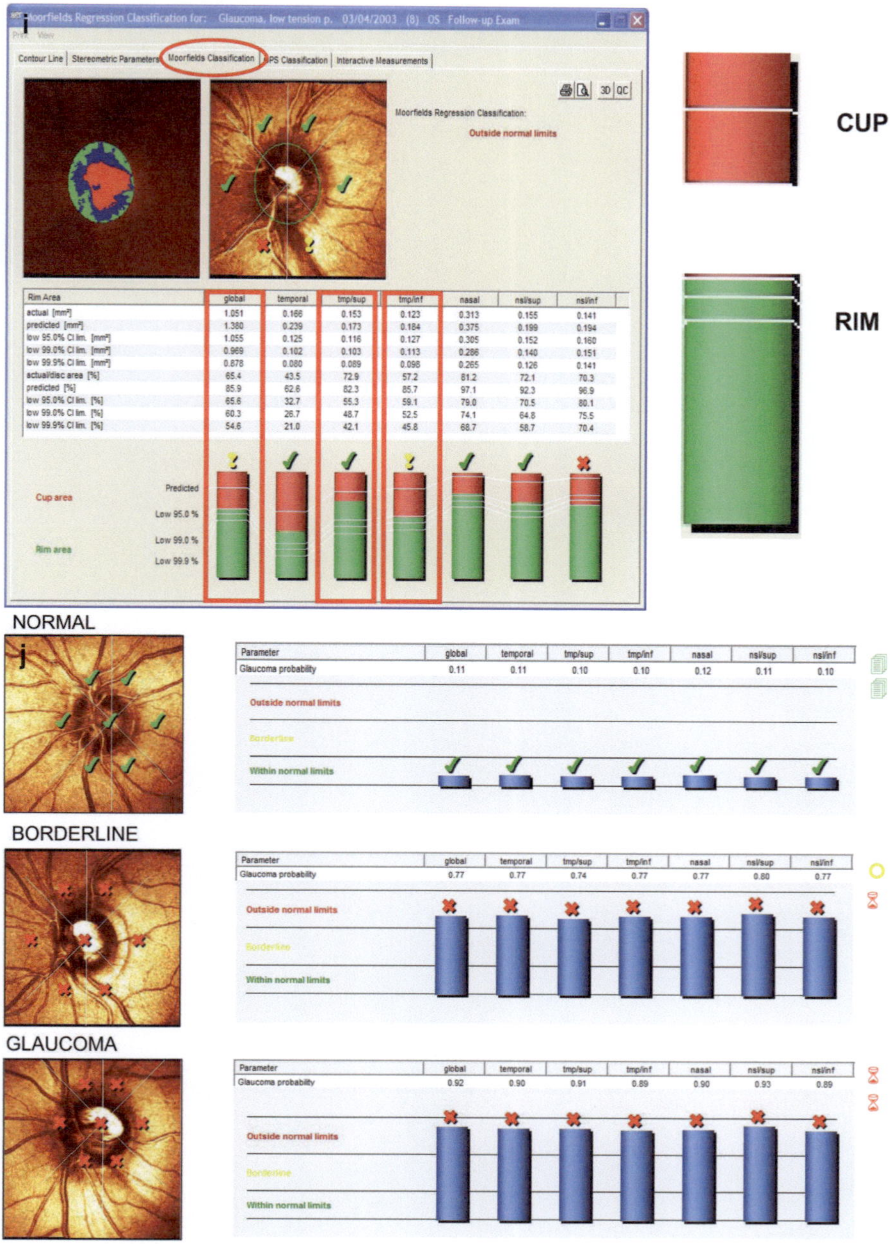

Fig. 7.3 (continued)

k

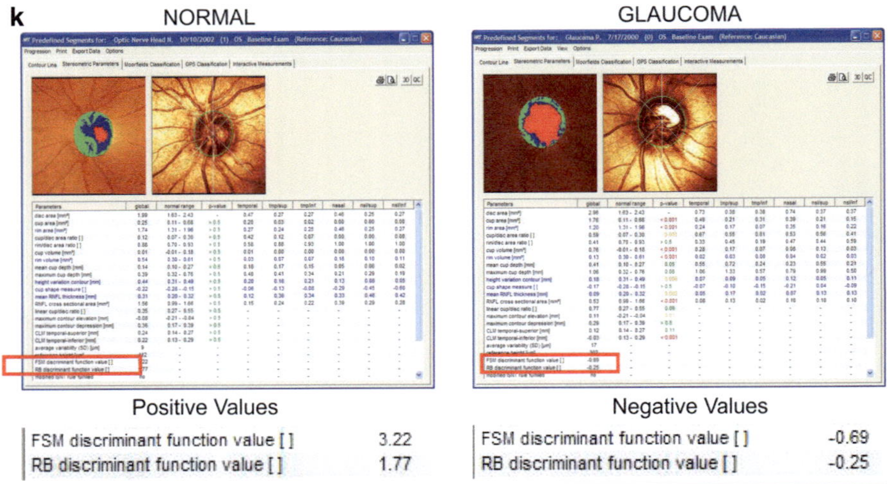

l

Parameters	global	normal range	p-value	temporal	tmp/sup	tmp/inf	nasal	nsl/sup	nsl/inf
disc area [mm²]	2.61	1.63 - 2.43	-	0.65	0.33	0.34	0.66	0.32	0.31
cup area [mm²]	1.22	0.11 - 0.68	0.01	0.39	0.15	0.21	0.20	0.16	0.12
rim area [mm²]	1.39	1.31 - 1.96	0.01	0.26	0.18	0.13	0.47	0.16	0.19
cup/disc area ratio [ ]	0.47	0.07 - 0.30	0.04	0.60	0.45	0.61	0.30	0.50	0.39
rim/disc area ratio [ ]	0.53	0.70 - 0.93	> 0.5	0.40	0.55	0.39	0.70	0.50	0.61
cup volume [mm³]	0.52	-0.01 - 0.18	< 0.001	0.13	0.08	0.10	0.07	0.07	0.07
rim volume [mm³]	0.27	0.30 - 0.61	0.04	0.02	0.04	0.02	0.10	0.03	0.05
mean cup depth [mm]	0.40	0.10 - 0.27	0.03	0.36	0.52	0.52	0.28	0.42	0.50
maximum cup depth [mm]	0.95	0.32 - 0.76	0.12	0.86	0.99	0.89	0.89	0.95	0.98
height variation contour [mm]	0.30	0.31 - 0.49	0.21	0.14	0.15	0.13	0.06	0.07	0.14
cup shape measure [ ]	-0.13	-0.28 - -0.15	0.35	-0.11	0.05	0.09	-0.27	-0.10	-0.05
mean RNFL thickness [mm]	0.21	0.20 - 0.32	0.38	0.09	0.29	0.14	0.26	0.25	0.30
RNFL cross sectional area [mm²]	1.19	0.99 - 1.66	0.30	0.12	0.21	0.10	0.37	0.18	0.21
linear cup/disc ratio [ ]	0.68	0.27 - 0.55	0.16	-	-	-	-	-	-
maximum contour elevation [mm]	0.05	-0.21 - -0.04	0.06	-	-	-	-	-	-
maximum contour depression [mm]	0.35	0.17 - 0.39	> 0.5	-	-	-	-	-	-
CLM temporal-superior [mm]	0.21	0.14 - 0.27	> 0.5	-	-	-	-	-	-
CLM temporal-inferior [mm]	0.06	0.13 - 0.29	0.05	-	-	-	-	-	-
average variability (SD) [µm]	11	-	-	-	-	-	-	-	-
reference height [µm]	402	-	-	-	-	-	-	-	-
FSM discriminant function value [ ]	-0.10	-	-	-	-	-	-	-	-
RB discriminant function value [ ]	0.01	-	-	-	-	-	-	-	-
modified ISNT rule fulfilled	no	-	-	-	-	-	-	-	-

m

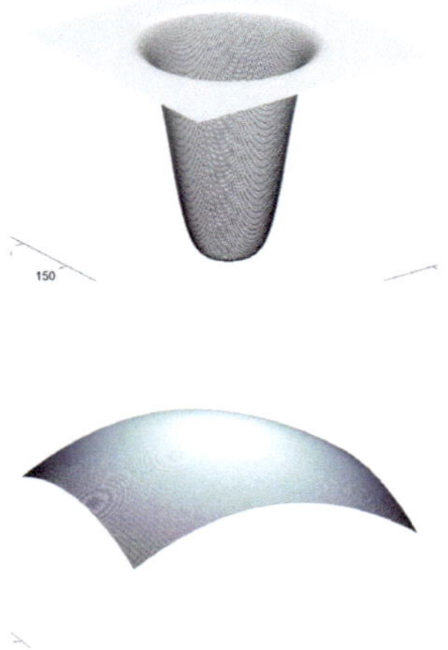

Fig. 7.3 (continued)

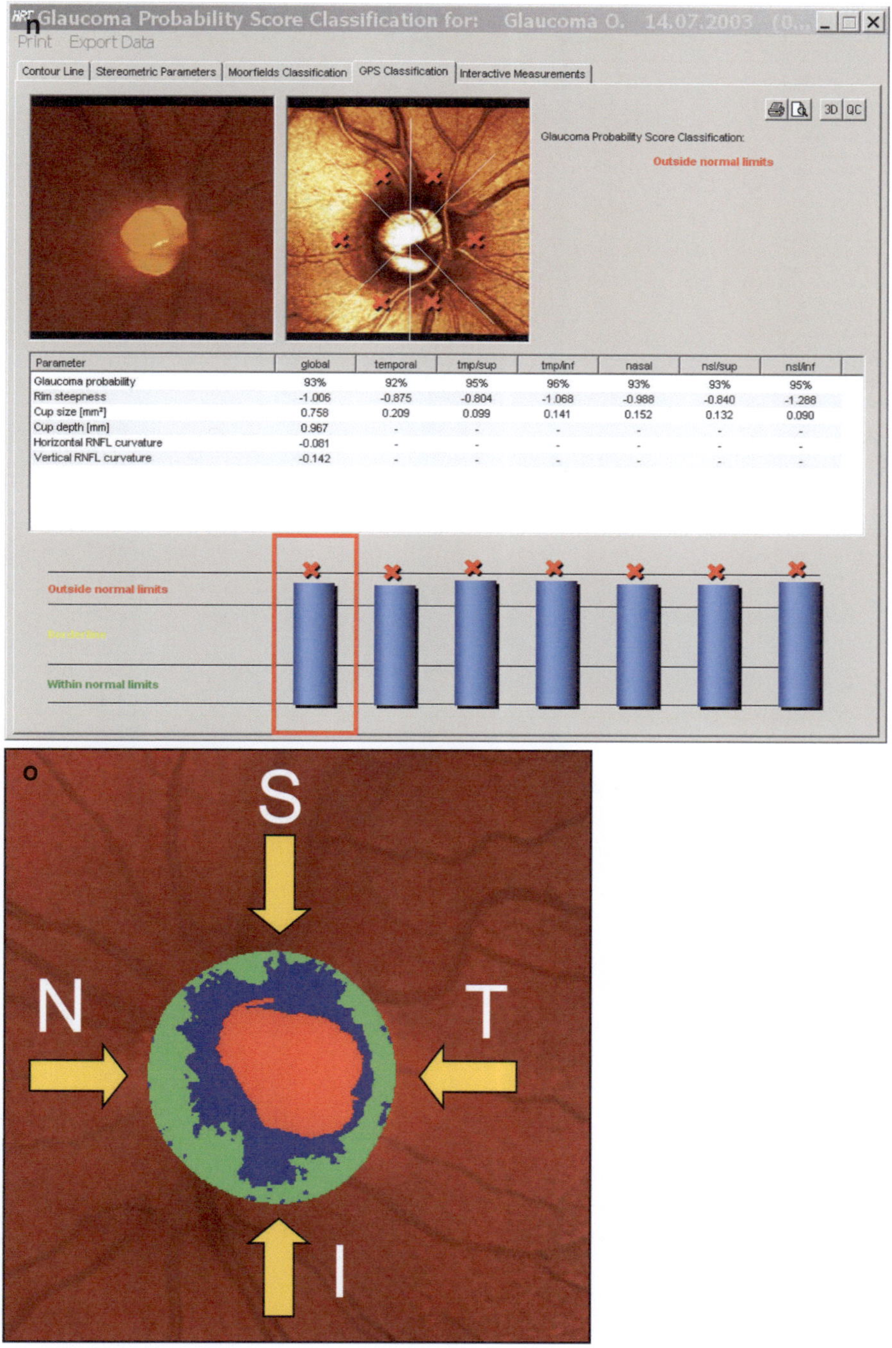

Parameter	global	temporal	tmp/sup	tmp/inf	nasal	nsl/sup	nsl/inf
Glaucoma probability	93%	92%	95%	96%	93%	93%	95%
Rim steepness	-1.006	-0.875	-0.804	-1.068	-0.988	-0.840	-1.288
Cup size [mm²]	0.758	0.209	0.099	0.141	0.152	0.132	0.090
Cup depth [mm]	0.967	-	-	-	-	-	-
Horizontal RNFL curvature	-0.081	-	-	-	-	-	-
Vertical RNFL curvature	-0.142	-	-	-	-	-	-

Fig. 7.3 (continued)

p

Parameters	global	normal range	p-value	temporal	tmp/sup	tmp/inf	nasal	nsl/sup	nsl/inf
disc area [mm²]	2.61	1.63 - 2.43	-	0.65	0.33	0.34	0.66	0.32	0.31
cup area [mm²]	1.22	0.11 - 0.68	0.01	0.39	0.15	0.21	0.20	0.16	0.12
rim area [mm²]	1.39	1.31 - 1.96	0.01	0.26	0.18	0.13	0.47	0.16	0.19
cup/disc area ratio [ ]	0.47	0.07 - 0.30	0.04	0.60	0.45	0.61	0.30	0.50	0.39
rim/disc area ratio [ ]	0.53	0.70 - 0.93	> 0.5	0.40	0.55	0.39	0.70	0.50	0.61
cup volume [mm³]	0.52	-0.01 - 0.18	< 0.001	0.13	0.08	0.10	0.07	0.07	0.07
rim volume [mm³]	0.27	0.30 - 0.61	0.04	0.02	0.04	0.02	0.10	0.03	0.05
mean cup depth [mm]	0.40	0.10 - 0.27	0.03	0.36	0.52	0.52	0.28	0.42	0.50
maximum cup depth [mm]	0.95	0.32 - 0.76	0.12	0.86	0.99	0.89	0.89	0.95	0.98
height variation contour [mm]	0.30	0.31 - 0.49	0.21	0.14	0.15	0.13	0.06	0.07	0.14
cup shape measure [ ]	-0.13	-0.28 - -0.15	0.35	-0.11	0.05	0.09	-0.27	-0.10	-0.05
mean RNFL thickness [mm]	0.21	0.20 - 0.32	0.38	0.09	0.29	0.14	0.26	0.25	0.30
RNFL cross sectional area [mm²]	1.19	0.99 - 1.66	0.30	0.12	0.21	0.10	0.37	0.18	0.21
linear cup/disc ratio [ ]	0.68	0.27 - 0.55	0.16	-	-	-	-	-	-
maximum contour elevation [mm]	0.05	-0.21 - -0.04	0.06	-	-	-	-	-	-
maximum contour depression [mm]	0.35	0.17 - 0.39	> 0.5	-	-	-	-	-	-
CLM temporal-superior [mm]	0.21	0.14 - 0.27	> 0.5	-	-	-	-	-	-
CLM temporal-inferior [mm]	0.06	0.13 - 0.29	0.05	-	-	-	-	-	-
average variability (SD) [µm]	11	-	-	-	-	-	-	-	-
reference height [µm]	402	-	-	-	-	-	-	-	-
FSM discriminant function value [ ]	-0.10	-	-	-	-	-	-	-	-
RB discriminant function value [ ]	0.01	-	-	-	-	-	-	-	-
modified ISNT rule fulfilled	no	-	-	-	-	-	-	-	-

I = 0.32 > ?
S = 0.34 > ?
N* = 0.47> ?
T = 0.26

*Nasal rim includes vessels

q

- Statistically compares parameters to database for automatic classification

p > 0.05 Within Normal Limits
p < 0.05 Borderline
p < 0.001 Outside Normal Limits

- All parameters adjusted for optic disc size and age

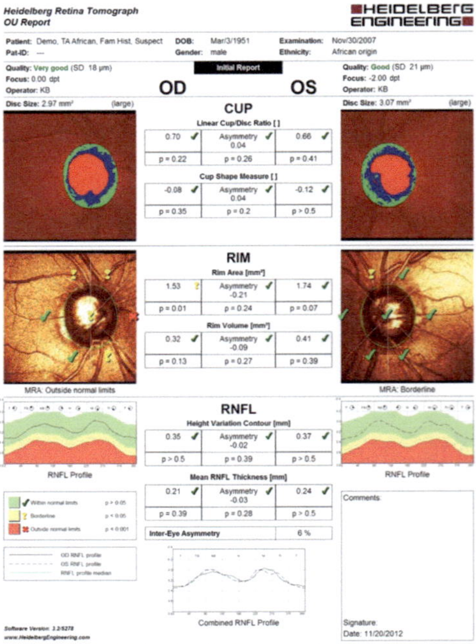

Fig. 7.3 (continued)

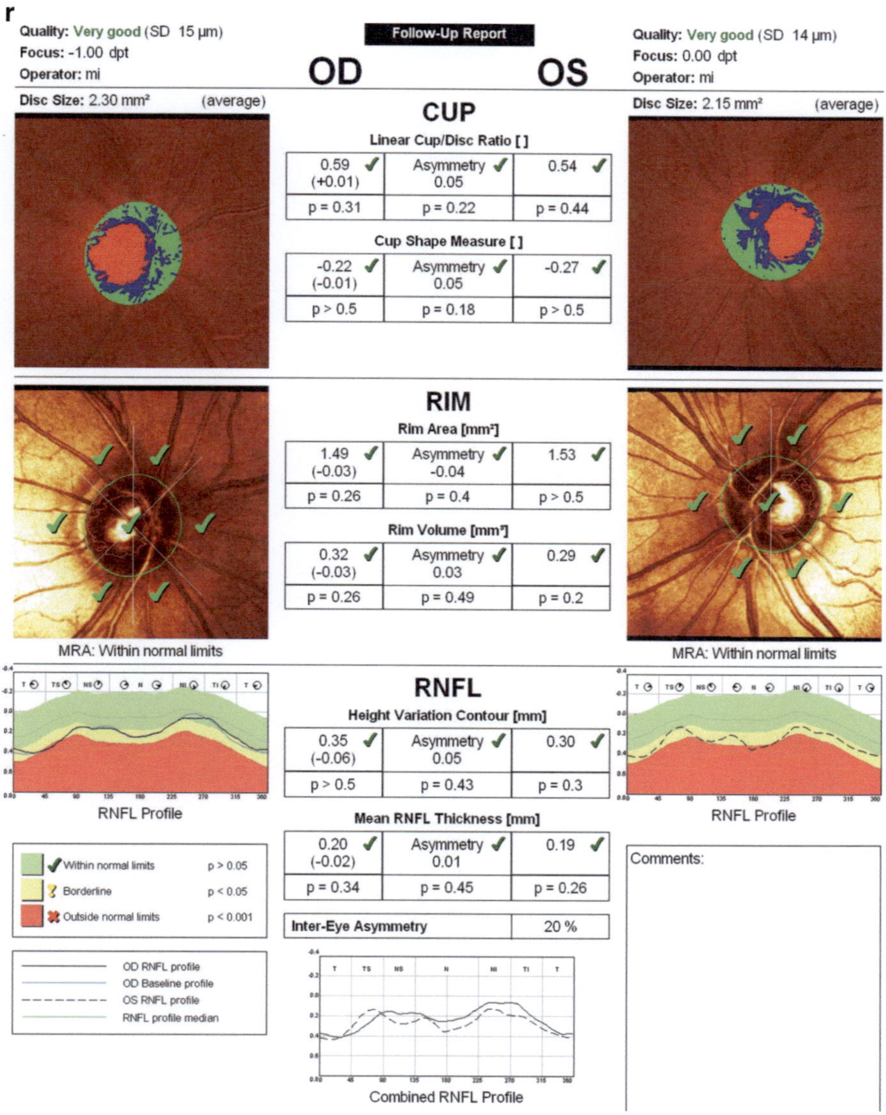

Fig. 7.3 (continued)

s

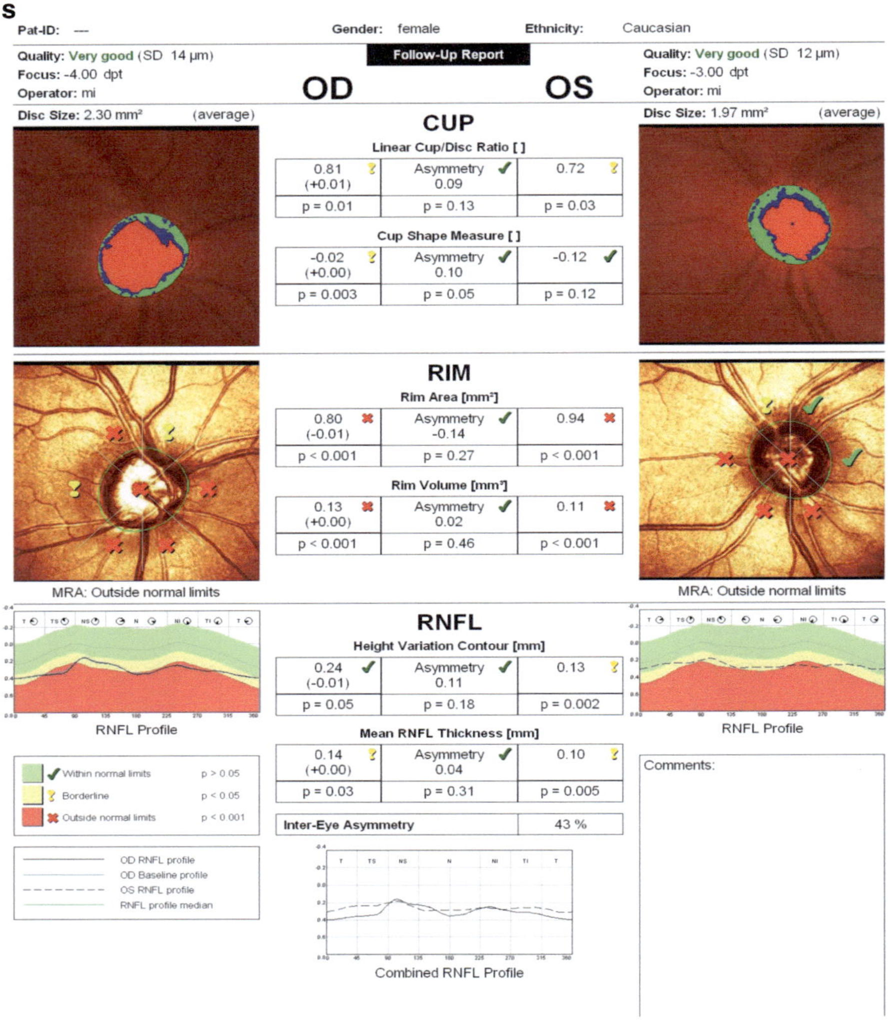

Fig. 7.3 (continued)

t

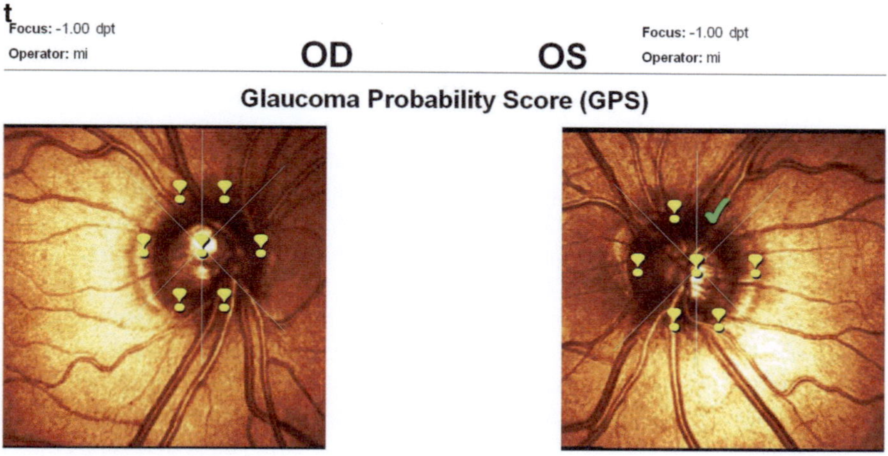

global	temporal	tmp/sup	tmp/inf	nasal	nsl/sup	nsl/inf	Parameter	global	temporal	tmp/sup	tmp/inf	nasal	nsl/sup	nsl/inf
0.46	0.44	0.41	0.47	0.44	0.41	0.42	Glaucoma prob.	0.34	0.35	0.25	0.39	0.40	0.30	0.29
-0.58	-0.68	-0.76	-0.52	-0.53	-0.43	-0.55	Rim steepness	0.04	-0.21	-0.10	-0.55	0.56	-0.07	0.12
0.46	0.14	0.05	0.09	0.11	0.05	0.05	Cup size [mm²]	0.38	0.14	0.04	0.10	0.04	0.06	0.02
0.90	---	---	---	---	---	---	Cup depth [mm]	0.62	---	---	---	---	---	---
-0.04	---	---	---	---	---	---	H. RNFL curv.	-0.04	---	---	---	---	---	---
-0.16	---	---	---	---	---	---	V. RNFL curv.	-0.19	---	---	---	---	---	---

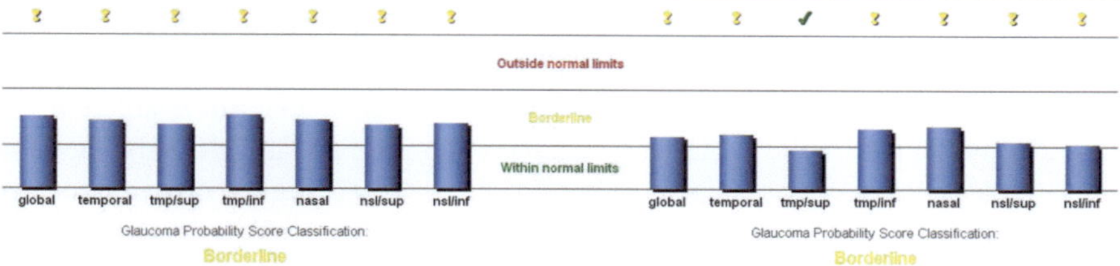

Fig. 7.3 (continued)

7.3 Discriminant Analysis Formulas

The HRT software produces a large number of ONH measurements, and discriminant analysis is a method of predicting group membership from the optimally weighted combination of variables. The mathematical approach to distinguish between healthy and glaucomatous eyes is based on generating a discriminant function from a linear discriminant analysis of measurement data derived from healthy and glaucomatous eyes or on an analysis which derives limits for normality for the considered parameter (Fig. 7.3k).

The analysis determines a subset of variables that is most discriminating and the weights (positive or negative) for each variable. For the HRT, this means finding a combination of ONH parameters that predict the presence or absence of a glaucomatous VF. The first reported discriminant analysis was by Mikelberg et al. [13, 14]. Their analysis included a number of global parameters and subject age. Since then, more discriminant analyses have been developed. The HRT software provides the discriminant analyses of Mikelberg et al. [14] and Burk et al. [15] (Fig.7.3l).

The differences between the various formulas are likely to reflect differences in the subject groups, caused by factors such as subject selection, ONH size and disease definitions.

It has been shown that the discriminant analysis classification differed in small (disc area <2 mm^2), intermediate and large (disc area >3 mm^2) ONHs [14]. In the small ONH subgroup, the Mikelberg et al. and Bathija et al. analyses resulted in the best discrimination. In the subgroups with medium-sized and large ONHs, the sector formula of Iester et al. obtained the best results [15–19]. Slightly different results have been found by Ford et al.[20].

The type of glaucoma, subject gender and refractive error do not markedly affect the performance of the analyses [21].

7.4 Glaucoma Probability Score

Furthermore, all the HRT images were analysed by the *glaucoma probability score* (GPS) classification which involves the use of a geometric model to approximate the shape of the ONH topography with a three-dimensional surface described by five parameters derived from ONH and peripapillary retinal morphology (cup size, cup depth, rim steepness, horizontal and vertical RNFL curvature) (Fig. 7.3lj, m). The details of this method have been already published elsewhere [22]. The GPS is able to classify ONHs in three different groups: normal, borderline or suspect and 'outside normal limit' group based on the value obtained (within normal limits, 0–28; borderline, 28–64; outside normal limits, 64–100). Using the HRT GPS, it was possible to differentiate normal from glaucomatous with a diagnostic capacity similar to DAF, but without any observer input (Fig. 7.3n).

Iester et al. obtained similar results between discriminant formulas and GPS. However, the agreement between techniques was not so high as we supposed. At this moment the GPS has a too high sensitivity, but it is a way to analyse ONHs without any input. As for DFAs, in average DA size subgroup, the GPS had the best diagnostic capacity [23–25] (Fig. 7.3t).

Zangwill et al. found that GPS could differentiate between glaucomatous and healthy eyes with relatively good sensitivity and specificity; however, using the manufacturer's suggested cut-off values for classification as abnormal, the GPS tended to have higher sensitivities and lower specificities and likelihood ratios than did the MRA. Disc size influences the diagnostic accuracy of both the GPS and MRA [26]. Also Coops et al. found that in few patients with glaucoma (7 %) and control subjects (11 %), the GPS failed to provide a complete global and sectorial optic disc classification. They could not identify a single distinct cause of this failure in the glaucoma group, but failures in the control subjects occurred most often with small and crowded optic discs. In subjects who were successfully classified at least globally by the GPS, the diagnostic performances of GPS and MRA were similar and the areas under the receiver operating characteristic curve found values of 0.78 for GPS and 0.77 for MRA [27]. Similar results were obtained by Ferreras et al. who found a sensitivity and specificity of 73.9 and 91.5 % for MRA and a sensitivity and specificity of 58.2 and 94.4 % for GPA. They found that GPS had a slightly higher sensitivity and a lower specificity than MRA when there was a mild glaucoma damage. Both methods had lower sensitivity and higher specificity for small ONHs compared to medium and large ONHs [28]. In a different study also Burgansky-Eliash Z et al. found that the ROC areas for discrimination between glaucomatous and healthy eyes of the overall classification by HRT 2 Moorfields regression analysis (MRA), HRT 3 MRA, and GPS were 0.927, 0.934 and 0.880, respectively [29].

7.5 ISNT Rule

Some years ago, Jonas et al. introduced a very interesting method to distinguish normal from glaucomatous by just observing the optic rim area ophthalmoscopically. In particular, in a cross-sectional study, they observed that the inferior sector RA was greater than superior, nasal and temporal sectors (inferior RA > superior RA > nasal RA > temporal RA) [30, 31] (Fig. 7.3o). They divided the entire rim area into four special segments: temporal (337.5–22.5°), superior (22.5–112.5°), nasal (112.5–247.5°) and inferior (247.5– 337.5°). This rule was applied also in glaucoma clinic just by using the thickness of the rim at the four poles of the optic disc. In particular the physicians observed the ONH, and when the ONH was oval with a great vertical axis, the RA width was calculated in the main four positions: temporal (0°), superior (90°), nasal (180°) and inferior (270°). If the inferior RA > superior RA > nasal RA > temporal RA, the ONH was classified as normal (Fig. 7.3p).

This formula has been introduced in the HRT software to distinguish normal ONH from glaucomatous ones. Harizman et al. found that the ISNT rule was useful in differentiating normal from glaucomatous ONHs and was unaffected by race [32]. Different results were obtained by Sihota et al. who showed that the inferior rim area was wider than the superior one in 2/3 of the normal eyes; furthermore, they found that this rule was maintained in most patients with early glaucoma [33]. Iester et al. applied the 'ISNT Rule' to the ONH parameters obtained by the HRT system, and RA in the superior, inferior fads and nasal sectors was wider than temporal one, but only 12.44 % of the included patients confirmed the 'ISN'T rule' [34]. In a different study on paediatric healthy subjects, Larsson et al. found that ISNT rule was fulfilled in 56 % of the eyes [35]. Violation of ISNT rule was found more frequently in paediatric population with large optic disc cup of nonglaucomatous origin compared with normal cup discs [36].

At the end of the analysis, the statistical approach you can use is different. In the final printout: SD, DA, 6 stereometric parameters, MRA and RNFL height profile are shown (Fig. 7.3q–s).

7.6 Follow-Up

A potentially important clinical application of the HRT is the detection of glaucomatous progression from a baseline image.

7.6.1 Stereometric Parameters

Stereometric parameters, such as rim area and cup area, could be used to monitor for changes. The advantages of this approach are that change is measured in parameters that are clinically familiar (such as neuroretinal rim) and that have an easily comprehended anatomic correlate (such as the ganglion cell axons and supporting tissues). Relative disadvantages are that only a proportion of the topographical data in the images is used and the measurements are dependent on reference plane position. The potential benefit of identifying change in stereometric parameters was first demonstrated by Kamal et al. in 1999 [37]. They estimated 95 % confidence limits for change from the differences in stereometric parameters measured in sequential HRT images acquired from normal eyes (normal variability) [38]. Tan et al. avoided this problem by deriving limits for change for each eye from the three single topography images acquired at the baseline visit. When rim area change exceeded the confidence limits on one occasion, 'tentative' progression was ascribed. 'Definite progression' required confirmation in at least two out of three consecutive tests. This strategy accounted for the possibility that isolated events may be spurious or reverse on subsequent testing by [39, 40].

A different, simple approach is to perform a linear regression of rim area over time. Rate of change may be expressed as a percentage of the baseline rim area lost per year.

7.6.2 Topographic Change Analysis (TCA)

TCA is a statistical method to compare the topographic height values in discrete areas of the image, called super-pixels (an array of 4 by 4 pixels), at two points in time. After a series of image over time has been obtained, each follow-up image is aligned to the baseline image and the topography images are compared [41] (Fig. 7.4a).

The TCA computes, at each super-pixel, the probability of the difference in height values between the two time points occurring by chance alone. Hence, a high probability value (when P is high) indicates that the likelihood of a change is low. On the other hand, a low probability (when $P<0.05$) indicates that there is little chance that the difference was due to chance alone and that the change was likely to be real (Fig. 7.4b).

The analysis requires the mean of a set of three topographic images at each point in time, so that each pixel in the image will have three height values (Fig. 7.4c). The key determinant in the TCA is the variability in topographic height values within the superpixel over the two sets of three images for each comparison (three at baseline, three at follow-up). If the local variability is high, a much larger height difference between the two time points will be required to reach statistical significance and vice versa. Typically the variability of measurements is highest at the edge of the ONH cup and along the blood vessels and lowest in the topographically flatter parapapillary retina. Therefore, relatively larger changes will be required to reach significance in the former case and relatively smaller changes in the latter (Fig. 7.4d, e).

The main analysis from the TCA is contained in the change probability maps. These show each of the follow-up images, either in a single display with all reflectivity and topography images in the series (Fig. 7.4c, d) or the baseline and single follow-up images individually. In the latter format, it is possible to display the baseline reflectivity or topography image and the follow-up images one at a time. In addition, a greyscale of the P-values at changing locations and a map of the absolute change values are displayed. The reflectivity map is overlaid with red and green symbols that highlight superpixels in which the P-values are significant, with red demonstrating depression and green demonstrating elevation (Figs. 7.4b, d, f). By default, only those superpixels where the P-values are significant over three consecutive examinations are shown.

The TCA is an analysis that has been demonstrated to detect small changes in ONH and parapapillary retinal topography. There are, however, no rules regarding when the change detected becomes clinically significant. The criterion for significant change was the presence of a cluster of 20 superpixels within the ONH margin

[42]. Furthermore, the following criteria of progression [43] could improve agreement amongst graders:

- Reproducible clusters of red spots in follow-up exams.
- Red clusters must be within the ONH margin.
- Red spots located along the blood vessels should be ignored.
- Red spots occurring on steep slopes along the optic rim edge should be judged with caution as the reliability of the surface detection of the device is low at these locations.
- Alternating clusters of red and green areas are typically artefacts and should not be considered progression.

In a series of images with very little variability, small changes may reach statistical significance. Conversely, in an image series with high variability, even large changes may not reach statistical significance. It is, therefore, important to examine the magnitude of change and the image variability when interpreting the TCA analysis.

Unfortunately to date, there are no proven guidelines on what degree or rate of change in absolute units (i.e. microns or microns per year) is clinically significant, principally because we do not have an independent standard for progression.

7.7 Correlation with Visual Field

Several studies have demonstrated significant correlation between structural parameters obtained with the HRT and VF indices, either globally [44–50] or sectorially [44, 48, 49]. The data from these studies confirm the complexity of the relationship between structural and functional changes in glaucoma. Recently it has been shown that inter-individual variability in both the quantitative and the topographical relationships between structure and function could be related to a different anatomical position of the fibres (Fig. 7.5a, b, c).

However many parameters from HRT significantly correlate with visual field indices [44–48], among these cup area, cup/disk area ratio, rim area, rim volume, cup shape measure, RNFL thickness and RNFL cross-sectional area. Rim area and cup shape measure are the best predictors of SAP VF indices [45, 47, 48, 50]. Correlations appears to be stronger between HRT global parameters and MD than between HRT and CPSD. There is also a topographical relationship between ONH structure and visual function in patients with glaucoma. Inferior and superior HRT parameters are significantly more correlated with corresponding VF hemifield indices.

Furthermore, there is some indication that the relationship between HRT rim area and VF sensitivity is non-linear [51, 52].

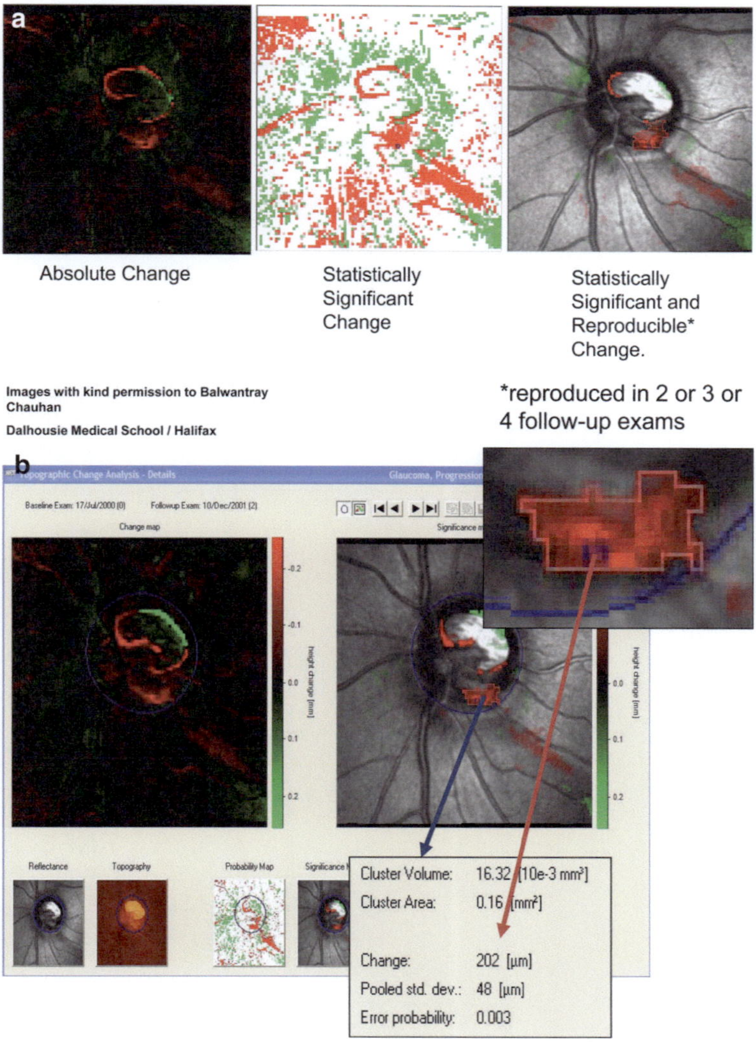

Fig. 7.4 (**a**) Presentation of follow-up exams. The three images show the absolute change, the statistically significant change and the reproducible change (Images with kind permission to Balwantray Chauhan. Dalhousie Medical School/Halifax). (**b**) Cluster and pixel analysis. TCA is able to align sequential exams and objectively compare all height measurements to tell you exactly where the progression is for the complete optic nerve, how the structure is changing both by area and depth. This is a totally objective method and covers the entire optic nerve head structure. (**c**) Presentation of follow-up exams. TCA analysis: Baseline and F/U, it is easy to detect a change in the inferior sector (Images with kind permission to Balwantray Chauhan, Dalhousie Medical School/Halifax). (**d**) Glaucomatous change in the eye. There is an obvious wedge defect, but the changes outside the disc are on average only 50 µm. However, within the disc they are 3 times the level – 150 µm and so this is why you need to evaluate the whole optic nerve head structure to be sure of assessing all the different appearance of glaucoma. (**e**) Cluster analysis. In this graph the data (area and volume of cluster) are shown in the follow-up. (**f**) Cluster analysis. In this graph the data (area and volume of cluster) are shown in the follow-up together with the topographic maps

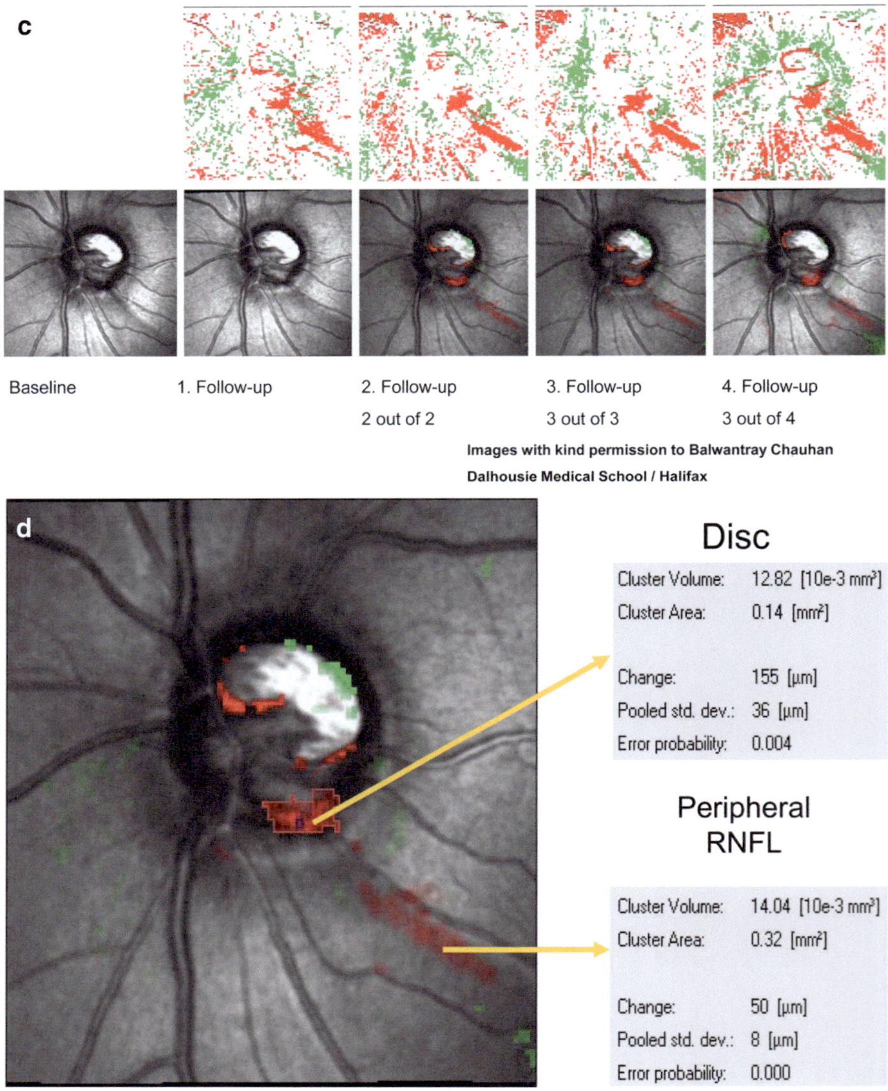

Fig. 7.4 (continued)

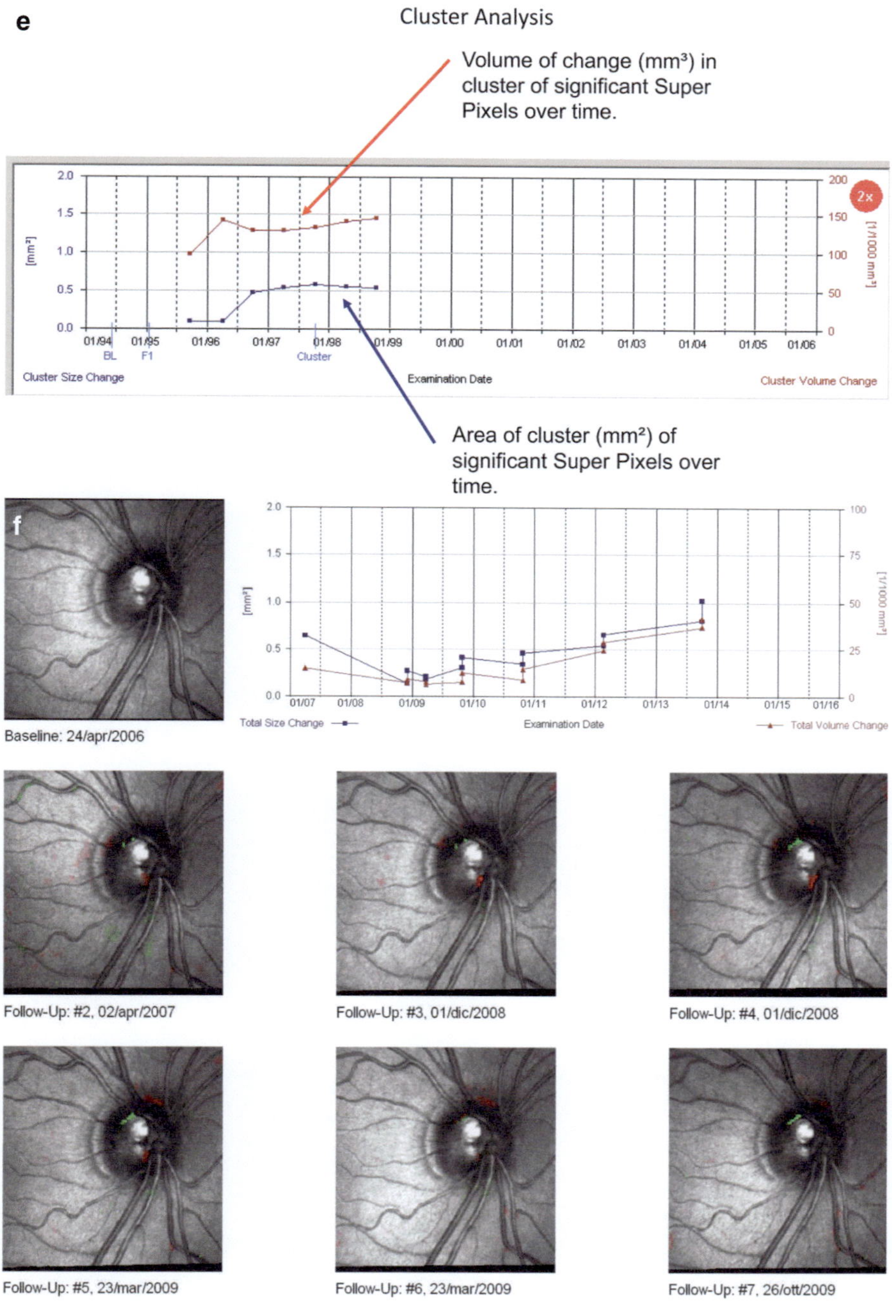

Fig. 7.4 (continued)

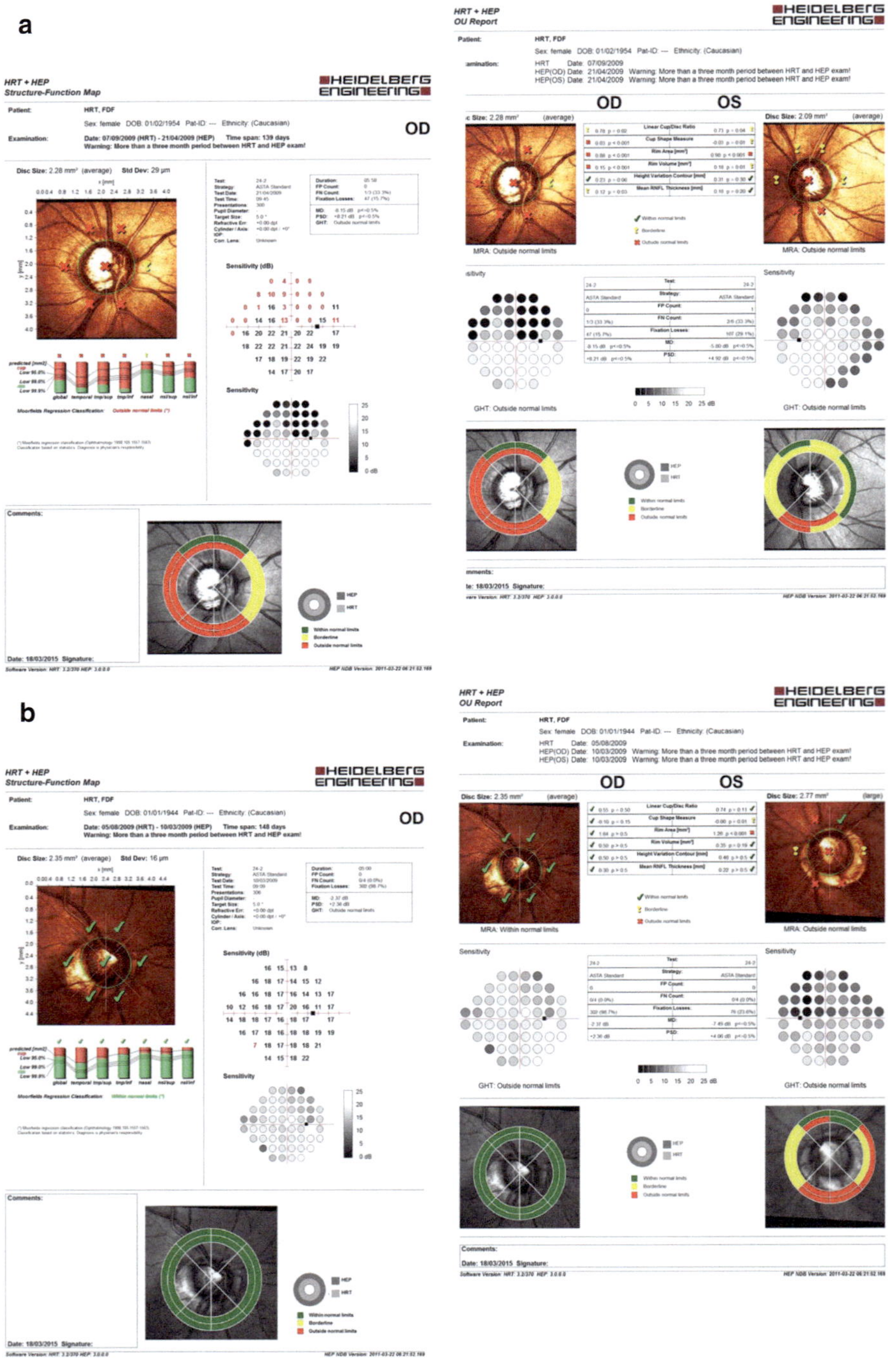

Fig. 7.5 Structure and function correlation. (**a**) On the left OD printout where there is the MRA analysis together with the HEP (sensitivity and probability map). On the bottom, the schematic function-structure graph is shown, where MRA and HEP results are displayed together. (**b**) Patient with normal ONH and VF on the right eye and abnormal ONH and VF on the left eye. (**c**) Patient with a glaucoma suspect right eye and a glaucomatous left eye

c

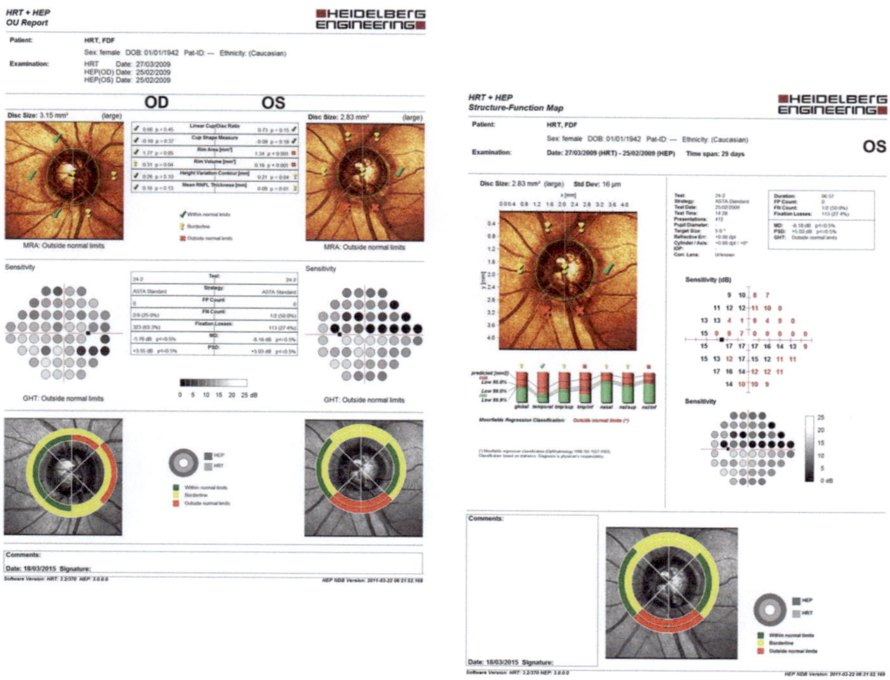

Fig. 7.5 (continued)

References

1. Kruse FE, Burk RO, Volcker HE, Zinser G, Harbarth U (1989) 3-dimensional biomorphometry of the papilla using a laser tomography scanning procedure–initial experiences with pathologic papillary findings. Fortschr Ophthalmol 86:710–713
2. Burk RO, Rohrschneider K, Noack H, Volcker HE (1991) Volumetric analysis of the optic papilla using laser scanning tomography. Parameter definition and comparison of glaucoma and control papilla. Klin Monatsbl Augenheilkd 198:522–529
3. Sihota R, Gulati V, Agarwal HC et al (2002) Variables affecting test-retest variability of Heidelberg Retina Tomograph II stereometric parameters. J Glaucoma 11:321–328
4. Yücel YH, Gupta N, Kalichman M, Mizisin AP, Hare W, de Souza Lima M, Zangwill L, Weinreb RN (1998) Relationship of optic disc topography to optic nerve fiber number in glaucoma. Arch Ophthalmol 116:493–497
5. Burk RO, Vihanninjoki K, Bartke T, Tuulonen A, Airaksinen PJ, Volcker HE, Konig JM (2000) Development of the standard reference plane for the Heidelberg retina tomograph. Graefes Arch Clin Exp Ophthalmol 238:375–384
6. Chen E, Gedda U, Landau I (2001) Thinning of the papillomacular bundle in the glaucomatous eye and its influence on the reference plane of the Heidelberg retinal tomography. J Glaucoma 10:386–389
7. Tan JC, Garway-Heath DF, Fitzke FW, Hitchings RA (2003) Reasons for rim area variability in scanning laser tomography. Invest Ophthalmol Vis Sci 44:1126–1131
8. Tan JC, Hitchings RA (2003) Reference plane definition and reproducibility in optic nerve head images. Invest Ophthalmol Vis Sci 44:1132–1137
9. Iester M, Mariotti V, Lanza F, Calabria G (2009) The effect of contour line position on optic nerve head analysis by Heidelberg Retina Tomograph. Eur J Ophthalmol 19:942–948
10. Wollstein G, Garway-Heath DF, Hitchings RA (1998) Identification of early glaucoma cases with the scanning laser ophthalmoscope. Ophthalmology 105:1557–1563
11. Garway-Heath DF, Wollstein G, Hitchings RA (1997) Aging changes of the optic nerve head in relation to open angle glaucoma. Br J Ophthalmol 81:840–845
12. Zangwill LM, Weinreb RN, Beiser JA et al (2005) Baseline topographic optic disc measurements are associated with the development of primary open-angle glaucoma: the Confocal Scanning Laser Ophthalmoscopy Ancillary Study to the Ocular Hypertension Treatment Study. Arch Ophthalmol 123(9):1188–1197
13. Mikelberg FS, Parfitt CM, Swindale NV, Graham SL, Drance SM, Gosine R (1995) Ability of the Heidelberg Retina Tomograph to detect early glaucomatous visual field loss. J Glaucoma 4:242–247
14. Iester M, Mikelberg FS, Drance SM (1997) The effect of optic disc size diagnostic precision with the Heidelberg Retina Tomograph. Ophthalmology 104:545–548
15. Burk ROW, Noack H, Rohrschneider K, Volcker HE (1999) Prediction of glaucomatous visual field defects by reference plane independent three-dimensional optic nerve head parameters. In: Wall M, Wild JM (eds) Perimetry update 1998/1999: Proceedings of the XIII International Perimetric Society Meeting, Gardone Riviera (BS), 1998. The Hangue, Kugler, The Netherlands, pp 463–474
16. Iester M, Parfitt CM, Swindale NV, Mikelberg FS (1997) Sector-based analysis of Heidelberg Retina Tomograph (HRT) parameters in normal and glaucomatous eyes. Invest Ophthalmol Vis Sci 38(Suppl):S835
17. Iester M, Jonas JB, Mardin CY, Budde WM (2000) Discriminant analysis models for early detection of glaucomatous optic disc changes. Br J Ophthalmol 84:464–468
18. Mardin CY, Horn FK, Jonas JB, Budde WM (1999) Preperimetric glaucoma diagnosis by confocal scanning laser tomography of the optic disc. Br J Ophthalmol 83:299–304
19. Iester M, Oddone F, Prato M, Centofanti M, Fogagnolo P, Rossetti L, Vaccarezza V, Manni G, Ferreras A (2013) Linear discriminant functions to improve the glaucoma probability score analysis to detect glaucomatous optic nerve heads: a multicenter study. J Glaucoma 22:73–79

20. Ford BA, Artes PH, McCormick TA, Nicolela MT, LeBlanc RP, Chauhan BC (2003) Comparison of data analysis tools for detection of glaucoma with the Heidelberg Retina Tomograph. Ophthalmology 110:1145–1150
21. Iester M, Mardin CY, Budde WM, Junemann AG, Hayler JK, Jonas JB (2002) Discriminant analysis formulas of optic nerve head parameters measured by confocal scanning laser tomography. J Glaucoma 11:97–104
22. Swindale NV, Stjepanovic G, Chin A, Mikelberg FS (2000) Automated analysis of normal and glaucomatous optic nerve head topography images. Invest Ophthalmol Vis Sci 41:1730–1742
23. Iester M, Perdicchi A, Capris E, Siniscalco A, Calabria GA, Recupero SM (2008) Comparison between discriminant analysis models and 'glaucoma probability score' for the detection of glaucomatous optic nerve head changes. J Glaucoma 17:535–540
24. Oddone F, Centofanti M, Iester M, Rossetti L, Fogagnolo P, Michelessi M, Capris E, Manni G (2009) Sector-based analysis with the Heidelberg retinal tomograph 3 across disc sizes and glaucoma stages a multicenter study. Ophthalmology 116:1106–1111
25. Oddone F, Centofanti M, Rossetti L, Iester M, Fogagnolo P, Capris E, Manni GL (2008) Exploring the Heidelberg Retinal Tomograph 3 diagnostic accuracy across disc sizes and glaucoma stages: a multicenter study. Ophthalmology 115:1358–1365
26. Zangwill LM, Jain S, Racette L, Ernstrom KB, Bowd C, Medeiros FA, Sample PA, Weinreb RW (2007) The effect of disc size and severity of disease on the diagnostic accuracy of the Heidelberg Retina Tomograph glaucoma probability score. Invest Ophthalmol Vis Sci 48: 2653–2660
27. Coops A, Henson DB, Kwartz AJ, Artes PH (2006) Automated analysis of Heidelberg Retina Tomograph optic disc images by glaucoma probability score. Invest Ophthalmol Vis Sci 47:5348–5355
28. Ferreras A, Pajarín AB, Polo V, Larrosa JM, Pablo LE, Honrubia FM (2007) Diagnostic ability of Heidelberg Retina Tomograph 3 classifications. Glaucoma probability score versus moorfields regression analysis. Ophthalmology 114:1981–1987
29. Burgansky-Eliash Z, Wollstein G, Bilonick RA, Ishikawa H, Kagemann L, Schuman JS (2007) Glaucoma Detection with the Heidelberg Retina Tomograph 3. Ophthalmology 114:466–471
30. Jonas JB et al (1998) Neuroretinal rim width ratios in morphological glaucoma diagnosis. Br J Ophthalmol 82:1366–1371
31. Jonas JB, Gusek GC, Naumann GOH (1988) Optic disc, cup and neuroretinal rim size, configuration and correlation in normal eyes. Invest Ophthalmol Vis Sci 29:1151–1158
32. Harizman N, Oliveira C, Chiang A, Tello C et al (2006) The ISNT rule and differentiation of normal form glaucomatous eyes. Arch Ophthalmol 124:1579–1583
33. Sihota R, Srinivasan G, Dada T, Gupta V et al (2008) Is the ISNT rule violated in early primary open angle glaucoma – a scanning laser tomography study. Eye 22:819–824
34. Iester M, Bertolotto M, Recupero SM, Perdicchi A (2011) The "ISN'T Rule" in healthy participant optic nerve head by confocal scanning laser ophthalmoscopy. J Glaucoma 20:350–354
35. Larsoson E, Nuija E, Alm A (2011) The optic nerve head assessed with HRT in 5-16–year-old normal children: normal values, repeatability and interocular difference. Acta Ophthalmol 89(8):755–758
36. Pogrebniak AE, Webrung B, Pogrebniak KL, Shetty RK, Crawford P (2010) Violation of the ISNT rule in nonglaucomatous pediatric optic disc cupping. Invest Ophthalmol Vis Sci 51:890–895
37. Kamal DS, Viswanathan AC, Garway-Heath DF, Hitchings RA, Poinoosawmy D, Bunce C (1999) Detection of optic disc change with the Heidelberg retina tomograph before confirmed visual field change in ocular hypertensives converting to early glaucoma. Br J Ophthalmol 83:290–294
38. Kamal DS, Garway-Heath DF, Hitchings RA, Fitzke FW (2000) Use of sequential Heidelberg retina tomograph images to identify changes at the optic disc in ocular hypertensive patients at risk of developing glaucoma. Br J Ophthalmol 84:993–998
39. Tan JC, Hitchings RA (2003) Approach for identifying glaucomatous optic nerve progression by scanning laser tomography. Invest Ophthalmol Vis Sci 44:2621–2626

40. Tan JC, Poinoosawmy D, Hitchings RA (2004) Tomographic identification of neuroretinal rim loss in high-pressure, normal-pressure, and suspected glaucoma. Invest Ophthalmol Vis Sci 45:2279–2285
41. Chauhan BC, Blanchard JW, Hamilton DC, LeBlanc RP (2000) Technique for detecting serial topographic changes in the optic disc and peripapillary retina using scanning laser tomography. Invest Ophthalmol Vis Sci 41:775–782
42. Chauhan BC, McCormick TA, Nicolela MT, LeBlanc RP (2001) Optic disc and visual field changes in a prospective longitudinal study of patients with glaucoma: comparison of scanning laser tomography with conventional perimetry and optic disc photography. Arch Ophthalmol 119:1492–1499
43. Iester MM, Wollstein G, Bilonick RA, Xu J, Ishikawa H, Kagemann L, Schuman JS (2015) Agreement among graders on Heidelberg retina tomograph (HRT) topographic change analysis (TCA) glaucoma progression interpretation. Br J Ophthalmol 99(4):519–523
44. Weinreb RN, Shakiba S, Sample PA, Shahrokni S, van Horn S et al (1995) Association between quantitative nerve fiber layer measurement and visual field loss in glaucoma. Am J Ophthalmol 120:732–738
45. Iester M, Mikelberg FS, Courtright P, Drance SM (1997) Correlation between the visual field indices and Heidelberg retina tomograph parameters. J Glaucoma 6:78–82
46. Tole DM, Edwards MP, Davey KG, Menage MJ (1998) The correlation of the visual field with scanning laser ophthalmoscope measurements in glaucoma. Eye 12:686–690
47. Teesalu P, Vihanninjoki K, Airaksinen PJ, Tuulonen A (1998) Hemifield association between blue-on-yellow visual field and optic nerve head topographic measurements. Graefe's Arch Clin Exp Ophthalmol 236:339–345
48. Lan YW, Henson DB, Kwartz AJ (2003) The correlation between optic nerve head topographic measurements, peripapillary nerve fibre layer thickness, and visual field indices in glaucoma. Br J Ophthalmol 87:1135–41
49. Iester M, Swindale NV, Mikelberg FS (1997) Sector-based analysis of optic nerve head shape parameters and visual field indices in healthy and glaucomatous eyes. J Glaucoma 6:371–6
50. Brigatti L, Caprioli J (1995) Correlation of visual field with scanning confocal laser optic disc measurements in glaucoma. Arch Ophthalmol 113:1191–4
51. Bartz-Schmidt KU, Thumann G, Jonescu-Cuypers CP, Krieglstein GK (1999) Quantitative morphologic and functional evaluation of the optic nerve head in chronic open-angle glaucoma. Surv Ophthalmol 44(Suppl 1):S41–53
52. Garway-Heath DF, Holder GE, Fitzke FW, Hitchings RA (2002) Relationship between electrophysiological, psychophysical, and anatomical measurements in glaucoma. Invest Ophthalmol Vis Sci 43:2213–20

Chapter 8
Detection of Glaucoma Using Scanning Laser Polarimetry

Patricio G. Schlottmann and Pilar Calvo

8.1 Evolution

Scanning laser polarimetry (SLP) is an imaging technology that measures the thickness of the retinal nerve fiber layer (RNFL) based on the birefringent properties of this tissue. SLP has been developed since early 1990 by Laser Diagnostic Technologies (LDT). The most widely used version of SLP was the GDx with variable corneal compensation (GDx VCC; Fig. 8.1). Nevertheless, the ultimate edition of this device is the GDx with enhanced corneal compensation (ECC), which is currently manufactured by Carl Zeiss Meditec (Dublin, Ca, USA). The GDx ECC includes a software image processing method by which image quality is improved in eyes with atypical patterns of retardation.

P.G. Schlottmann (✉)
Department of Ophthalmology, Organizacion Medica de Investigacion, Autonomous City of Buenos Aires, Argentina
e-mail: schlottp@yahoo.com.ar

P. Calvo
Department of Ophthalmology, Miguel Servet university hospital, Zaragoza, Spain
e-mail: xenatrance@yahoo.es

A. Ferreras (ed.), *Glaucoma Imaging*, DOI 10.1007/978-3-319-18959-8_8

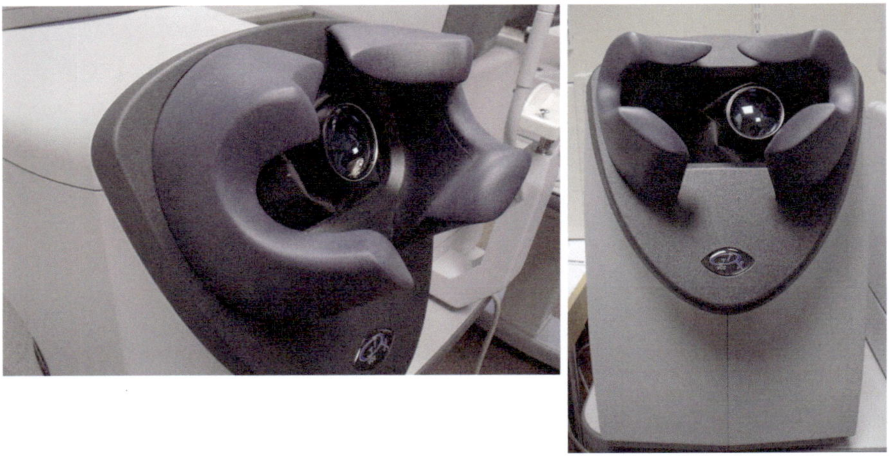

Fig. 8.1 The SLP device (patient side). Image courtesy of DF Garway Heath

8.2 Technology

The GDx ECC is a confocal scanning laser device that quantitatively measures the thickness of the peripapillary retinal nerve fiber layer (RNFL). Measurements are based on the assumption that the parallel arrangement of the microtubules within ganglion cell axons causes a change in the state of polarization of an incident laser beam. This is known as birefringence and it is a common property of anisotropic or birefringent structures. The change in polarization status (phase shift) is known as retardation and is measured on the reflected beam after double passing the RNFL [1–4].

When the incident beam passes through the RNFL, it is affected by two different refractive indices (common property of birefringent structures), splitting light into two refracted rays. One of the rays is affected by the lower of the two refractive indices and travels with the same velocity of the incident beam along the optical axis of the tissue and is called ordinary or fast axis. The other ray travels with a velocity that is affected by the highest refractive index of the birefringent structure (RNFL in this case) and is called the slow or extraordinary axis. The difference in speed between the two rays is called retardation (Fig. 8.2). Retardation values are then used to calculate the thickness of the structure as retardation increases with greater tissue thickness.

The RNFL is not the only birefringent structure in the eye. The Henle fiber layer in the macula is made of elongated photoreceptor axons radially arranged around the fovea. Because of this arrangement of the fibers, it exhibits significant birefringence. The cornea due to its particular structure made of collagen fibers is also a highly birefringent structure. The lens and the vitreous exhibit very little birefringence.

The incident beam passes through the cornea, lens, vitreous, RNFL, and the rest of the retina to reach the retinal pigmentary epithelium (RPE) where it is reflected back. After being reflected it passes again through the mentioned structures to finally reach the device's sensors. As the incident beam is affected by all birefringent structures in the eye, producing polarization changes, the final retardation will consist largely of contributions from the RNFL and the cornea. To accurately measure RNFL originated retardation the device needs to subtract corneal retardation from the total retardation measurement. The way to achieve this is by measuring first, corneal retardation, then measuring total retardation and subtracting them.

Individual corneal compensation is achieved by calculating the specific axis and magnitude of the anterior segment birefringence. This is determined by first imaging the eye without any compensation. The uncompensated image presents total retardation from the eye and includes retardation from the cornea, lens, and RNFL. The macular region of this image is then analyzed to determine the axis and magnitude of the anterior segment birefringence. Macular birefringence is uniform and symmetric due to the radial distribution of Henle's fiber layer. However, in uncompensated scans, a non-uniform retardation pattern is present in the macula due to the birefringence from the anterior segment. The axis and magnitude values from the anterior segment can be calculated by analyzing the non-uniform retardation profile around the macula. The axis of the anterior segment birefringence is determined by the orientation of the "bow-tie" birefringent pattern in the macula, and the magnitude of the anterior segment birefringence is calculated by analyzing the circular profile of the birefringence in the macula according to specific equations.

Once the anterior segment birefringence axis and magnitude values are determined, the retardation signal from the anterior segment can be compensated. The VCC consists of two linear retarders in rotating mounts; as a result, both the magnitude and the axis can be adjusted to match the values to compensate for the anterior segment birefringence for each eye. When the anterior segment has been successfully compensated, the RNFL image will have a uniform retardation (thickness) profile around the macula.

In the case of macular pathology present at the moment of scanning the patient, the GDX VCC provides an alternative algorithm to accurately compensate anterior segment birefringence analyzing the birefringence pattern over a large area centered on the fovea (6° × 6° square region). This method assumes the birefringence in this macula region preserves the birefringence from the anterior segment. By averaging the signal from a large area, the impact of local irregularities of the retinal birefringence is greatly reduced and corneal birefringence can be extracted.

This method for calculating anterior segment birefringence is accurate, even in eyes with macular pathology where the original method failed due to an indeterminate macular "bow-tie" pattern [4–9].

Once the device acquires an image and it is compensated, the final results are then compared against an age-matched normative database. This database is made of glaucoma patients and normal subjects. It includes a wide range of ages and racial backgrounds. The data were collected in the United States of America and it is made of 70 % Caucasian and Hispanic derived subjects, 12 % of Asian derived subjects and 18 % of African derived subjects of a total of more than 800 patients (540 normals, 92 pre-perimetric, 70 early, 60 moderate, 49 advanced). The glaucoma patient data were used to train a machine learning classifier that gives an overall score to each patient, representing the likelihood of that subject to have glaucoma.

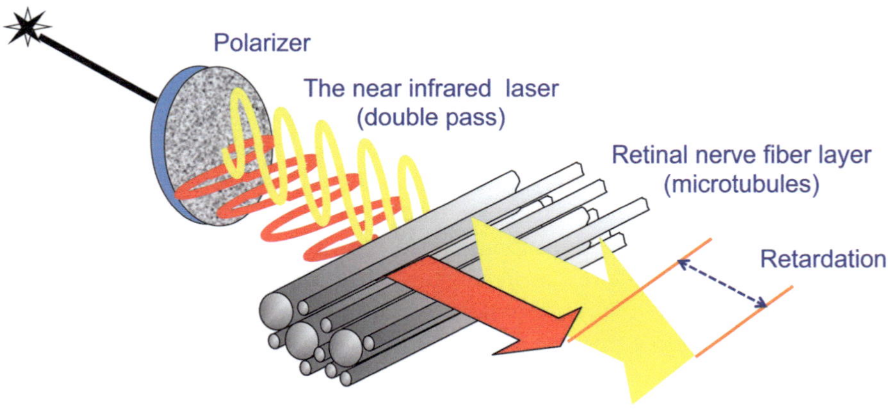

Fig. 8.2 Polarized light passing through the RNFL. The GDx VCC uses a fixed conversion factor of 0.67 nm of retardation per μm of thickness

8.3 Enhanced Corneal Compensation

In some patients, when images are acquired using the VCC, a pattern of noise can be obtained covering the whole image, being more visible in the nasal and temporal areas (Fig. 8.3). This noise arises from extra retardation being detected but not filtered.

Eyes more susceptible to produce this atypical pattern are those with poor pigmentation, advanced glaucoma or high fundus depolarization. Total retardance in the measurement beam path is relatively low, particularly in the temporal and nasal regions, as well as in eyes with advanced glaucoma damage.

SLP measurements are inherently less sensitive and more susceptible to system noise at low retardance. To improve the ability of SLP to detect small changes at low retardance, a large bias retardation is introduced during image acquisition. This bias method ensures that the total retardance in the measurement beam path is relatively high. After capturing the image, the bias is measured from the total retardance image and mathematically removed, point by point, to produce the final RNFL image (Fig. 8.4). Individualized corneal compensation is well achieved and with compensation residual comparable to or less than that of the VCC method (Figs. 8.5, 8.6, and 8.7) [10–18].

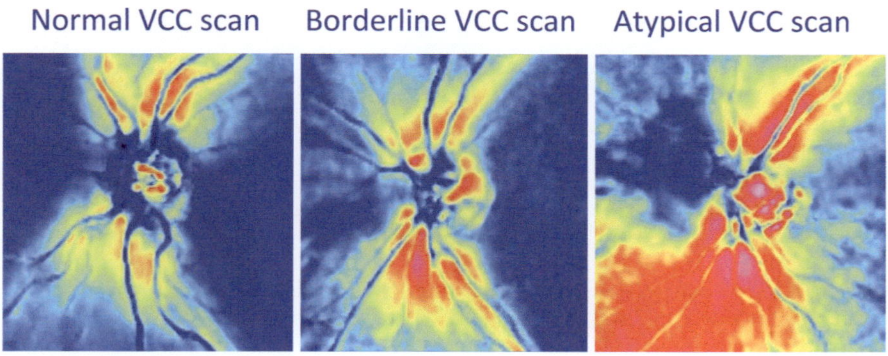

Fig. 8.3 In some cases, atypical scan patterns can be obtained by using the VCC mode (Image courtesy of DF Garway Heath)

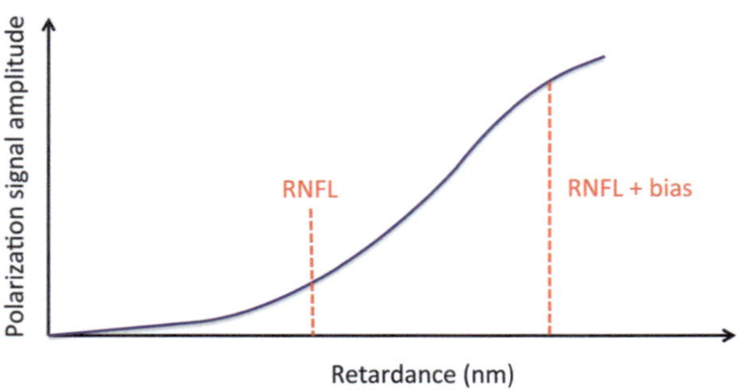

Fig. 8.4 To increase the signal to noise ratio, the software of GDx ECC adds a large bias to the original scan and then mathematically subtracts it from the resultant scan

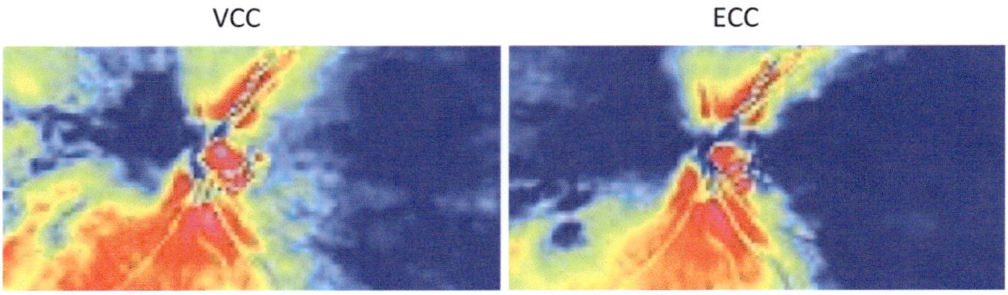

Fig. 8.5 The ECC mode reduces artifactual measurement in areas of poor signal-to-noise ratio, compared to the VCC mode (Image courtesy of DF Garway Heath)

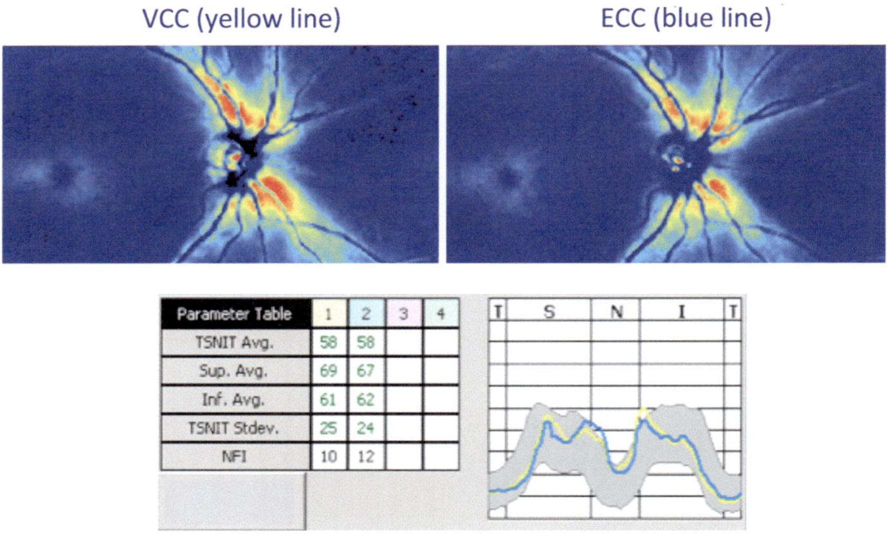

Parameter Table	1	2	3	4
TSNIT Avg.	58	58		
Sup. Avg.	69	67		
Inf. Avg.	61	62		
TSNIT Stdev.	25	24		
NFI	10	12		

Fig. 8.6 Comparison of VCC and ECC modes. The RNFL retardance measurements were similar in a healthy individual eye (Image courtesy of DF Garway Heath)

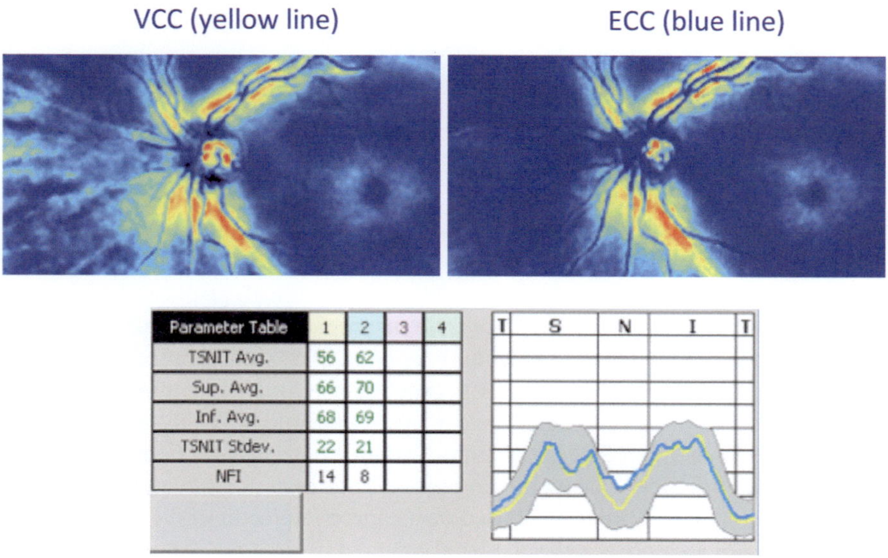

Parameter Table	1	2	3	4
TSNIT Avg.	56	62		
Sup. Avg.	66	70		
Inf. Avg.	68	69		
TSNIT Stdev.	22	21		
NFI	14	8		

Fig. 8.7 Comparison of VCC and ECC modes. The ECC mode reduces the measurement noise in the nasal region (Image courtesy of DF Garway Heath)

8.4 Specifications

The GDx VCC measurements are taken by scanning the beam of a near-infrared laser (780 nm) in a raster pattern. The raster scan captures an image with a field 40° horizontally by 20° vertically, and including both the peripapillary and the macular region. Total scan time is 0.8 s per scan. Two scans are acquired per eye one for corneal compensation and one for RNFL measurement. Overall scanning a patient demands 5–10 min considering data entry, scanning and printing.

Each image is made up of 256 (horizontal) × 128 (vertical) pixels, or 32,768 total pixels. Each pixel subtends 0.156°. For an emmetropic eye, 1 pixel is 0.0465 mm in size, and the total scan field is 11.9 mm (horizontal) × 5.9 mm (vertical).

For each measurement, the GDx VCC generates two images: a reflectance image and a retardation image. The reflectance image is generated from the light reflected directly back from the surface of the retina, and is displayed as the Fundus Image on the device and printouts. The retardation image is the map of retardation values and is converted into RNFL thickness based on a conversion factor of 0.67 nm/μm55.

The calculation circle is a circular band centered in the optic nerve with an inner diameter of 2.4 mm and an outer diameter of 3.2 mm. The width of the band is therefore 0.4 mm (Fig. 8.8).

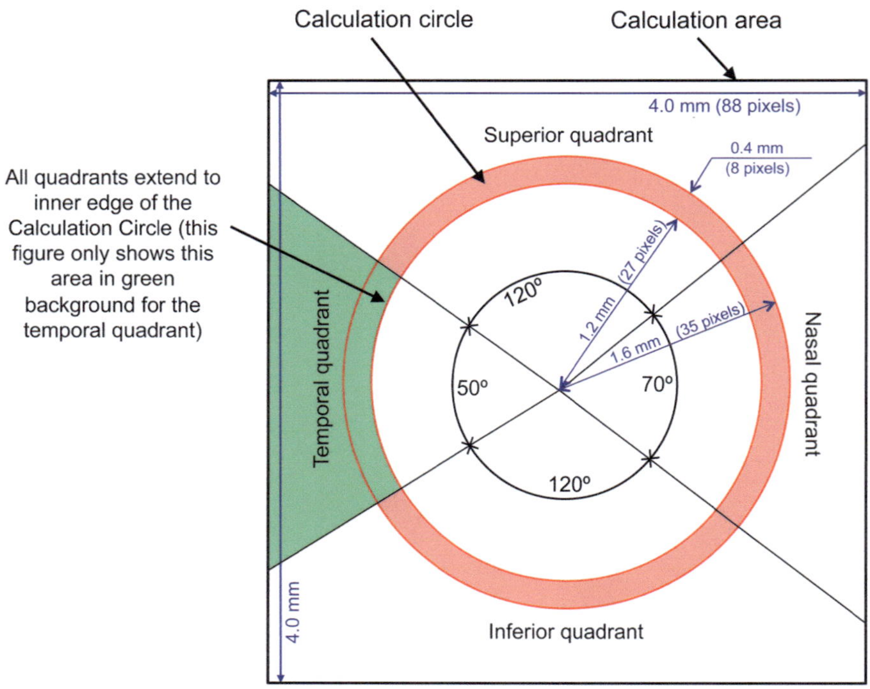

Fig. 8.8 All measurements are based on measurements within the calculation circle

8.5 The Printout

After scanning a patient with the GDx you decide whether to save the scans or save and print them.

At the top of the report, name, surname, date of birth, gender, ancestry, ID number, and print date and time are presented (Fig. 8.9). Then for each eye extra data are presented as quality of scan (graded between 1 and 10), operator initials, horizontal and vertical size of the optic nerve head (measured by an ellipse that is automatically placed and can be adjusted by the operator), and time/date of the scan.

The parameter table is presented centrally in the report providing information for both eyes (Fig. 8.10).

The default calculation circle is a fixed size centered on the optic nerve head. The inner diameter of the band is 2.4 mm, the outer diameter of the band is 3.2 mm, and the band is 0.4 mm wide. There is an option to choose larger calculation circle sizes if needed to avoid peripapillary atrophy.

OD: Right eye; *OS*: Left eye.

TSNIT: Temporal-Superior-Nasal-Inferior-Temporal.

TSNIT Average represents the average RNFL thickness around the entire calculation circle.

Superior Average represents the RNFL thickness of the superior 120° of the calculation circle (Fig. 8.11).

Inferior Average represents the RNFL thickness of the inferior 120° of the calculation circle.

TSNIT Standard Deviation represents the modulation (peak to trough difference) of the measurement. Large modulation is found in normal subjects while low modulation is found in subjects with RNFL loss (Fig. 8.12).

Inter-eye Symmetry represents the degree of symmetry between the right and left eyes by correlating the TSNIT functions from the two eyes. Values range from −1 to 1, where values near one represent good symmetry. Normal eyes have good symmetry with values around 0.9. The parameter is very useful because in glaucoma, one eye is often more advanced than the fellow eye. This measure is the Pearson product correlation coefficient (r-value) from the correlation of the TSNIT curves of the two eyes.

NFI is a single output value that represents the likelihood of that patient to have glaucoma. It is calculated using an advanced form of neural network, called a Support Vector Machine (SVM) and is a global measure based on the entire RNFL thickness map. Output values range from 1 to 100, with classification based on the ranges:

1–30 represents normal RNFL
31–50 represents borderline RNFL
51–100 represents abnormal RNFL

Values presented in the parameter table are color coded according to probability of the measurement to be found in an age-matched normal control population.

White background means that values can be found in more than 5 % of the population. Dark blue background means that values can only be found in less than 5 % of the population and the same for the rest of the colors.

In the printout three images of the peripapillary area are provided for each eye. The three images are the *Fundus Image* (*reflectance*), the *RNFL Thickness Map* (*retardation*), and the *Deviation Map* (*probability*).

The *Fundus Image* is used to check for image quality. To see if the image is well focused and evenly illuminated with the optic disc well centered, and the ellipse properly placed around the optic disc (Fig. 8.14).

The *RNFL Thickness Map* (GDx VCC) or Nerve Fiber Layer Map (GDx ECC) is a color-coded representation of the RNFL thickness (Fig. 8.15).

The *Deviation Map:* The Deviation Map reveals the location and magnitude of RNFL defects over the entire thickness map (Fig. 8.16). The Deviation Map analyzes a 128 × 128 pixel region (20° × 20°) centered on the optic disc. To reduce variability due to slight anatomical deviations between individuals, the 128 × 128 pixel thickness map is averaged into a 32 × 32 square grid, where each square is the average of a 4 × 4 pixel region (called super pixels). For each scan, the RNFL thickness at each super pixel is compared to the age-matched normative database, and the super pixels that fall below the normal range are flagged by colored squares based on the probability of normality. Dark blue squares represent areas where the RNFL thickness is below the fifth percentile of the normative database. This means that there is only a 5 % probability that the RNFL thickness in this area is within the normal range, determined by an age-matched comparison to the normative database. Light blue squares represent deviation below the 2 % level, yellow represents deviation below 1 %, and red represents deviation below 0.05 %. The Deviation Map uses a grayscale fundus image of the eye as a background, and displays abnormal grid values as colored squares over this image. This helps the user determine precisely the location of the abnormalities.

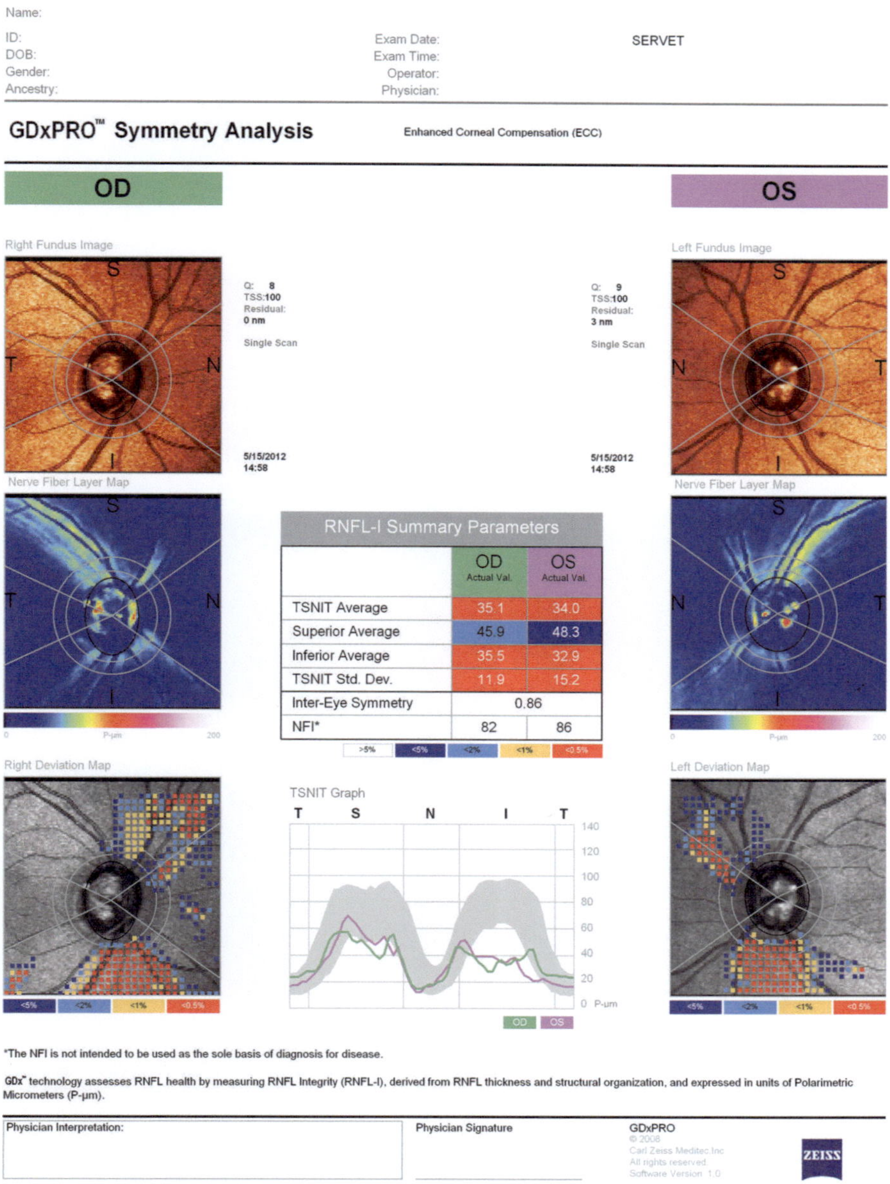

Fig. 8.9 An original GDx-ECC printout of a patient with advanced RNFL loss (Image courtesy of A Ferreras)

RNFL-I Summary Parameters		
	OD Actual Val.	OS Actual Val.
TSNIT Average	35.1	34.0
Superior Average	45.9	48.3
Inferior Average	35.5	32.9
TSNIT Std. Dev.	11.9	15.2
Inter-Eye Symmetry	0.86	
NFI*	82	86

>5%	<5%	<2%	<1%	<0.5%

Fig. 8.10 The Parameter Table for a glaucoma patient. Abnormal values are color-coded based on their probability value, similar to the super pixels in the Deviation Map. The NFI values are not color-coded (see below for a description of the NFI)

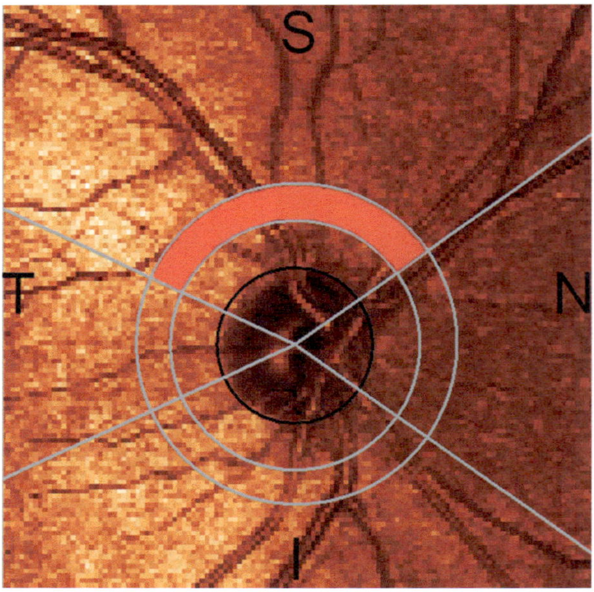

Fig. 8.11 The superior average corresponds to the superior 120° of the calculation circle (*red area*) (Image courtesy of A Ferreras)

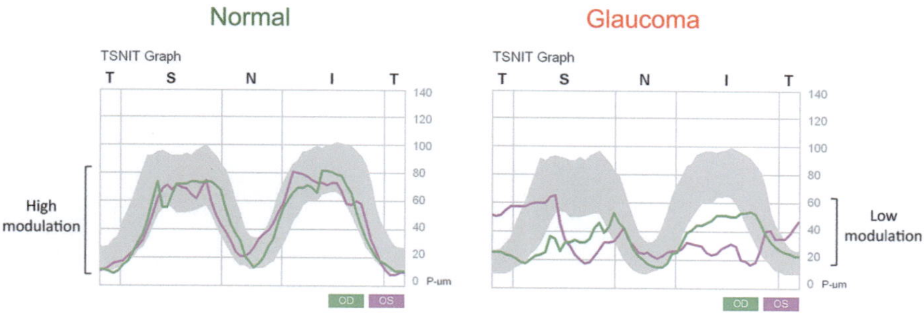

Fig. 8.12 Standard Deviation (modulation) examples in normal and glaucoma subjects (Image courtesy of A Ferreras)

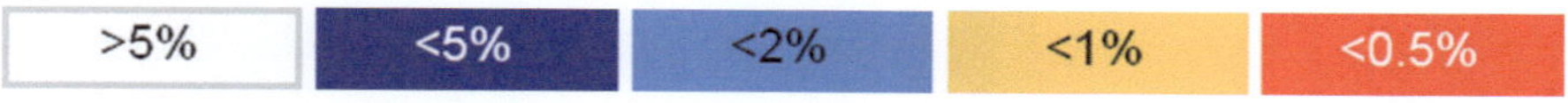

Fig. 8.13 Color-coded probability table

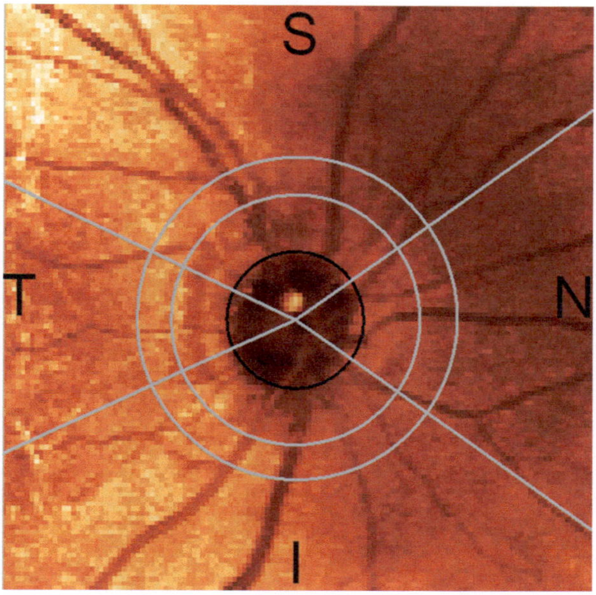

Fig. 8.14 Fundus Image (reflectance) with a correctly centered calculation circle

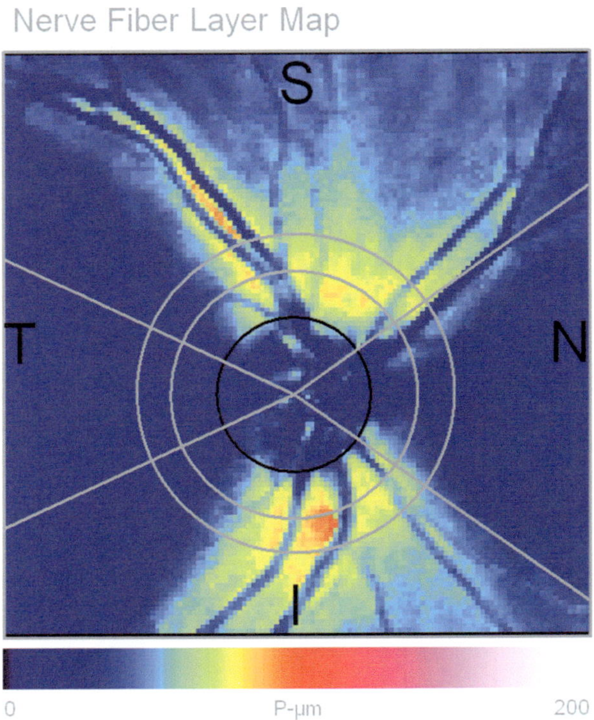

Fig. 8.15 The nerve fiber layer map is a false color retardation (thickness) map with the corresponding color-thickness legend

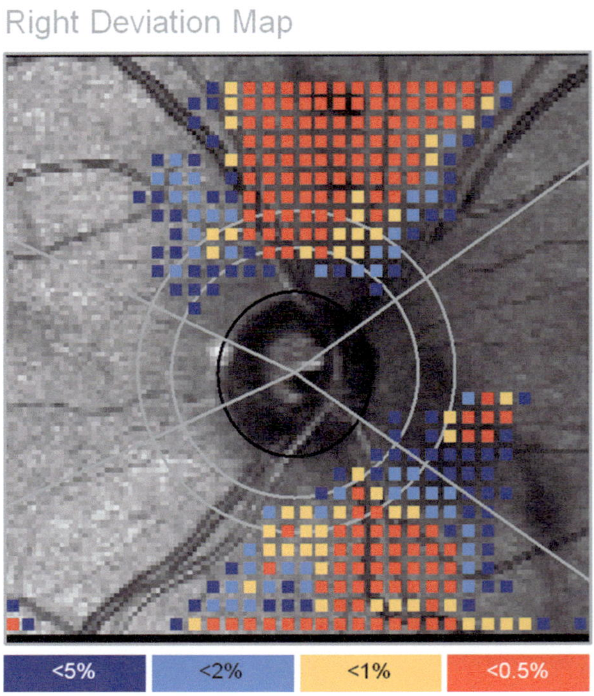

Fig. 8.16 Deviation from normal map in a color-coded representation of probability

8.6 Examples

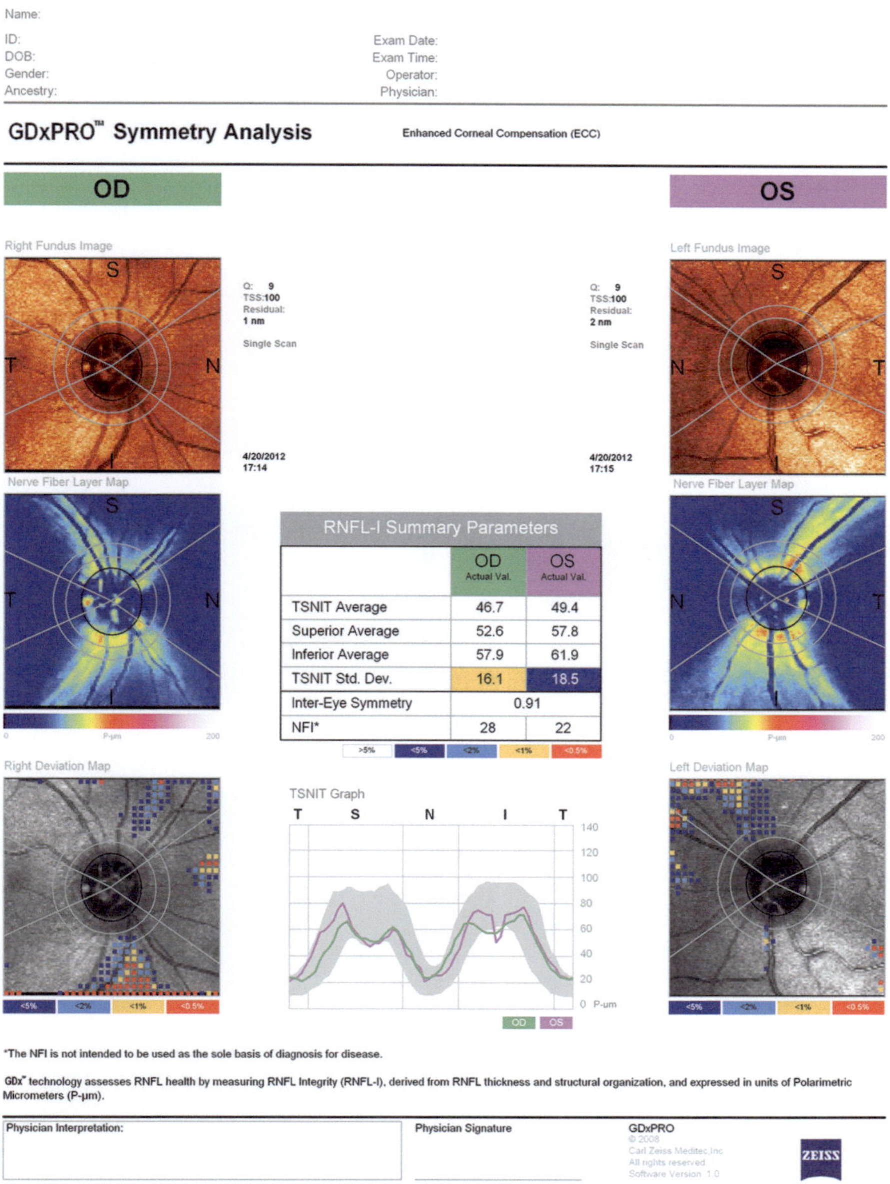

Fig. 8.17 Focal RNFL defects in the superior and inferior poles of the optic disc in the right eye, and superior area in the left eye (GDx ECC report) (Image courtesy of A Ferreras)

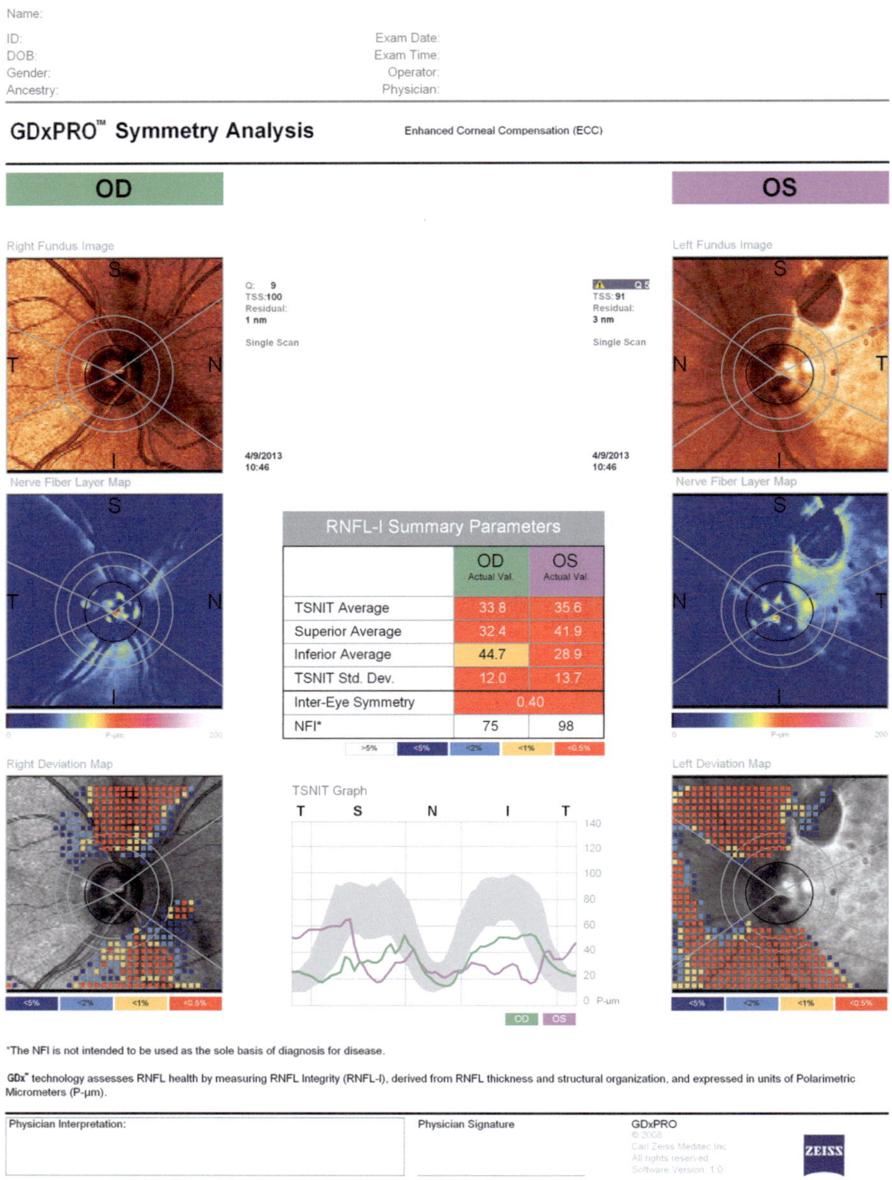

Fig. 8.18 Diffuse damage on the RNFL in both eyes (GDx ECC report) (Image courtesy of A Ferreras)

References

1. Weinreb RN, Dreher AW, Coleman A, Quigley HA, Shaw B, Reiter K (1990) Histopathologic validation of Fourier-ellipsometry measurements of retinal nerve fiber layer thickness. Arch Ophthalmol 108:557–560
2. Morgan JE, Waldock A, Jeffery G, Cowey A (1998) Retinal nerve fiber layer polarimetry: histological and clinical comparison. Br J Ophthalmol 82:684–690
3. Reus NJ, Lemij HG (2004) Diagnostic accuracy of the GDx VCC for glaucoma. Ophthalmology 111:1860–1865
4. Medeiros F, Zangwill LM, Bowd C, Mohammadi K, Weinreb RN (2004) Comparison of scanning laser polarimetry using variable corneal polarization compensation and retinal nerve fiber layer photography for detection of glaucoma. Am J Ophthalmol 138:592–601
5. Garway-Heath DF, Greaney MJ, Caprioli J (2002) Correction for the erroneous compensation of anterior segment birenfringence with the scanning laser polarimeter for glaucoma diagnosis. Invest Ophthalmol Vis Sci 43(5):1465–1474
6. Zhou Q, Weinreb RN (2002) Individualized compensation of anterior segment birefringence during scanning laser polarimetry. Invest Ophthalmol Vis Sci 43:2221–2228
7. Greenfield DS, Knighton RW, Feuer W, Schiffman J, Zangwill L, Weinreb RN (2002) Correction for corneal polarization axis improves the discriminating power of scanning laser polarimetry. Ophthalmology 108:1065–1069
8. Reus NJ, Colen TP, Lemij HG (2003) Visualization of localized retinal nerve fiber layer defects with the GDX with individualized and with fixed compensation of anterior segment birefringence. Ophthalmology 110:1512–1516
9. Ferreras A, Pablo LE, Pajarín AB, García-Feijoo J, Honrubia FM (2009) Scanning laser polarimetry: logistic regression analysis for perimetric glaucoma diagnosis. Eye 23(3):593–600
10. Tóth M, Holló G (2005) Enhanced corneal compensation for scanning laser polarimetry on eyes with atypical polarisation pattern. Br J Ophthalmol 89(9):1139–1142
11. Sehi M, Guaqueta DC, Greenfield DS (2006) An enhancement module to improve the atypical birefringence pattern using scanning laser polarimetry with variable corneal compensation. Br J Ophthalmol 90(6):749–753
12. Reus NJ, Zhou Q, Lemij HG (2006) Enhanced imaging algorithm for scanning laser polarimetry with variable corneal compensation. Invest Ophthalmol Vis Sci 47(9):3870–3877
13. Bowd C, Tavares IM, Medeiros FA, Zangwill LM, Sample PA, Weinreb RN (2007) Retinal nerve fiber layer thickness and visual sensitivity using scanning laser polarimetry with variable and enhanced corneal compensation. Ophthalmology 114(7):1259–1265
14. Sehi M, Guaqueta DC, Feuer WJ, Greenfield DS, Advanced Imaging in Glaucoma Study Group (2007) Scanning laser polarimetry with variable and enhanced corneal compensation in normal and glaucomatous eyes. Am J Ophthalmol 143(2):272–279
15. Medeiros FA, Bowd C, Zangwill LM, Patel C, Weinreb RN (2007) Detection of glaucoma using scanning laser polarimetry with enhanced corneal compensation. Invest Ophthalmol Vis Sci 48(7):3146–3153
16. Mai TA, Reus NJ, Lemij HG (2007) Diagnostic accuracy of scanning laser polarimetry with enhanced versus variable corneal compensation. Ophthalmology 114(11):1988–1993
17. Grewal DS, Sehi M, Greenfield DS (2011) Detecting glaucomatous progression using GDx with variable and enhanced corneal compensation using Guided Progression Analysis. Br J Ophthalmol 95(4):502–508
18. Rao HL, Yadav RK, Begum VU, Addepalli UK, Senthil S, Choudhari NS, Garudadri CS (2015) Atypical birefringence pattern and the diagnostic ability of scanning laser polarimetry with enhanced corneal compensation in glaucoma. Acta Ophthalmol 93(2):e105–e110

Chapter 9
Optical Coherence Tomography

Paolo Frezzotti

Optical coherence tomography (OCT) is the most sensitive and promising diagnostic technique for detecting damage to optic nerve fibres. OCT is a modern imaging technique based on analysis of semicoherent radiation reflected by the structure of the tissue analysed. The high resolution possible with OCT (about 2 μm versus 150 μm with ultrasonometry) enables noninvasive imaging of the anterior chamber, retinal layers, choriocapillaris, retinal pigmented epithelium (RPE) and optic nerve/lamina cribrosa. The method is based on light, which unlike sound waves used in B-mode ultrasonography does not require contact with the tissue to be examined. It measures the delay in the echo and the intensity of diffused light, that is, the light reflected by tissue microstructure, using a wavelength of about 820 nm. This low coherence, near-infrared beam is projected by a superluminescent diode. The echo propagation times of the light reflected by the tissue are compared with those of the same beam reflected from a reference mirror at a known distance. The OCT system combines the pulses of light reflected by the eye (e.g. the retina) and the mirror, creating interference that is measured with a photodetector. Although the light reflected by the tissue is composed of multiple echoes, the distance travelled is determined by changes in mirror distance. The lag time of the reference light is used to deduce the thickness of the structures through which the light passed. Time-domain OCT is a technique by which movement of the mirror enables repeated scans at different depths (a single coherence measurement on a single structure at a given depth is called an A-scan). Maximum scan rate can be 17,000 A-scans/s, providing a one-dimensional measurement, which is then processed in two dimensions (B-scan) giving an image of the different tissue layers at the point analysed. The resulting section is called a "tomogram" (Fig. 9.1), visualised in real time using a scale of false colours representing the degree of backscattering of the light by the tissues at different depths.

P. Frezzotti
Ophthalmology Unit, University of Siena, Siena, Italy
e-mail: paolofrezzotti@paolofrezzotti.it

A. Ferreras (ed.), *Glaucoma Imaging*, DOI 10.1007/978-3-319-18959-8_9

The image is captured in a few seconds and requires steady fixation by the patient. A major advance consisted in analysing (by Fourier transform) the interference spectrum of the two reflected broad-spectrum beams, instead of measuring beam coherence. This Fourier spectral domain technique is much faster (simultaneous analysis at different depths), more accurate (2 μm) and therefore greatly reduces imaging times. Its main disadvantages are that the light cannot reach the retina if there are lens opacities and fixation must be extremely steady. However, it is worth bearing in mind that OCT images are not images of structure but a mathematical reconstruction built on a photograph of the fundus. The structures visualised are the result of selective absorption and selective reflection by the structure or the interface illuminated by the laser. This can depend on the type of structures (the most reflective are the retinal nerve fibre layer (RNFL), retinal pigmented epithelium and interplexiform cells) and on the direction of the incident ray (when structures are perpendicular to the ray, reflectivity is greater, indicated in red in OCT images).

Since 2001, analysis of the anterior segment using a wavelength of 1310 nm has been combined with analysis of eye fundus structures. This wavelength makes it possible also to examine the iris-corneal angle. The OCT-Visante® instrument we used for this chapter performs 2048 scans/s with axial and transverse optical resolution of 18 and 60 μm, respectively, and an imaging time of 0.125 s. In any case, OCT enables qualitative, morphological (anterior chamber, retina and optic nerve head) and quantitative analysis providing thickness mapping in various sectors. It is reliable, easy to perform, contact-free, pain-free and has a short learning curve. The images can be analysed, quantified, compared with later images or with other images obtained, for example, by fluoroangiography or ICG. In this chapter, we consider the information that OCT offers for studying, classifying and monitoring glaucoma patients through:

1. Anterior pole evaluation
2. Retinal nerve fibre layer and optic nerve head analysis
3. Ganglion cell analysis
4. Lamina cribrosa assessment

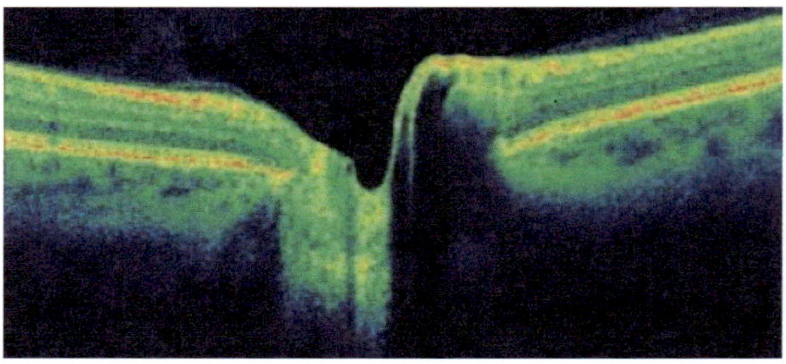

Fig. 9.1 Tomogram based on scale of false colours

9.1 Anterior Pole Evaluation

The Visante OCT instrument enables visualisation of the form, site and position of anterior chamber components and defines and measures the distances between them. The software automatically eliminates distortion induced by optical transmission factors. Various measurements can be obtained from the images: CA depth, angle to angle, chamber angle amplitude, pupil diameter and lens curvature.

In glaucoma, OCT of the anterior chamber is of special interest for assessing the amplitude and conformation of the angle, complementing gonioscopic evaluation. The anterior chamber angle is the junction between the iris root and the cornea. An important anatomical landmark for evaluating the angle is the scleral spur, which is the connecting point between the posterior curvature of the cornea and the curvature of the sclera. The trabecular meshwork and Schwalbe's line are located anterior to the scleral spur, whereas the iris root and the ciliary body are located posterior to it. Once the scleral spur is identified, the position of the iris relative to the scleral spur is checked. If the iris is posterior to the scleral spur, the angle is open, whereas if the iris is anterior to the spur, the angle is either narrow or closed.

The following figures show different clinical conditions detected by Visante OCT:

OCT is a useful tool for evaluating filtering blebs or glaucoma drainage devices in the postoperative period. Clinically, blebs can be described as diffuse, cystic, encapsulated or flat. However, these descriptions are subjective and there may be cases in which clinical appearance does not correlate with bleb function. Visualising intrableb morphology with anterior segment imaging may therefore enhance our understanding of different surgical outcomes and wound healing. The following figures show certain aspects of conjunctival blebs after trabeculectomy.

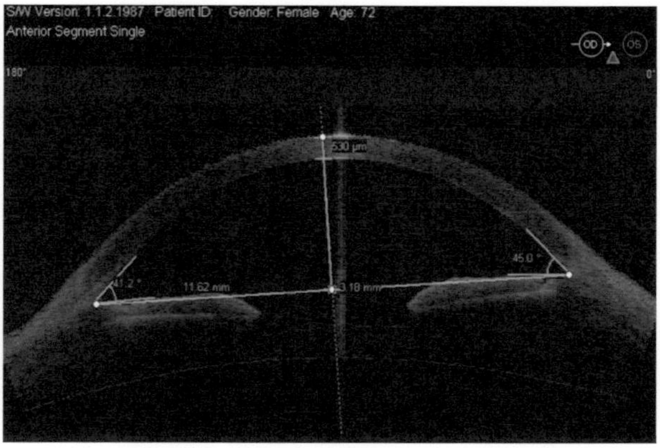

Fig. 9.2 Measurement of horizontal and vertical anterior chamber diameters, angle amplitude and corneal thickness

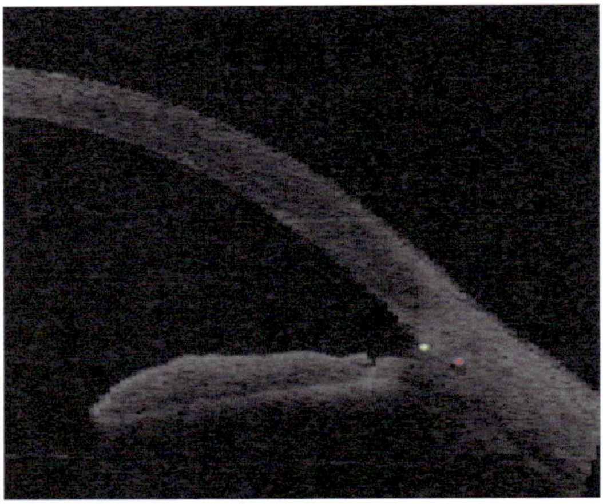

Fig. 9.3 Anatomical aspects of the anterior chamber angle. *Red dot*: scleral spur connecting point between the posterior curvature of the cornea and the curvature of the sclera. *Yellow dot*: linear distance of 500 μm anterior to the scleral spur marking the site of the trabecular meshwork

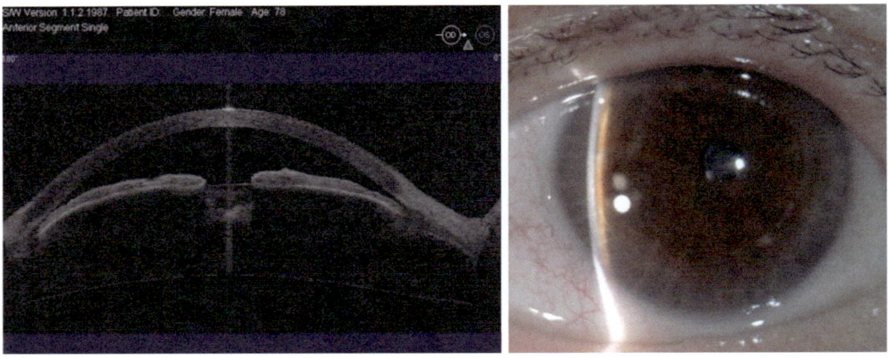

Fig. 9.4 Narrow angle. Clinical feature with Van Herick sign. OCT image shows temporal and nasal closure of the angle

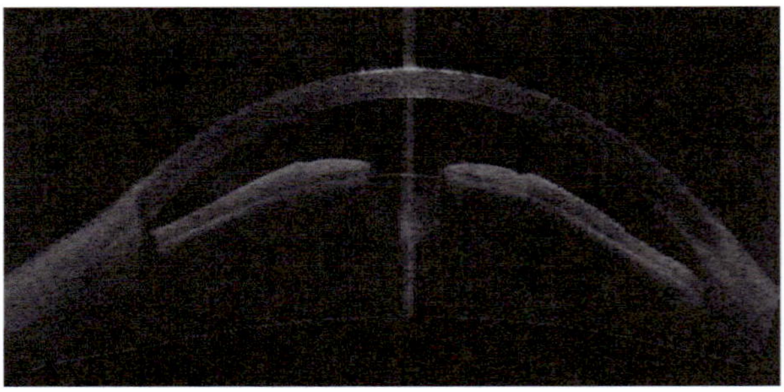

Fig. 9.5 Narrow angle. The chamber angle is closed. Note synechia at the base of the angle caused by inflammation arising during closure crises

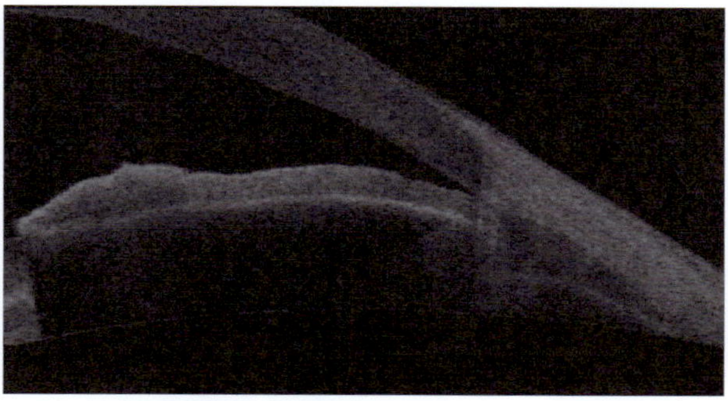

Fig. 9.6 Narrow angle. The angular recess is present. The situation worsens during midriasis and progressive apposition will lead to chronic closure (Mapstone's hypothesis of two-stage closure of the angle)

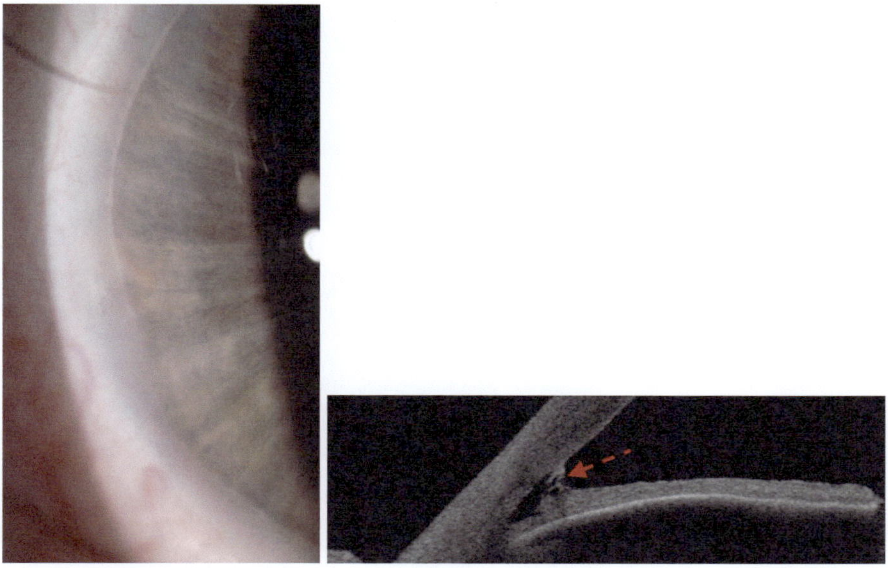

Fig. 9.7 Anxenfeld's anomaly. Anterior segment photo and OCT image showing posterior embryotoxon with iris processes that extend to Schawalbe's line (*red dotted arrow*). The changes to the angle affect the entire angle and the iris usually inserts anteriorly and obscures the scleral spur

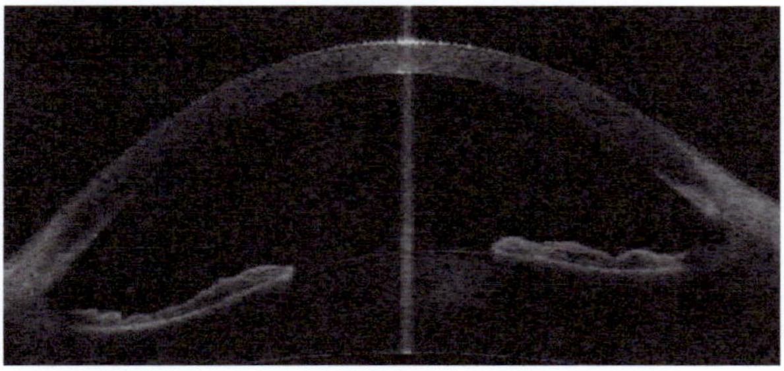

Fig. 9.8 Pigment dispersion glaucoma. OCT image showing concave iris with underlying iris-zonula contact that during miosis-midriasis causes degranulation and dispersion of pigment. Indeed, the pathogenetic event of this syndrome has extensive close contact between iris and lens that by causing contact at the pupil leads to accumulation of aqueous humour in the anterior chamber, pressure imbalance and iris concavity (inverse pupillary block)

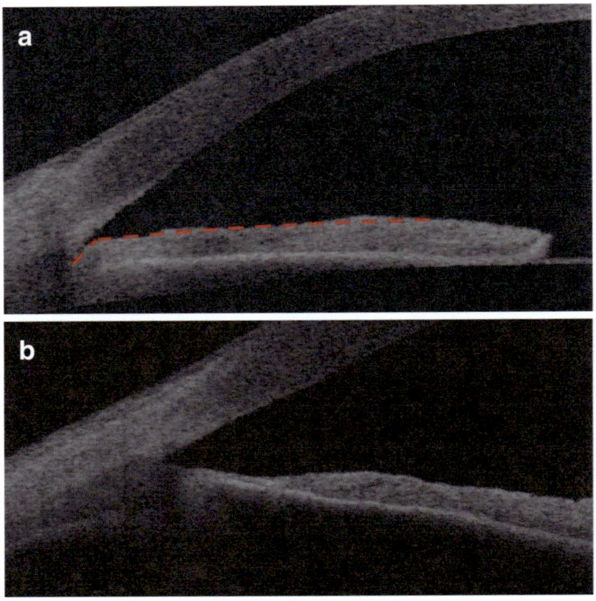

Fig. 9.9 (**a**) Plateau iris. OCT image showing a flat iris profile with anterior insertion (*red dotted line*) and anterior rotation of the ciliary bodies which raise and push the iris root towards the angle. (**b**) Plateau iris. OCT image showing the angle of (**a**) after Argon laser iridoplasty treatment. The angle appear open now

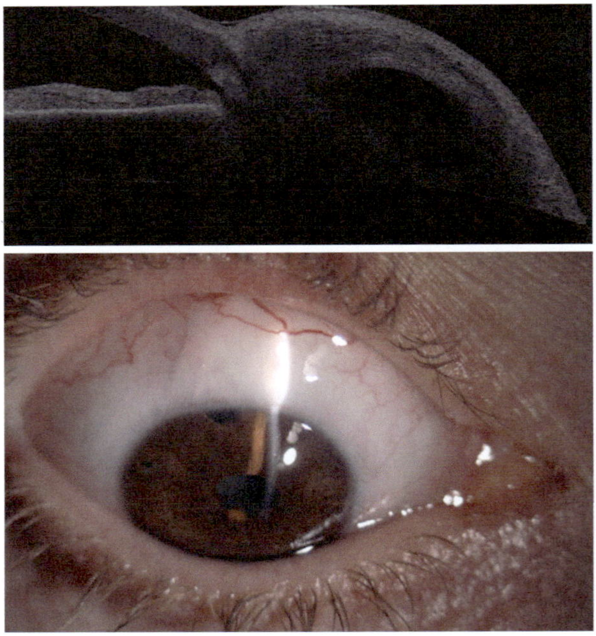

Fig. 9.10 Type L bleb (low reflectivity). OCT image showing surgical path from anterior chamber to the evident bleb. The low reflectivity of the conjunctiva indicates imbibition of aqueous humour by the bleb and success of the operation. The biomicroscope image shows a wide raised bleb

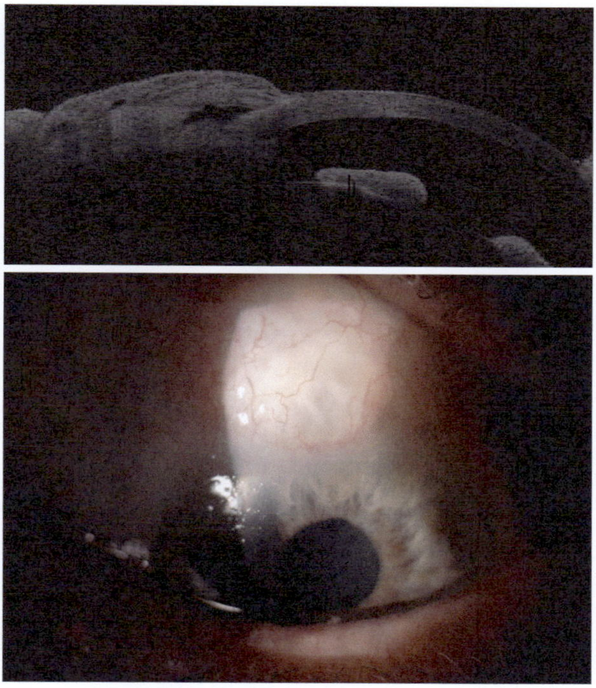

Fig. 9.11 Type H bleb (high reflectivity). OCT image showing that the bleb is functioning. The scleral surgical path is evident. The high reflectivity of the conjunctiva over the bleb indicates reduced imbibition. The biomicroscope image shows a wide functioning bleb

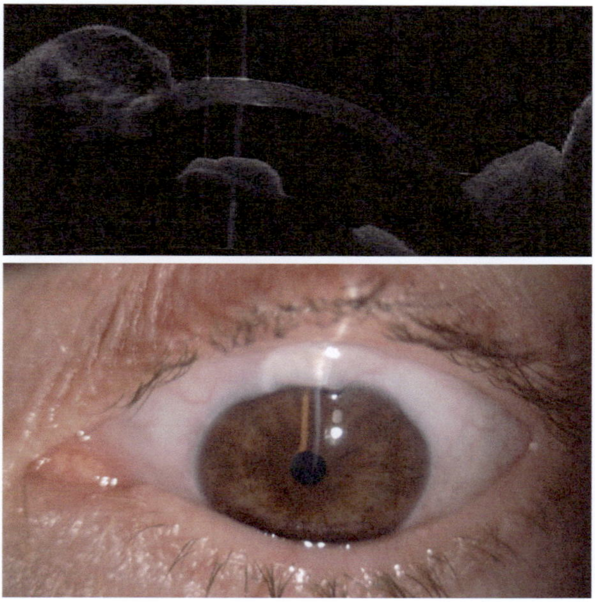

Fig. 9.12 Type E bleb (encapsulated or cystic). OCT image showing thin conjunctiva and iridectomy. Function may be relative and variable. The biomicroscope image shows a thin raised bleb with a cystic appearance; it maintains relative function in the nasal sector

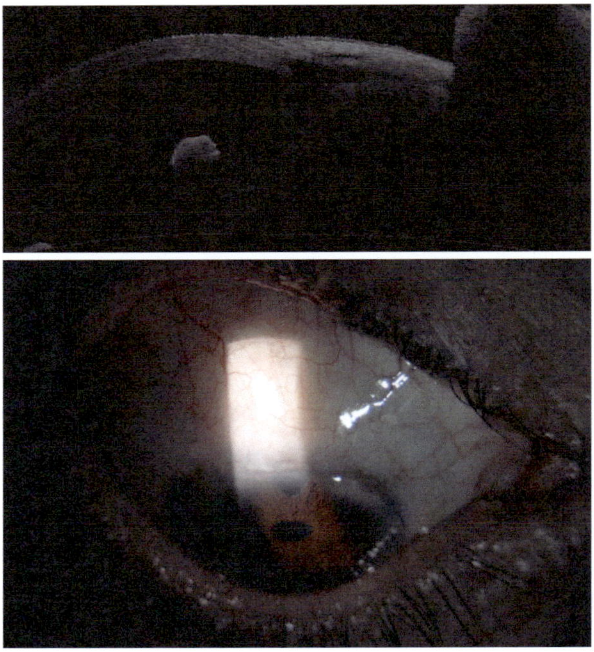

Fig. 9.13 Type F bleb (flat). OCT image showing opening of the anterior chamber but the surgical path is not visible. The bleb is absent and not functioning. The biomicroscope image shows a flat bleb with absence of filtration

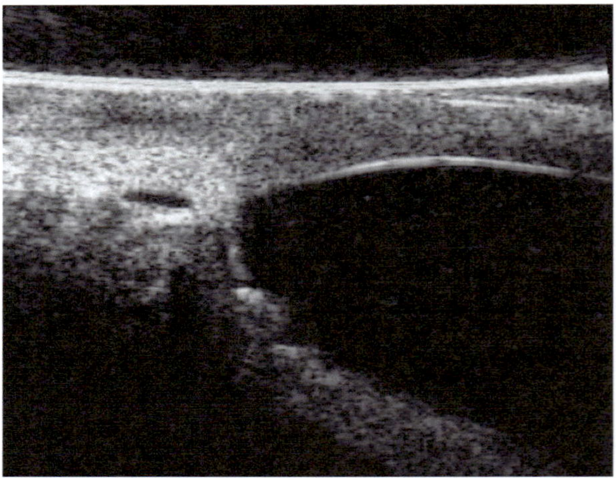

Fig. 9.14 Canaloplasty: detail of the Schlemm canal stretched by a prolene suture, which when correctly tensioned, improves its drainage capacity

9.2 Retinal Nerve Fibre Layer and Optic Nerve Head Analysis

The new generations of spectral-domain OCT have improved sensitivity in detecting structural changes in retinal nerve fibres and optic nerve head (ONH) morphology, achieving a resolution of 2 μm. The OCT software package includes 19 scan and 18 analysis protocols. Together they make it possible to analyse the optic disc, the nerve fibre layer and the macula with the same instrument. The video camera enables fundus examination in action and simultaneous saving of video images and scans. OCT of the optic nerve enables detection of retinal nerve fibre damage and changes in time by statistical comparison of different OCT images from the same patient.

OCT examination print-out consists of various parts (Fig. 9.15):

1. Table of parameters compared with a normative database
2. Topographic map of retinal nerve fibre layer (RNFL) thickness
3. Map of RNFL deviation from normal values
4. Neuroretinal rim thickness
5. RNFL TSINIT graph of measurements in the area analysed
6. Mean RNFL thickness in each quadrant
7. Horizontal and vertical B-scans
8. Calculation of RNFL thickness in the circle of interest

In the protocol, mean RNFL thickness is visualised using a white-green-yellow-red colour code. Colour coding indicates the particular position of the A-scan in the graph, the quadrant mean values and the clock-position in the circular graphs, and right and left eye columns of the table of data. In the age-matched normal population, the percentiles regard each specific measurement of RNFL thickness, in the following way:

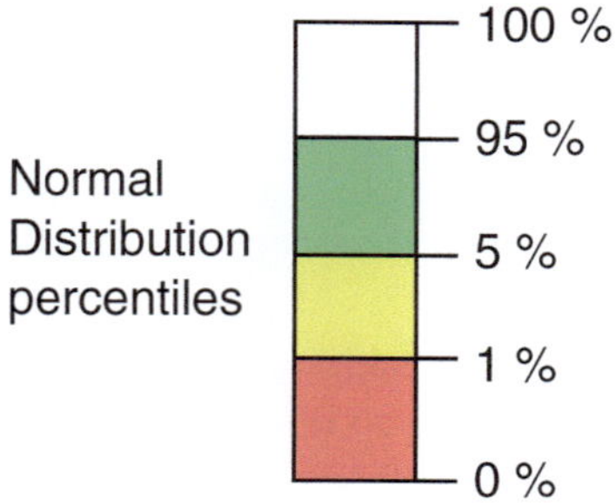

- The thinnest 1 % of measurements fall in the red area. Measurements in red are considered outside normal limits (red <1 %, outside normal limits).
- The thinnest 5 % of measurements fall in or below the yellow area (1 %<yellow<5 %, suspect).

- 90 % of measurements fall in the green area (5 % < green < 95 %).
- The thickest 5 % of measurements fall in the white area (white > 95 %).

Of the ONH parameters examined, those that revealed progressive changes in the manifestations of glaucoma were vertical thickness of the neuroretinal rim, overall area of the rim and vertical C/D ratio. However, these parameters do not help distinguish initial from advanced glaucoma. For this purpose, OCT measurements of RNFL parameters, especially average RNFL thickness, RNFL thickness in the lower temporal zone and RNFL in the lower quadrant (Fig. 9.16) were more useful.

Although diagnosis and follow-up assessments of glaucoma are based on anatomical and functional damage, the relationship between the two has not yet been clearly defined. Studies seeking a connection between visual field and anatomical damage have begun to link this data. An understanding of the relation between structure and function in glaucoma could facilitate efficacy evaluation of structural and functional tests for early diagnosis of glaucoma damage and for accurate staging. As damage progresses, there is a correlation between worsening of both the optic disc and the disease; structural changes seem to be detectable before functional ones. Rao et al. (2011) compared treated and untreated patients with POAG, finding that in the course of the disease most patients (>50 %) deteriorated prevalently from a structural point of view, about 30 % deteriorated only functionally and about 10 % deteriorated structurally and functionally. More recent studies showed that when applied to slight-moderate glaucoma, spectral-domain OCT ensures a better correlation between structure and function than time-domain OCT. However, one parameter explains only 30 % of the trend of the other. Thus it is possible to be faced with different clinical situations, as illustrated in the following examples.

Anatomical variations in the optic nerve are so numerous that they cannot all be included in the database used by OCT software. This may lead to classification of abnormal ONH parameters for absolutely normal RNF and white-on-white perimetry parameters. In such situations, the RNFL classification must be preferred, monitoring any changes through careful follow-up (Fig. 9.17).

When faced with altered anatomical ONH and RNFL parameters and high intraocular pressure without visual field damage according to conventional white-on-white perimetry, we have preperimetric glaucoma. Besides monitoring the patient we can consider beginning therapy, especially when anatomical damage is substantial (Figs. 9.18 and 9.19).

When structural damage is associated with functional visual field damage, we have initial glaucoma. In this stage, ONH and RNFL damage is greater than visual field damage, especially in young patients.

There are cases in which alteration of ONH parameters and visual field is associated with normal RNFL thickness. Indeed, one may encounter patients with OCT evidence of damage as well as visual field damage in one eye, but only visual field damage in the other eye. This is sufficient for a diagnosis of glaucoma in both eyes (Fig. 9.21).

When the severity of glaucoma increases to the stage of moderate, it can present with greater OCT evidence of structural damage than functional visual field damage. In this case, anatomical damage can provide important indications of how functional damage could evolve (Fig. 9.22). Another possible presentation shows greater concordance of structural ONH damage and RNFL thickness with visual field damage (Fig. 9.23).

Imaging of structural damage is also important in advanced forms of glaucoma, although assessment of clinical condition and progression are essentially based on functional visual field data. Structural damage to RNFL thickness does not go below 50 μm, which corresponds to visual field areas of absolute scotoma. In these forms of glaucoma, the concordance between anatomical and functional damage may vary, but unlike in the above situations, the visual field usually shows greater evidence of damage. Examples follow (Figs. 9.24 and 9.25).

Another major use of OCT in assessing progression of glaucoma is that proposed by guided progression analysis (GPA), a programme of analysis of progression based on data obtained from OCT images (Fig. 9.26). As shown in the figure, the upper part of the OCT print-out shows images of ONH fibre thickness, and below it images showing changes in fibre thickness between OCT examinations. When a first reduction (possible change) is detected, it is highlighted in yellow (Fig. 9.27); if it is confirmed in the next OCT (probable change) it is highlighted in red; if an increase is detected, it is highlighted in violet (Fig. 9.27). Further down we find graphs representing longitudinal changes in RNFL thickness and in the overall mean value for the upper and lower sectors; changes in mean cup/disc ratio during follow-up are represented in the same way. In the lower part of the print-out on the left, we have a graph with RNFL thickness profile with the same colour coding for changes over time; on the right we have a window in which progression probability is indicated in an immediate and readily understood manner by summary boxes containing parameters that may vary significantly. It is important to bear in mind that like other types of morphological analysis of fibres, OCT, too, is subject to certain artefacts: strong interference at the vitreous-retinal interface and intraretinal oedema can deceive the automatic segmentation algorithm, creating false measures and increasing test-retest variability.

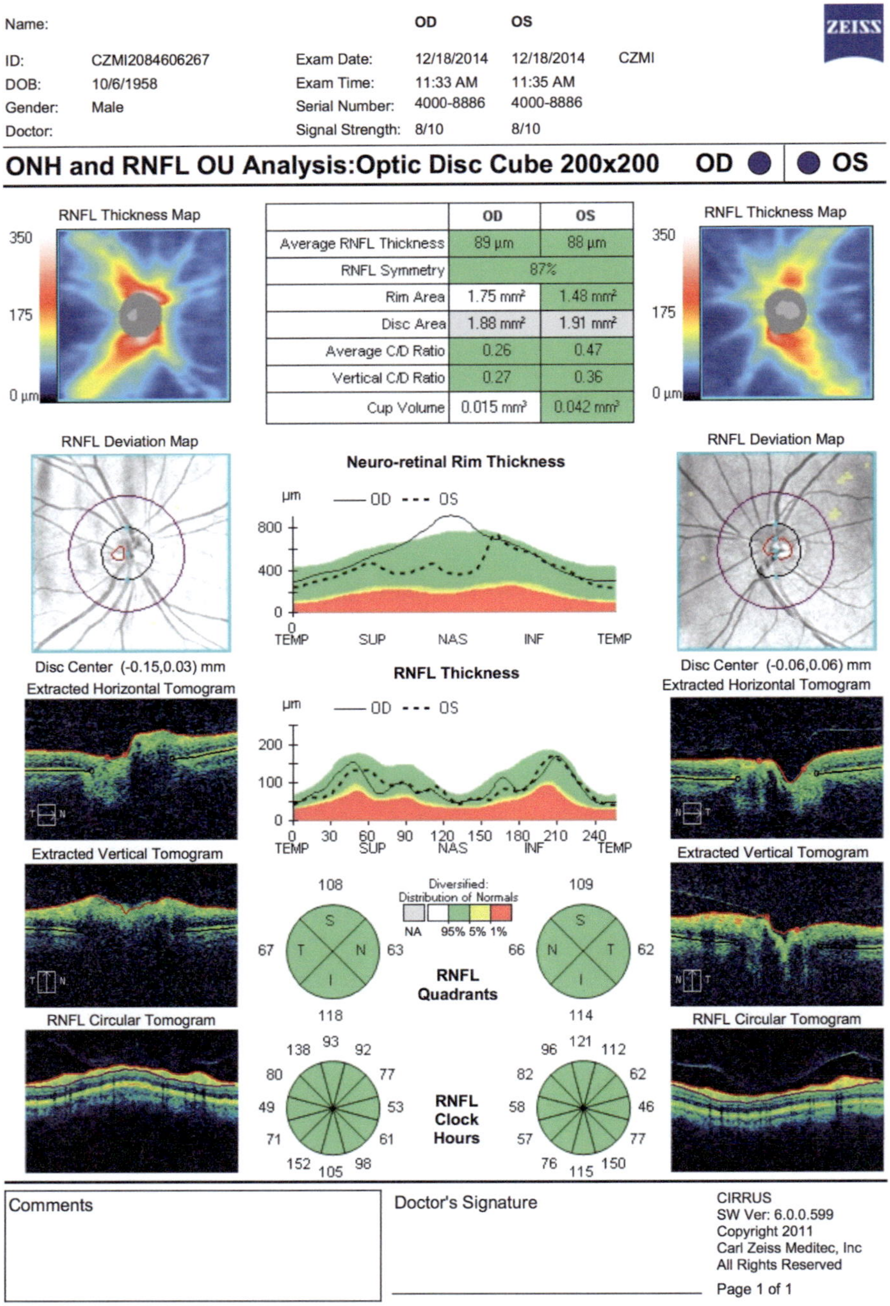

Fig. 9.15 Print-out of OCT examination of the optic nerve head and RNFL

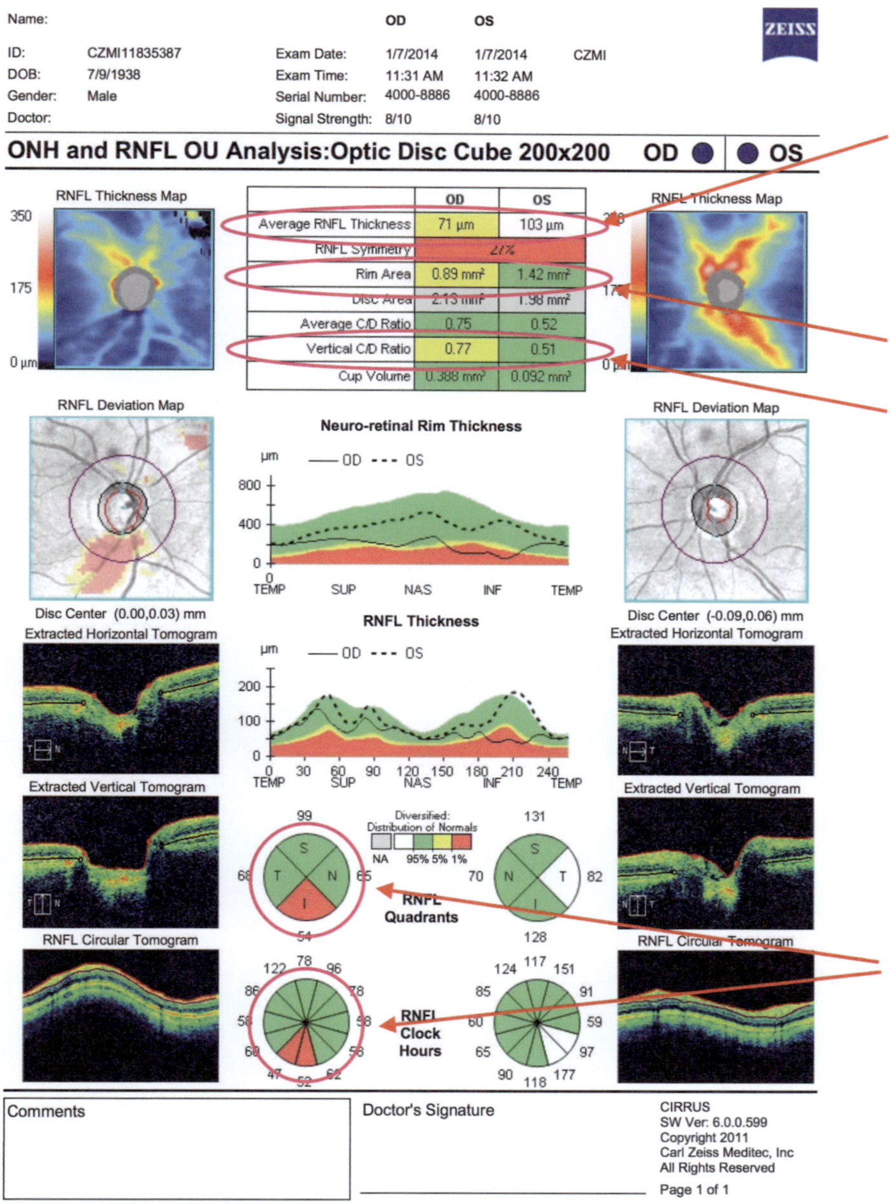

Fig. 9.16 OCT print-out – the most useful parameters (*circled*) for differentiating normal and glaucomatous patients are: vertical thickness of neuroretinal rim, overall area of rim, vertical C/D ratio, average RNFL thickness, RNFL thickness in lower temporal zone and in the lower quadrant

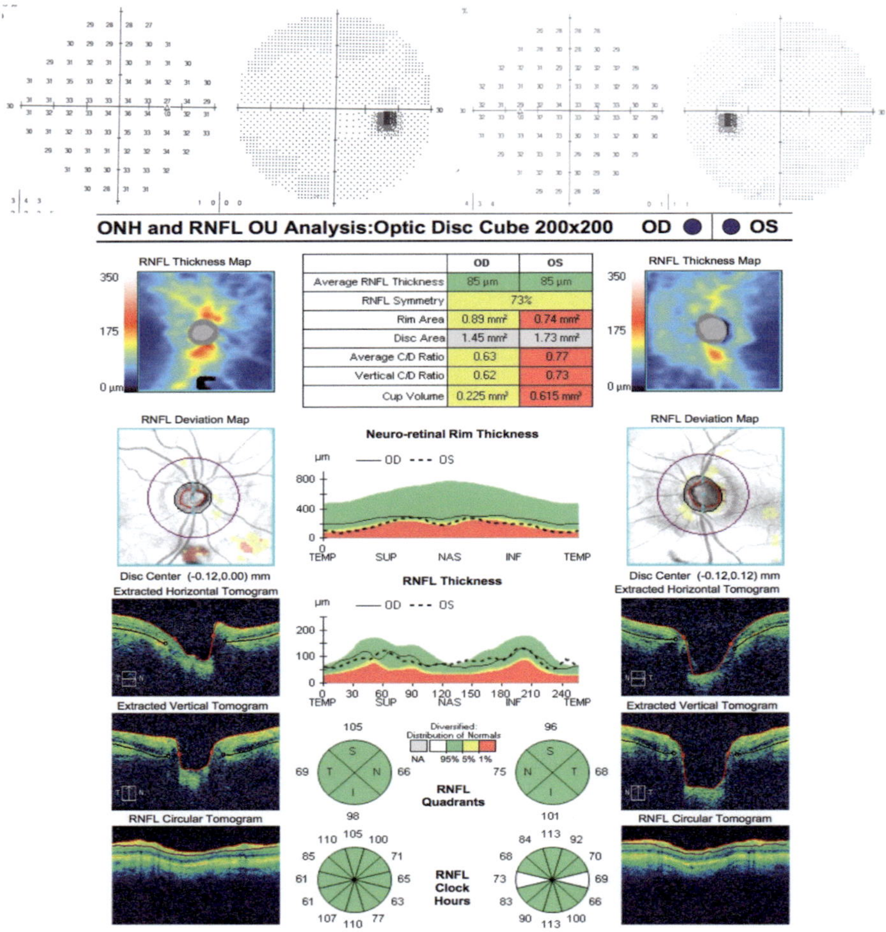

Fig. 9.17 RNFL parameters are normal, whereas ONH parameters (rim area, vertical and average C/D ratio, cup volume) are abnormal. In this case, it is sufficient to monitor the patient

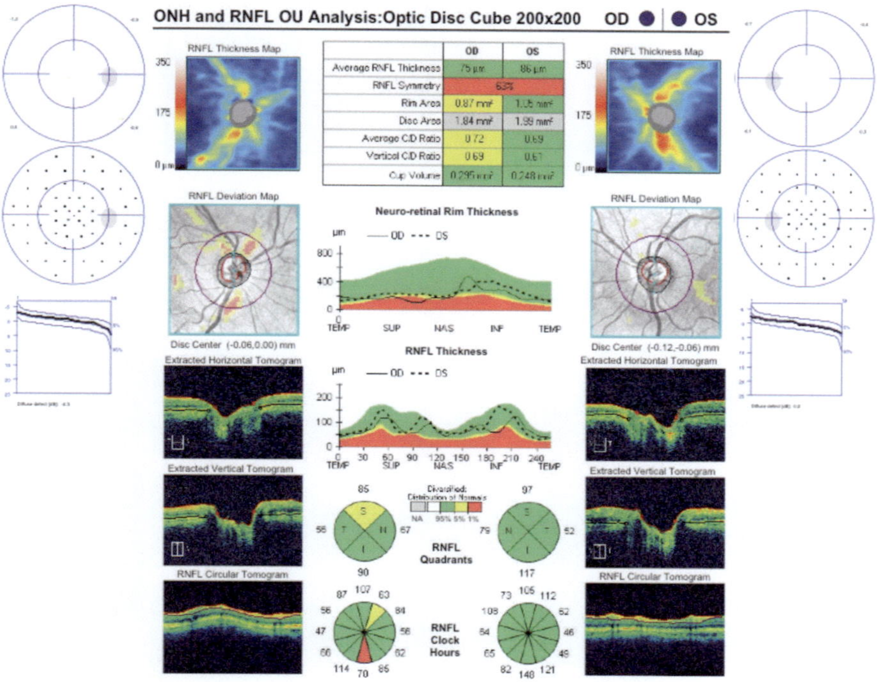

Fig. 9.18 ONH and RNFL parameters are slightly altered and Octopus perimetry seems normal. In deciding whether or not to begin therapy, it is also important to consider risk factors. The patient should be monitored

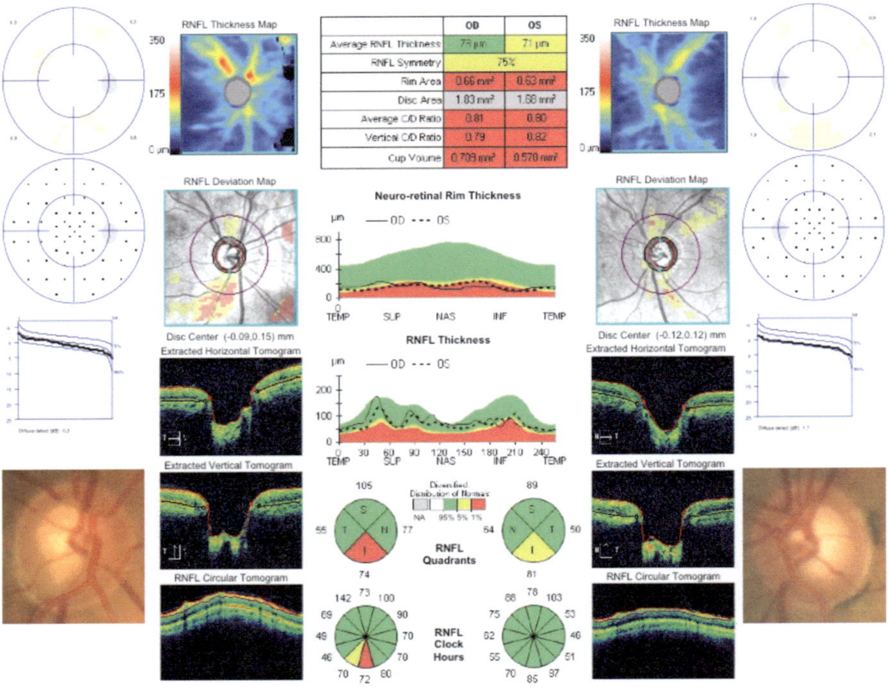

Fig. 9.19 ONH and RNFL parameters are altered in both eyes, especially in the right eye. Octopus perimetry is again normal. In this case with high intraocular pressure, we have preperimetric glaucoma and hypotonic therapy should be started

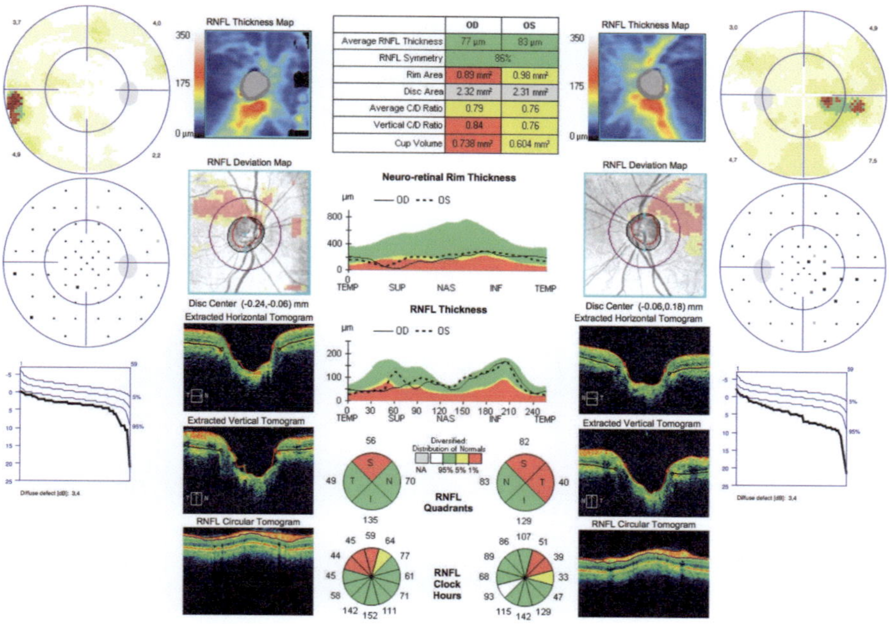

Fig. 9.20 ONH and RNFL parameters are altered in both eyes, especially in the left eye, and Octopus perimetry shows damage in both eyes. This case, in which there is good agreement between structural damage detected by OCT and perimetric damage, can be classified as initial glaucoma. In such patients, perfect concordance between the two is rare. Hypotonic therapy should be begun and the patient monitored periodically

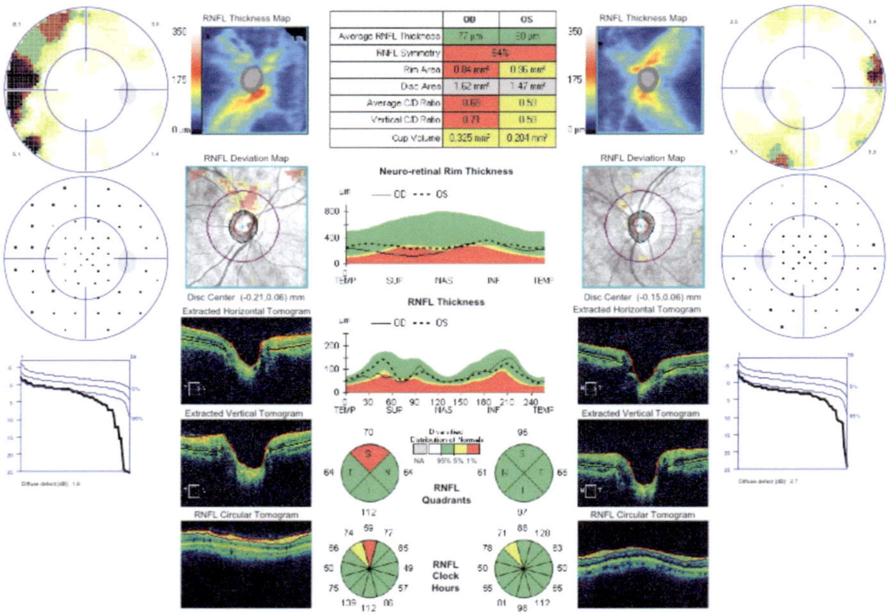

Fig. 9.21 ONH parameters are altered in both eyes, especially in the right eye, which also shows Octopus perimetry alterations. RNFL structural parameters detected by OCT are only altered in the right eye. In this case, we can also classify the left eye as glaucomatous due to perimetric damage, even in the absence of RNFL alterations

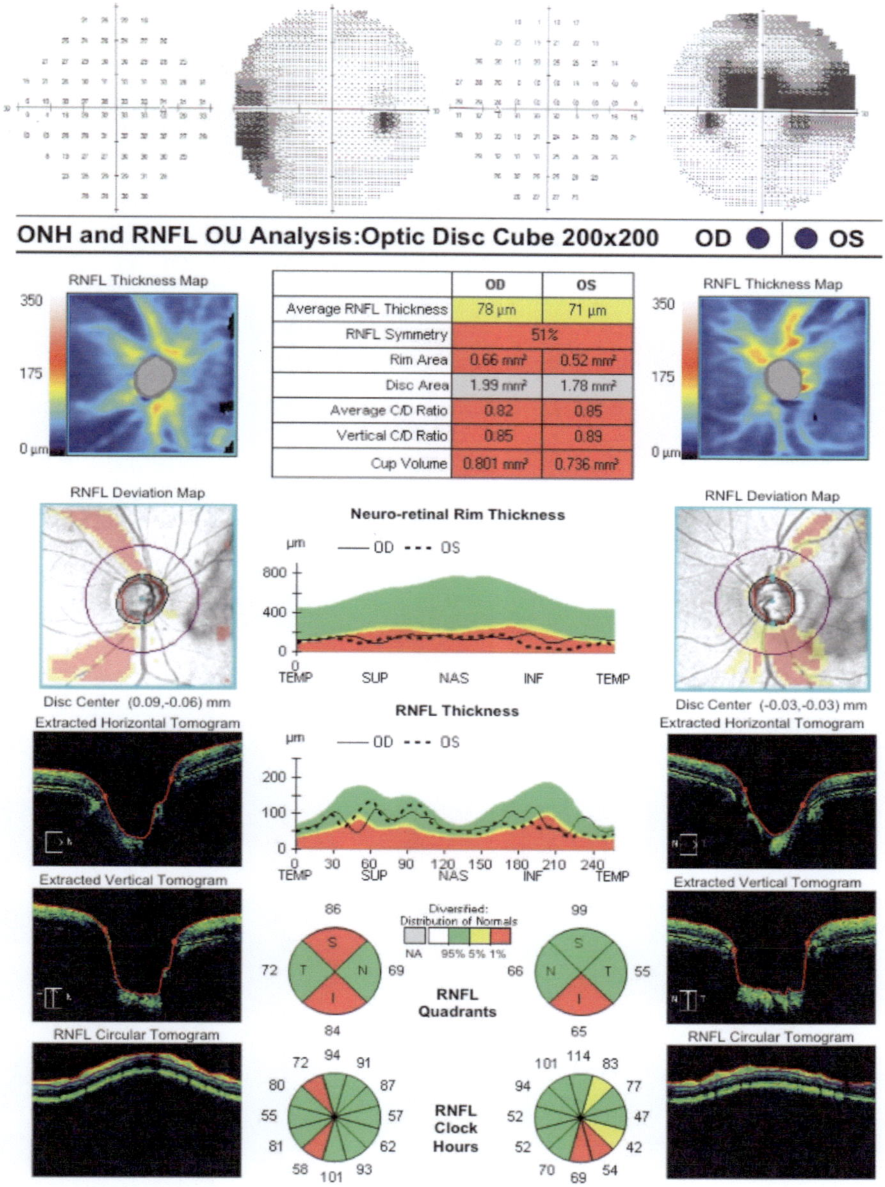

Fig. 9.22 ONH and RNFL parameters are altered in both eyes in more or less the same way. However, perimetry shows greater functional damage on the left. In such patients it is particularly useful to monitor regions that have structural damage but normal visual field

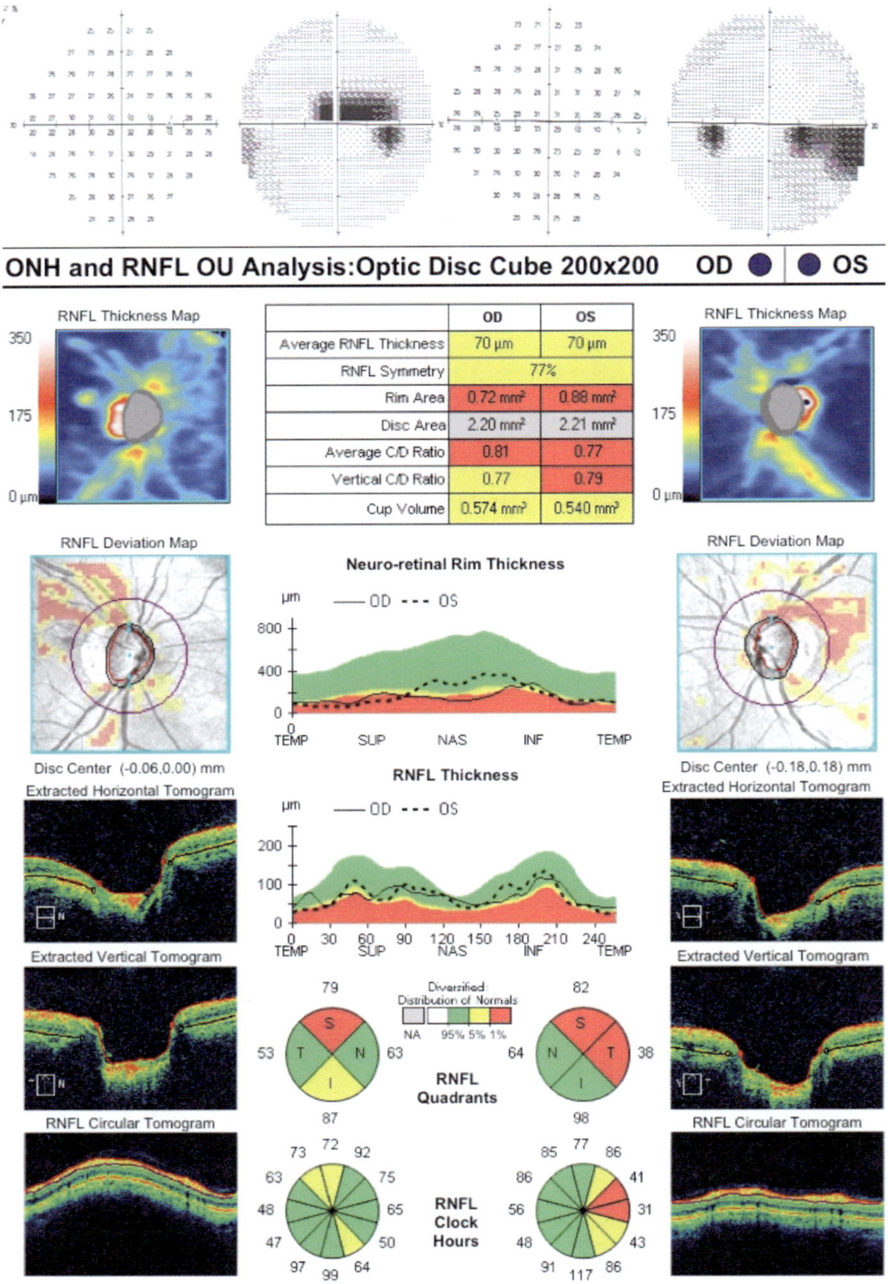

Fig. 9.23 ONH and RNFL parameters are altered in both eyes in more or less the same way. Perimetry confirms structural damage with good concordance. Progression of the disease should be carefully monitored by evaluating both anatomical and functional damage

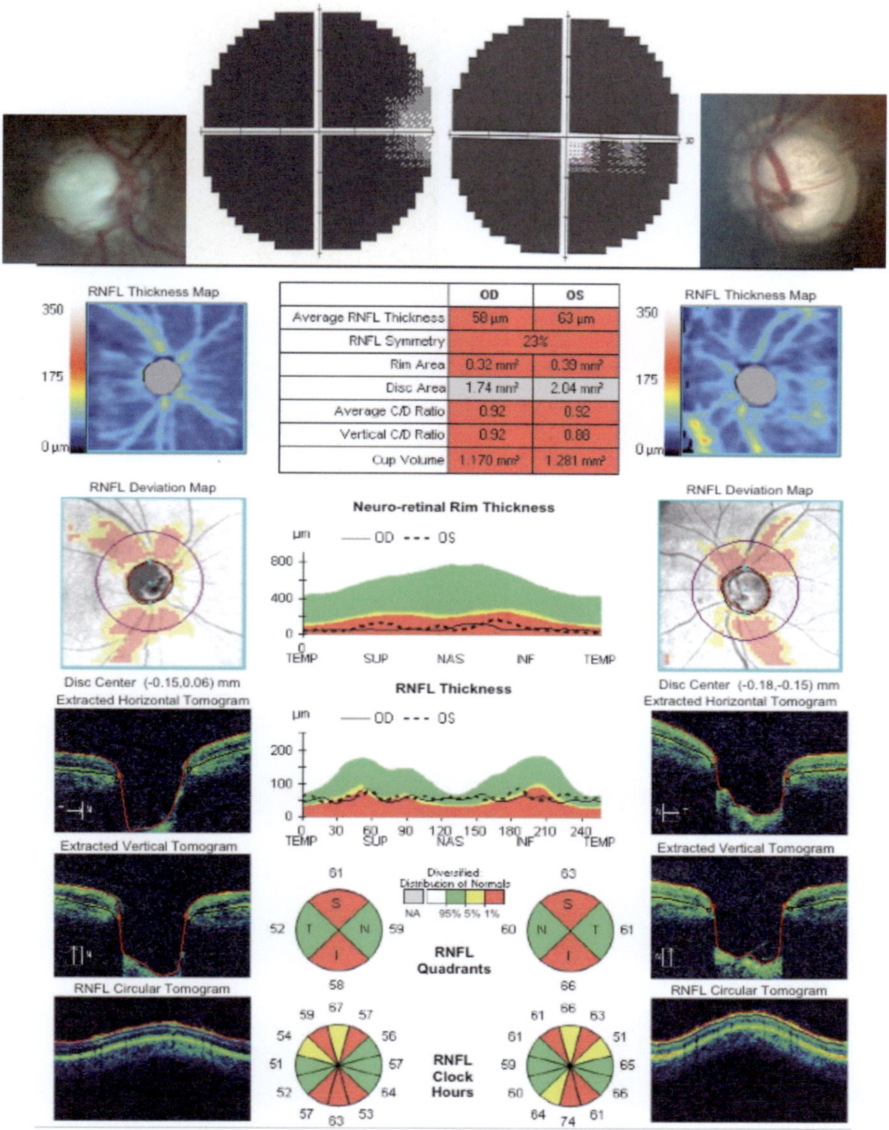

Fig. 9.24 Advanced glaucoma: ONH and RNFL parameters are severely altered in both eyes and more or less in the same manner. ONH morphological parameters are all pathological and average RNFL thickness of the right eye is 50 μm, although certain areas (nasal and temporal sectors) show RNFL thickness within normal limits. Perimetry amplifies the structural damage findings, showing visual field areas of the right and left eyes with VFIs of 1 % and 6 %, respectively. This is the terminal stage of the disease where functional damage outweighs OCT evidence of structural damage

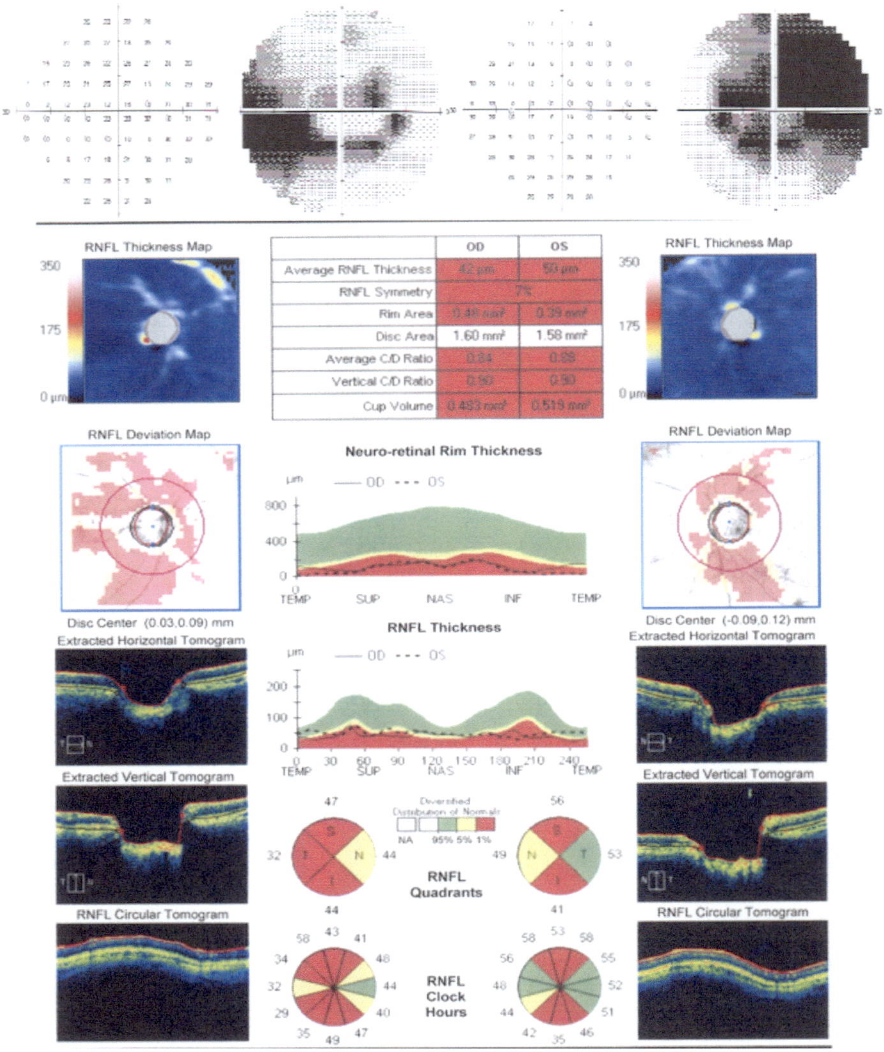

Fig. 9.25 Advanced glaucoma: ONH and RNFL parameters are severely altered in both eyes. ONH morphological parameters are all pathological and average RNFL thicknesses of the right and left eyes are 41 and 50 µm, respectively. Perimetry shows a good correlation with structural damage, revealing visual fields in line with clinical severity

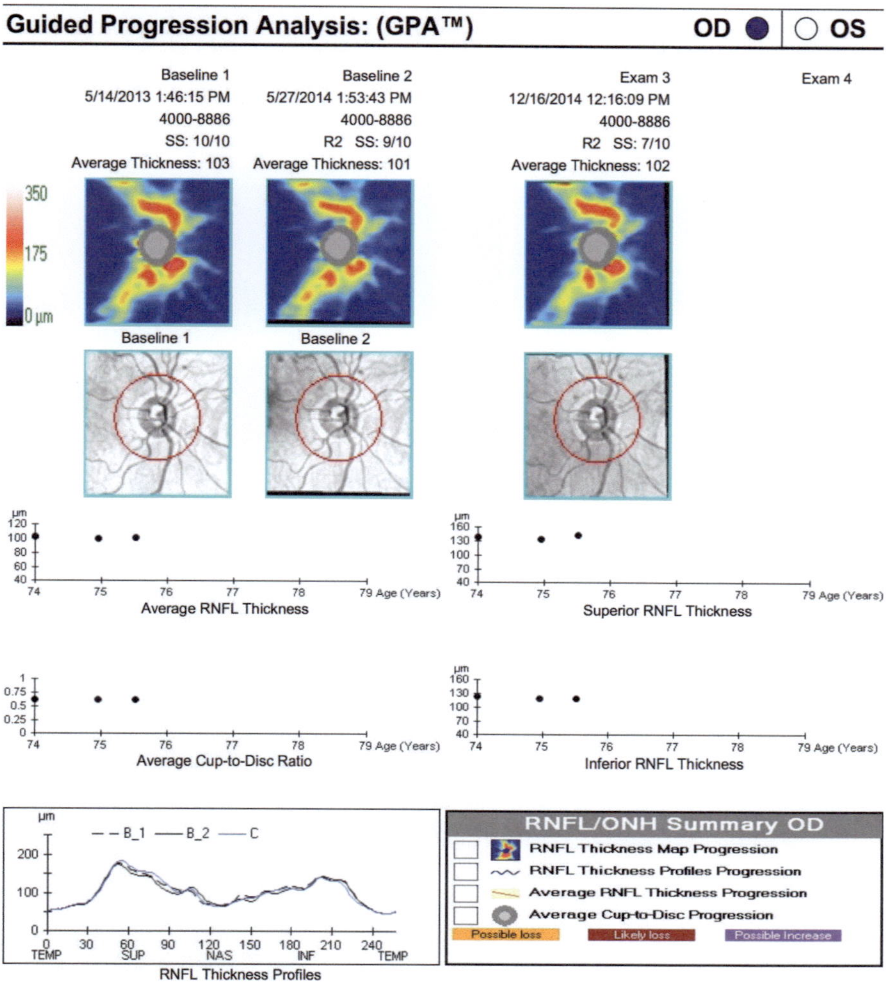

Fig. 9.26 Print-out of parameters used by GPA to monitor progression of glaucoma

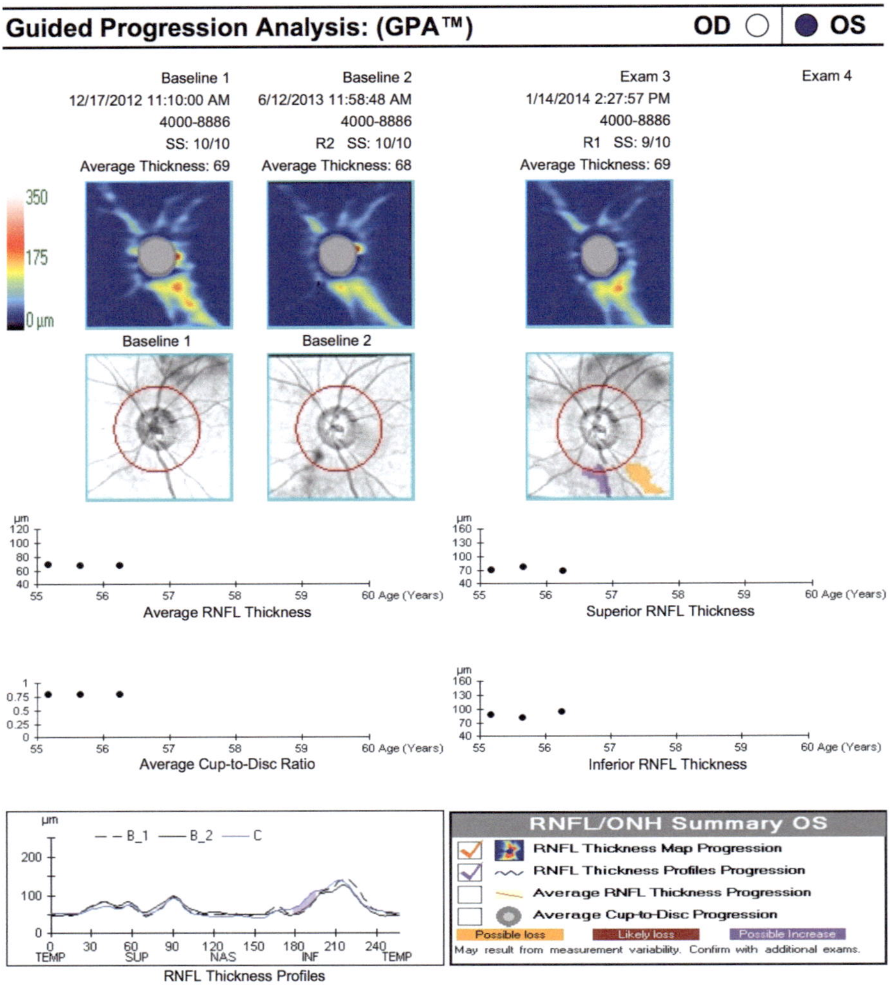

Fig. 9.27 Print-out of parameters used by GPA showing changes in fibre thickness during follow-up

9.3 Ganglion Cell Analysis

Spectral-domain OCT has proved useful for assessing glaucoma because it enables the ganglion cell complex (GCC) to be studied. The GCC consists of three layers (nerve fibre layer, ganglion cell layer and inner plexiform layer) containing axons, cell bodies and dendrites of ganglion cells, loss of which is typical of glaucoma optic neuropathy. Cross-sectional imaging of the macular area was performed using the Cirrus OCT macular cube (512×128). This acquisition protocol generates a cube through a 6 mm square grid of 128 B-scans, each consisting of 512 A-scans. A built-in GCC analysis algorithm detects and measures the thickness of the macular GCC in a 6×6×2 mm elliptical annulus centred on the fovea. The annulus has an inner vertical diameter of 1 mm, chosen to exclude parts of the fovea where the layers are very thin and difficult to detect accurately, and an outer vertical diameter of 4 mm, chosen to coincide with where the GCC again becomes thin and difficult to detect. The thickness values recorded are mean thickness, mean minimum thickness (thickness of the thinnest sector) and the topography of the macular region divided into six sectors: superior, inferior, superior and inferior temporal and superior and inferior nasal. Again, the data is first compared with a normative database in the form of maps, graphs and tables that use colours in the same manner as for the ONH protocol. GCC thicknesses in the normal range are represented by green backgrounds. The thinnest 5 and 1 % of measurements are represented by yellow and red backgrounds, respectively. The hypernormal (95th to 100th percentiles) pRNFL thicknesses are presented by a white colour (Fig. 9.28). Early glaucoma damage manifests with changes in the mean minimum thickness of the inferior temporal sector.

Continuous development and evolution of methods for measuring structure have helped researchers in their attempts to link structural evaluations with visual function. As already mentioned, many studies that examined the relation between structure and function in glaucoma have led to a simple linear (one-to-one) model linking structure (GCC thickness) and function (visual field sensitivity). However, other parameters such as wide anatomical variability, simultaneous presence of other local or systemic pathologies, or the entity of sight defects can influence structural measurements, such as RNFL and GCC thicknesses. We also have to consider that visual sensitivity expressed by the visual field reaches a plateau and does not increase indefinitely, even when GCC thickness is particularly large. Besides, a rapid decrease in visual sensitivity expressed by the visual field seems correlated with situations in which GCC thickness falls below a certain threshold. This indicates that nonlinear logistic analysis, as studied by many researchers, would be more appropriate for reliably linking this structural and functional data. Until this is achieved, I submit a series of conditions that can be useful in clinical practice.

When faced with high intraocular pressure and alterations in GCC anatomical parameters without conventional white-on-white perimetric evidence of visual field damage, we have preperimetric glaucoma. In such cases, besides monitoring the patient it is worth contemplating therapy, especially when anatomical damage is substantial (Fig. 9.29).

With progression of the disease, we have initial glaucoma when structural damage is associated with functional visual field damage. In this stage, one may be faced with situations in which GCC damage is congruous with functional damage as indicated by white-on-white perimetry (Fig. 9.30).

However, we are more likely to encounter cases in which ONH, RNFL and GCC damage is greater than visual field damage as detected by Humphrey perimetry (programme 30.2 and 10.2) or by Octopus perimetry (G1 and M), especially in young patients. Indeed, it is mainly in young patients that we find situations in which the difference between structure and function is much more accentuated. This is because young people have a high reserve of ganglion cells for the different areas of the visual field, so that structural damage may be greater than visual field damage (Fig. 9.31).

Also in more advanced forms of glaucoma, it is interesting to note that structural damage tends to be on average greater than perimetric damage. Patients with asymmetric damage, as shown in Figs. 9.32 and 9.33, are of special interest. Figure 9.30 showed a match between structure and function, both in the damaged and the undamaged (left) eye. In Fig. 9.31, structural and functional damages were congruous in both eyes. Indeed, MD was −17.6 dB and mean thickness 60 μm in the right eye, compared to −1.4 dB and 73 μm in the left eye.

In advanced forms of glaucoma, structural damage is also substantial, though assessment of clinical condition and progression are essentially based on functional visual field data. In fact it is often difficult to assess variations in structural damage when faced with major reductions in GCC thickness, as in the right eye shown below, in which structural damage is at a maximum and perfectly matches the functional damage detected by white-on-white Octopus perimetry. The major structural damage in the left eye provides an indication of the evolution of functional damage in time. In this example, we have extreme situations: MD −23.2 dB in the right eye coupled with a mean thickness of 44 μm, that is, correspondence of structural and functional damages, whereas MD 02.4 dB and 50 μm in the left eye show that structural damage is more evident than perimetric damage.

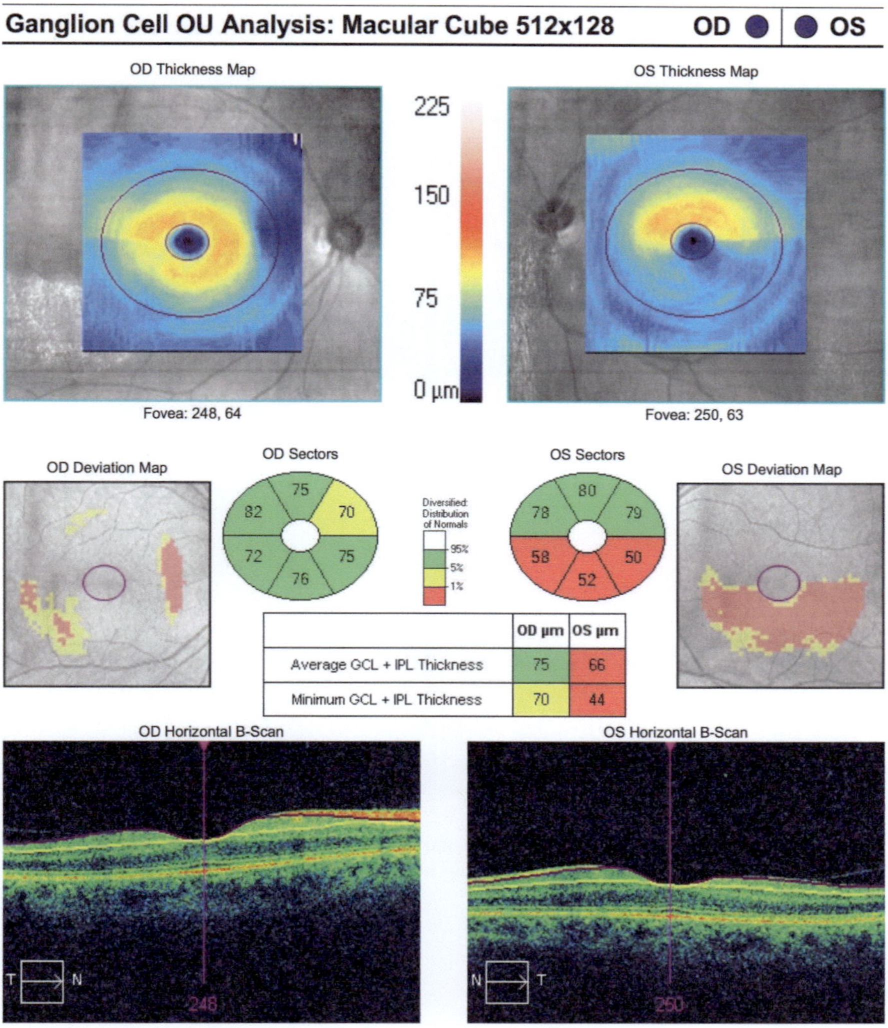

Fig. 9.28 Spectral-domain OCT analysis of retinal ganglion cells: thickness data is provided after comparison with a normative database in the form of maps, graphs and tables using colours in the same way as in the ONH protocol

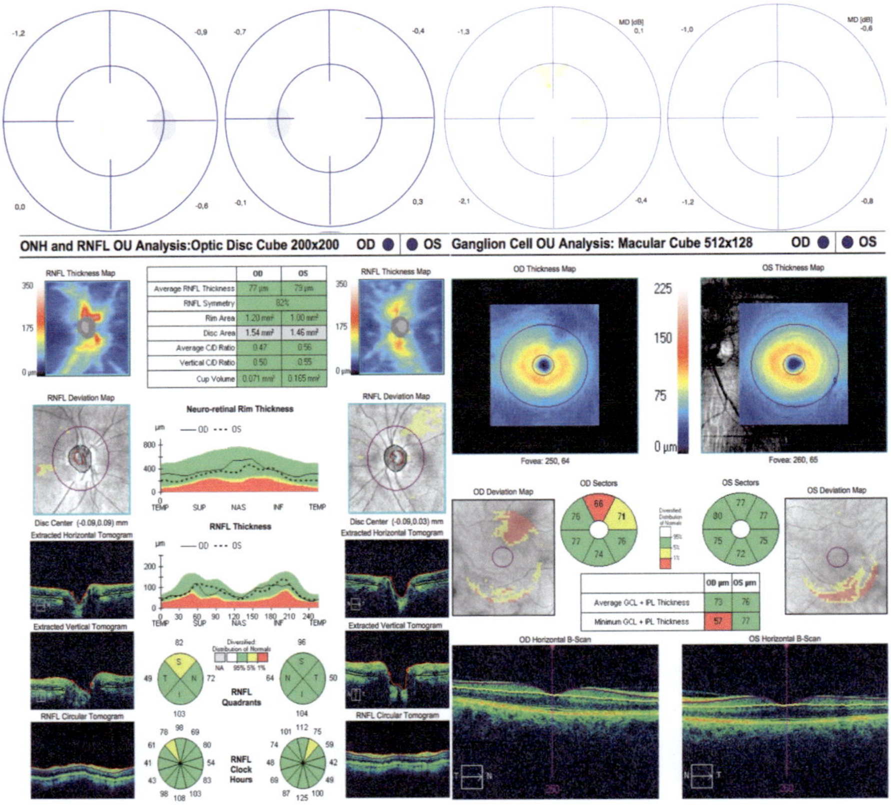

Fig. 9.29 GCC parameters are slightly altered and Octopus perimetry is normal. In this case, risk factors should also be considered when deciding whether to begin therapy. The patient should be monitored

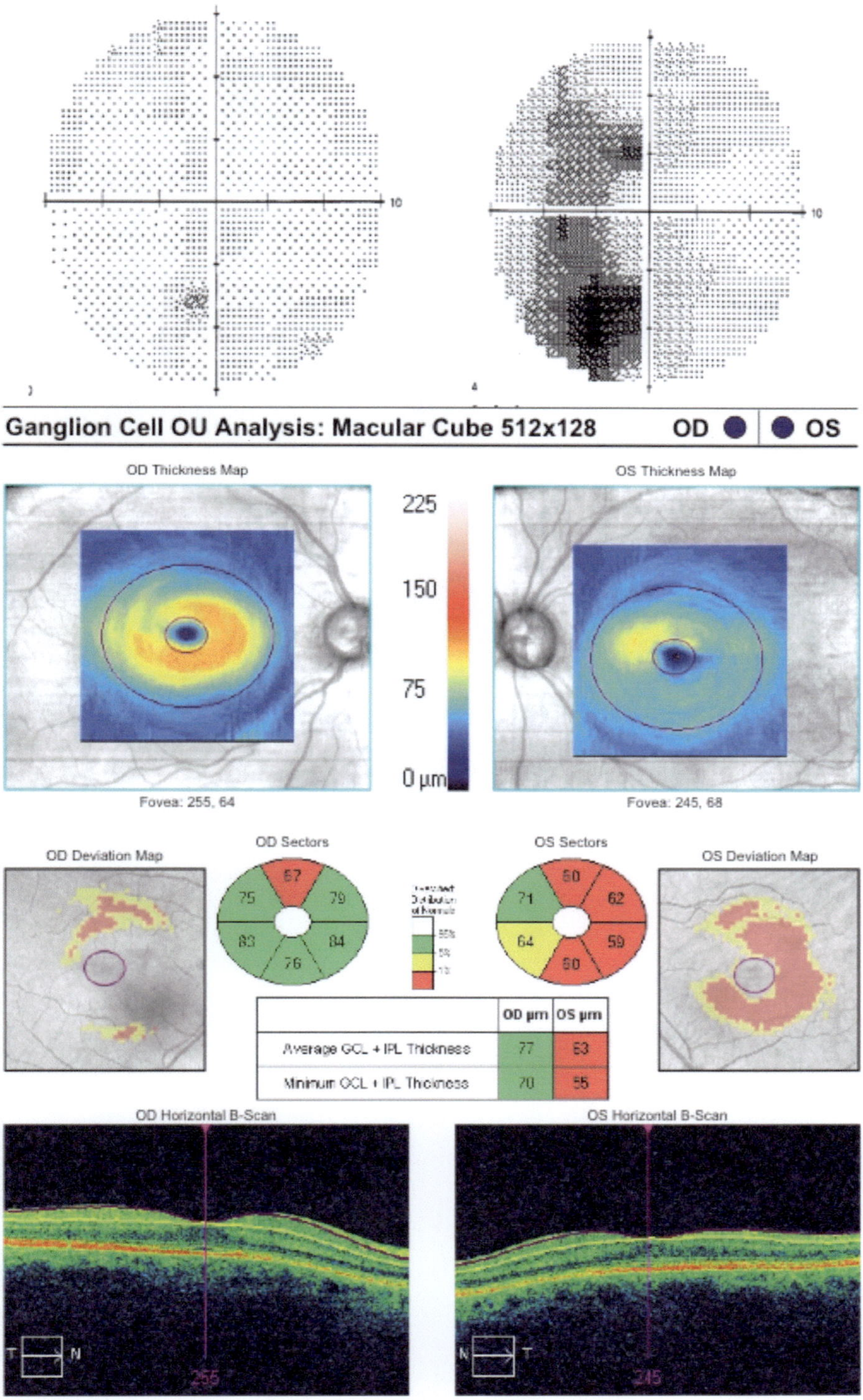

Fig. 9.30 GCC parameters are altered almost perfectly in line with severity and position indicated by Humphrey 10.2 perimetry. In these stages, structural damage can be detected earlier than functional damage

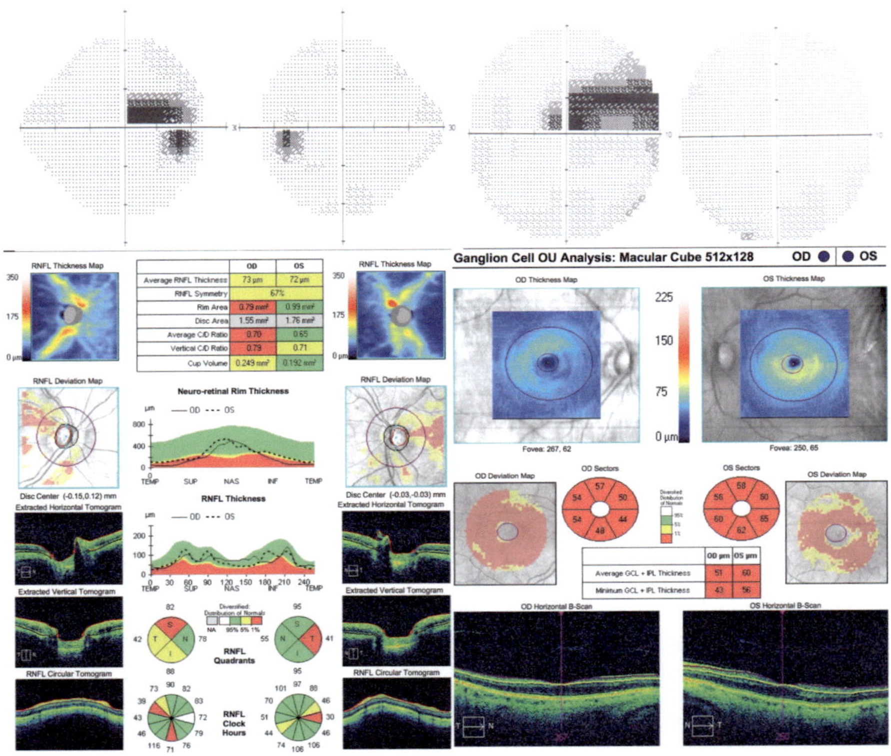

Fig. 9.31 ONH, RNFL and GCC parameters are altered more than those measured by Humphrey perimetry. Note that in the right eye there is structural and functional damage, though the former seems greater. In the left eye only structural damage is evident, and greatly precedes the appearance of functional damage as measured by Humphrey perimetry (24.2 and 10.2). In this case, it is important to begin therapy in both eyes, seeking an appropriate pressure target with patient risk factors in mind

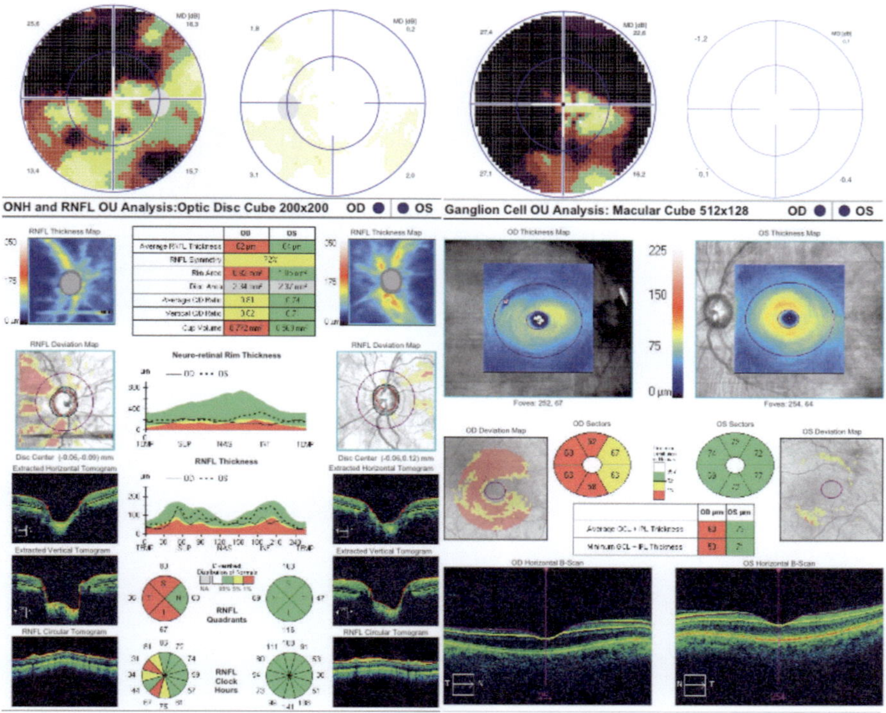

Fig. 9.32 Alterations in ONH, RNFL and GCC parameters matched functional damage as measured by Octopus perimetry. Note the interesting structural/functional congruence in both eyes

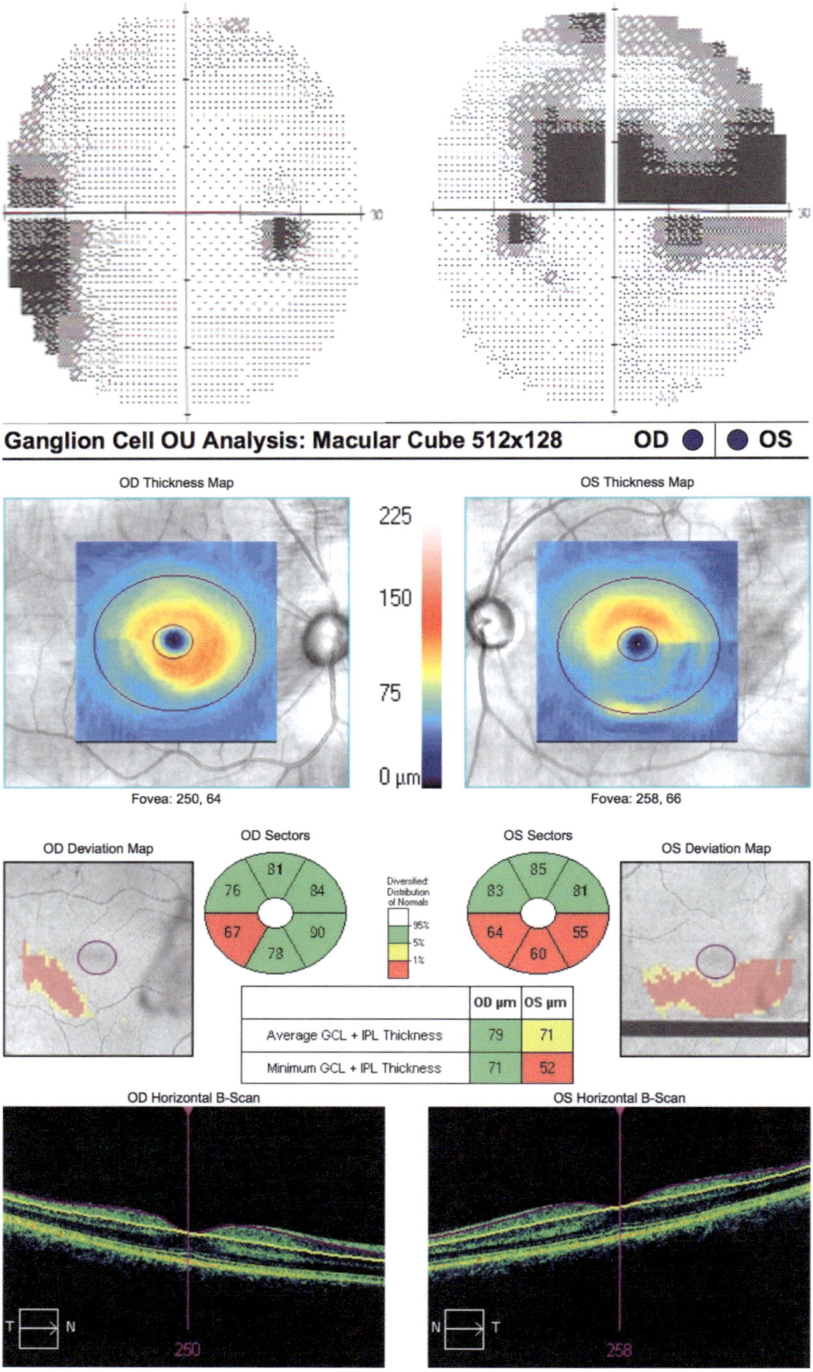

Fig. 9.33 GCC parameters are reduced and match evidence of functional damaged measured by Humphrey 30.2 perimetry in both eyes

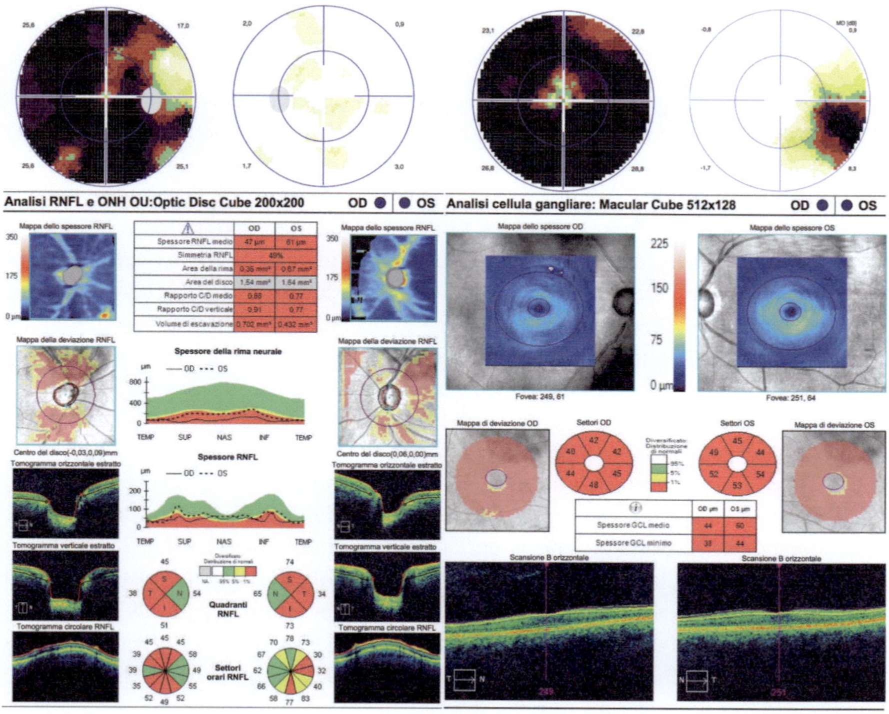

Fig. 9.34 Alterations of ONH, RNFL and GCC parameters in the right eye are at a maximum and congruous with damage detected by white-on-white Octopus perimetry. In the left eye, by contrast, structural damage is much more evident, providing an indication of the evolution of functional damage over time

9.4 Lamina Cribrosa Assessment

In glaucoma, functional damage affects the axons of retinal ganglion cells and this damage is thought to begin in the lamina cribrosa (LC). The pathology of the disease is not yet completely understood and to improve diagnosis and prognosis we need to know the effects of intraocular pressure on the biomechanics of the LC and the surrounding sclera. In recent years, OCT has been used to obtain in vivo images of deep ONH structures, especially the LC. OCT images of the LC are acquired with a deeper focal plane than the optimal plane for RNFL images. This means that traditional ONH images used to analyse RNFL thinning and thickness often do not give optimal visualisation of the LC. A technique known as enhanced depth imaging (EDI) has been developed to improve visualisation of deeper structures, such as the choroid and LC (Fig. 9.35). Available EDI-OCT instruments often use the mean of many photograms to see deeper tissue. To maintain reasonable image-acquisition times, these instruments use radial models and a certain distance between B-scans. In this way, it is possible to see posterior deformation of the LC and its posterior displacement with respect to the sclera. This technique is developing fast and will make it possible to visualise deep ONH components, though the resolution and contrast of OCT images are still less than those, for example, of RNFL images. Moreover, detection of the posterior surface of the LC is still highly variable even with EDI-OCT, as this surface is difficult to identify. Large areas of the LC also remain difficult to visualise. Much work is still necessary, comparing detection of the posterior surface of the LC by OCT with histological images from humans and primates. At the present time, the proliferation of articles on the topic could lead to premature introduction of LC thickness measures into clinical practice.

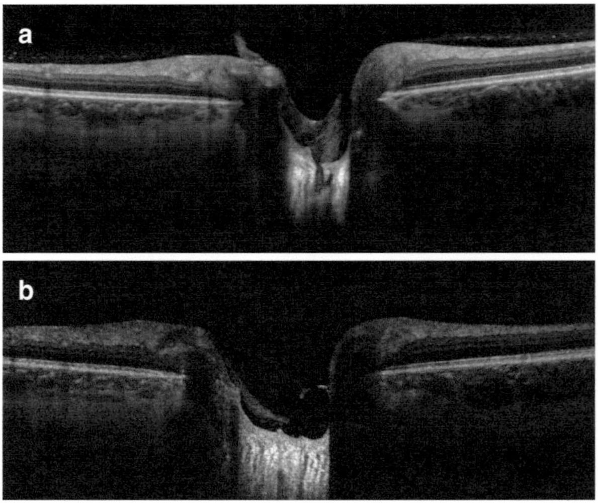

Fig. 9.35 EDI-OCT images use the mean of many photograms to see deeper tissue. In the image a is shown the lamina cribrosa of a normal subject; in the image b is shown a POAG patient with an evident deformation of the lamina cribrosa

Further Reading

1. Rao HL, Zangwill LM, Weinreb RN, Leite MT, Sample PA, Medeiros FA (2011) Structure-function relationship in glaucoma using spectral-domain optical coherence tomography. Arch Ophthalmol 129:864–871
2. Paunescu LA, Schuman JS, Price LL et al (2004) Reproducibility of nerve fiber thickness, macular thickness, and optic nerve head measurements using Stratus OCT. Invest Ophthalmol Vis Sci 45(6):1716–1724
3. Budenz DL, Chang RT, Huang X, Knighton RW, Tielsch JM (2005) Reproducibility of retinal nerve fiber thickness measurements using the Stratus OCT in normal and glaucomatous eyes. Invest Ophthalmol Vis Sci 46(7):2440–2443
4. Tzamalis A, Kynigopoulos M, Schlote T, Haefliger I (2009) Improved reproducibility of retinal nerve fiber layer thickness measurements with the repeat-scan protocol using the Stratus OCT in normal and glaucomatous eyes. Graefes Arch Clin Exp Ophthalmol 247(2):245–252
5. Smith M, Frost A, Graham CM, Shaw S (2007) Effect of pupillary dilatation on glaucoma assessments using optical coherence tomography. Br J Ophthalmol 91(12):1686–1690
6. Budenz DL, Fredette MJ, Feuer WJ, Anderson DR (2008) Reproducibility of peripapillary retinal nerve fiber thickness measurements with Stratus OCT in glaucomatous eyes. Ophthalmology 115(4):661–666
7. Barkana Y, Burgansky-Eliash Z, Gerber Y et al (2009) Interdevice variability of the Stratus optical coherence tomography. Am J Ophthalmol 147(2):260–266
8. Cheung CY, Leung CK, Lin D, Pang CP, Lam DS (2008) Relationship between retinal nerve fiber layer measurement and signal strength in optical coherence tomography. Ophthalmology 115(8):1347–1351
9. Mwanza JC, Chang RT, Budenz DL, Durbin MK, Gendy MG, Shi W, Feuer WJ (2010) Reproducibility of peripapillary retinal nerve fiber layer thickness and optic nerve head parameters measured with cirrus HD-OCT in glaucomatous eyes. Invest Ophthalmol Vis Sci 51(11):5724–5730
10. Vizzeri G, Weinreb RN, Gonzalez-Garcia AO, Bowd C, Medeiros FA, Sample PA, Zangwill LM (2009) Agreement between spectral-domain and time-domain OCT for measuring RNFL thickness. Br J Ophthalmol 93(6):775–781, 50. González-García AO, Vizzeri G, Bowd C, Medeiros FA, Zangwill LM, Weinreb RN (2009) Reproducibility of RTVue retinal nerve fiber layer thickness and optic disc measurements and agreement with Stratus optical coherence tomography measurements. Am J Ophthalmol 147(6):1067–1074
11. Kim JS, Ishikawa H, Sung KR et al (2009) Retinal nerve fiber layer thickness measure- ment reproducibility improved with spectral domain optical coherence tomography. Br J Ophthalmol 93(8):1057–1063, 52. Leung CK, Cheung CY, Weinreb RN et al (2009) Retinal nerve fiber layer imaging with spectral-domain optical coherence tomography: a variability and diagnostic per- formance study. Ophthalmology 116(7):1257–1263
12. Menke MN, Knecht P, Sturm V, Dabov S, Funk J (2008) Reproducibility of nerve fiber layer thickness measurements using 3D fourier-domain OCT. Invest Ophthalmol Vis Sci 49(12):5386–5391, 54. Garas A, Vargha P, Hollo G (2010) Reproducibility of RNFL and macular thickness meas- urements with RTVue-100 optical coherence tomograph. Ophthamology 117(4):738–746
13. Moreno-Montañés J, Olmo N, Alvarez A, García N, Zarranz-Ventura J (2010) Cirrus high-definition optical coherence tomography compared with Stratus optical coher- ence tomography in glaucoma diagnosis. Invest Ophthalmol Vis Sci 51(1):335–343
14. Seibold LK, Mandava N, Kahook MY (2010) Comparison of retinal nerve fiber layer thickness in normal eyes using time-domain and spectral-domain optical coherence tomography. Am J Ophthalmol 150(6):807
15. Sung KR, Kim DY, Park SB, Kook MS (2009) Comparison of retinal nerve fiber layer thickness measured by Cirrus HD and Stratus optical coherence tomography. Ophthalmology 116(7):1264–1270

16. Knight OJ, Chang RT, Feuer WJ, Budenz DL (2009) Comparison of retinal nerve fiber layer measurements using time domain and spectral domain optical coherent to- mography. Ophthalmology 116(7):1271–1277
17. Sehi M, Grewal DS, Sheets CW, Greenfield DS (2009) Diagnostic ability of Fourier- domain vs time-domain optical coherence tomography for glaucoma detection. Am J Ophthalmol 148(4):597–605
18. Mwanza JC, Oakley JD, Budenz DL et al (2011) Ability of Cirrus HD-OCT optic nerve head parameters to discriminate normal from glaucomatous eyes. Ophthalmology 118(2):241–248
19. Jeoung JW, Park KH (2010) Comparison of Cirrus OCT and Stratus OCT on the abil- ity to detect localized retinal nerve fiber layer defects in preperimetric glaucoma. Invest Ophthalmol Vis Sci 51(2):938–945
20. Park S, Sung K, Kang S et al (2009) Comparison of diagnostic glaucoma capabilities of Cirrus HD and stratus optical coherence tomograph. Arch Opththalmol 127(12):1603–1609
21. Sakata LM, Lavanya R, Friedman DS et al (2008) Comparison of gonioscopy and anterior segment ocular coherence tomography in detecting angle closure in different quadrants of the anterior chamber angle. Ophthalmology 115(5):769–774
22. Barkana Y, Dorairaj SK, Gerber Y, Liebmann JM, Ritch R (2007) Agreement between gonioscopy and ultrasound biomicroscopy in detecting iridotrabecular apposition. Arch Ophthalmol 125(10):1331–1335
23. Konstantopoulos A, Hossain P, Anderson DF (2007) Recent advances in ophthalmic anterior segment imaging: a new era for ophthalmic diagnosis?". Br J Ophthalmol 91(4):551–557
24. Radhakrishnan S, Rollins AM, Roth JE et al (2001) Realtime optical coherence tomography of the anterior segment at 1310 nm. Arch Ophthalmol 119(8):1179–1185
25. Radhakrishnan S, Goldsmith J, Huang D et al (2005) Comparison of optical coherence tomography and ultrasound biomicroscopy for detection of narrow anterior chamber angles. Arch Ophthalmol 123(8):1053–1059
26. Leung CKS, Li H, Weinreb RN et al (2008) Anterior chamber angle measurement with anterior segment optical coherence tomography: a comparison between slit lampOCT and visante OCT. Invest Ophthalmol Vis Sci 49(8):3469–3474
27. Sakata LM, Wong TTL, Wong HT et al (2010) Comparison of Visante and slit-lamp anterior segment optical coherence tomography in imaging the anterior chamber angle. Eye 24(4): 578–587
28. Li H, Leung CKS, Cheung CYL et al (2007) Repeatability and reproducibility of anterior chamber angle measurement with anterior segment optical coherence tomography. Br J Ophthalmol 91(11):1490–1497
29. Aptel F, Beccat S, Fortoul V, Denis P (2011) Biometric analysis of pigment dispersion syndrome using anterior segment optical coherence tomography. Ophthalmology 118(8):1563–1570
30. Singh M, Chew PTK, Friedman DS et al (2007) Imaging of trabeculectomy blebs using anterior segment optical coherence tomography. Ophthalmology 114(1):47–53
31. Leung CKS, Yick DWF, Kwong YYY et al (2007) Analysis of bleb morphology after trabeculectomy with Visante anterior segment optical coherence tomography. Br J Ophthalmol 91(3):340–344
32. Ishikawa H, Stein DM, Wollstein G, Beaton S, Fujimoto JG et al (2005) Macular segmentation with optical coherence tomography. Invest Ophthalmol Vis Sci 46:2012–2017
33. Tan O, Li G, Lu AT-H, Varma R, Huang D (2008) Mapping of macular substructures with optical coherence tomography for glaucoma diagnosis. Ophthalmology 115:949–956
34. Tan O, Chopra V, Lu AT-H, Schuman JS, Ishikawa H et al (2009) Detection of macular ganglion cell loss in glaucoma by Fourier-domain optical coherence tomography. Ophthalmology 116:2305–2314.e 2301–2302.
35. Kim NR, Lee ES, Seong GJ, Kim JH, An HG et al (2010) Structure-function relationship and diagnostic value of macular ganglion cell complex measurement using Fourier-domain OCT in glaucoma. Invest Ophthalmol Vis Sci 51:4646–4651
36. Raza AS, Cho J, de Moraes CGV, Wang M, Zhang X et al (2011) Retinal ganglion cell layer thickness and local visual field sensitivity in glaucoma. Arch Ophthalmol 129:1529–1536

37. Shin HY, Park HY, Jung KI, Park CK (2013) Comparative study of macular ganglion cell inner plexiform layer and retinal nerve fiber layer measurement: structure-function analysis. Invest Ophthalmol Vis Sci 54(12):7344–7353
38. Takahashi M, Omodaka K, Maruyama K, Yamaguchi T, Himori N et al (2013) Simulated visual fields produced from macular RNFLT data in patients with glaucoma. Curr Eye Res 38:1133–1141
39. Sato S, Hirooka K, Baba T, Tenkumo K, Nitta E et al (2013) Correlation between the ganglion cell-inner plexiform layer thickness measured with cirrus HD-OCT and macular visual field sensitivity measured with microperimetry. Invest Ophthalmol Vis Sci 54:3046–3051
40. Akagi T, Hangai M, Takayama K, Nonaka A, Ooto S et al (2012) In vivo imaging of lamina cribrosa pores by adaptive optics scanning laser ophthalmoscopy. Invest Ophthalmol Vis Sci 53:4111–4119
41. Inoue R, Hangai M, Kotera Y, Nakanishi H, Mori S et al (2009) Threedimensional high-speed optical coherence tomography imaging of lamina cribrosa in glaucoma. Ophthalmology 116:214–222
42. Ivers KM, Li C, Patel N, Sredar N, Luo X et al (2011) Reproducibility of measuring lamina cribrosa pore geometry in human and nonhuman primates with in vivo adaptive optics imaging. Invest Ophthalmol Vis Sci 52:5473–5480
43. Lee EJ, Kim T-W, Weinreb RN, Suh MH, Kang M et al (2012) Three-dimensional evaluation of the lamina cribrosa using spectral-domain optical coherence tomography in glaucoma. Invest Ophthalmol Vis Sci 53:198–204
44. Kiumehr S, Park SC, Syril D, Teng CC, Tello C et al (2012) In vivo evaluation of focal lamina cribrosa defects in glaucoma. Arch Ophthalmol 130:552–559
45. Nadler Z, Wang B, Wollstein G, Nevins JE, Ishikawa H et al (2013) Automated lamina cribrosa microstructural segmentation in optical coherence tomography scans of healthy and glaucomatous eyes. Biomed Opt Express 4:2596–2608

Chapter 10
Measuring Hemoglobin Levels in the Optic Nerve Head for Glaucoma Management

Manuel Gonzalez-de-la-Rosa, Marta Gonzalez-Hernandez, Carmen Mendez-Hernandez, Elena Garcia-Martin, Francisco Fumero-Bautista, Silvia Alayon, and Jose Sigut

10.1 Introduction

The color of the optic nerve head (ONH) is mainly due to its hemoglobin content. The ganglion cell axons may not have myelin at this level. Like the rest of the retina, this tissue is virtually transparent to radiation of the visible spectrum. In the rest of the retina, light is eventually absorbed by photoreceptors and the pigmentary epithelium, but in the ONH the light is reflected by the myelin in the lamina cribrosa. Part of it is absorbed by hemoglobin in the capillaries that nourish the axons, giving rise to the pink color of the ONH. The greater the thickness of the tissue or its concentration of hemoglobin, the more intense the color, and the thinner the tissue or the less abundance of blood, the whiter it will appear (Fig. 10.1).

In a color photograph of the ONH, the results also depend on additional factors such as the chromatic response of the camera's detector, the spectral composition of the illumination light and absorption by the lens, which is more pronounced in blue and increases with age or the presence of cataracts.

To determine the amount of hemoglobin present in the ONH, using a photographic color image, all these factors must be taken into account. Fortunately, we have a structure in the nerve itself that can serve as a reference; this structure is the network of

M. Gonzalez-de-la-Rosa (✉) • M. Gonzalez-Hernandez
Department of Ophthalmology, Hospital Universitario de Canarias, University of La Laguna, La Laguna, Spain
e-mail: mgdelarosa@telefonica.net

C. Mendez-Hernandez
Department of Ophthalmology, Hospital Clinico San Carlos, University Complutense of Madrid, Madrid, Spain

E. Garcia-Martin
Department of Ophthalmology, Hospital Universitario Miguel Servet, Zaragoza, Spain

F. Fumero-Bautista • S. Alayon • J. Sigut
Department of Systems Engineering, University of La Laguna, La Laguna, Spain

A. Ferreras (ed.), *Glaucoma Imaging*, DOI 10.1007/978-3-319-18959-8_10

central retinal vessels carrying hemoglobin. On comparing the color of neuronal tissue and that of these vessels, one can estimate the amount of hemoglobin in each region of tissue with little influence of the additional factors listed in the previous paragraph.

Hemoglobin absorbs more green radiation than red. It can be shown experimentally that for a relatively thin structure such as the ONH, the ratio of green component to red ((R-G)/R) is proportional to its thickness or its hematic content. Measuring this ratio in each zone of the tissue and taking the same measurement in the main vessels as a reference, one can obtain a representative map of local amounts of hemoglobin. This is very probably the most important factor for ONH perfusion. Other parameters to consider include the degree of oxygenation and the rate of blood circulation (Fig. 10.2).

The Laguna ONhE program (Optic Nerve Hemoglobin; insoftsl@gmail.com ©) allows measuring the amounts of hemoglobin present in the structures of the ONH, analyzing photographs captured by a fundus camera that has been appropriately calibrated. The program has demonstrated its capacity for the diagnosis and interpretation of glaucomatous damage, as well as other types of neurological damage such as that seen in multiple sclerosis or Parkinson's disease.

In the text that follows, we will describe the use of the program and provide some examples of practical results.

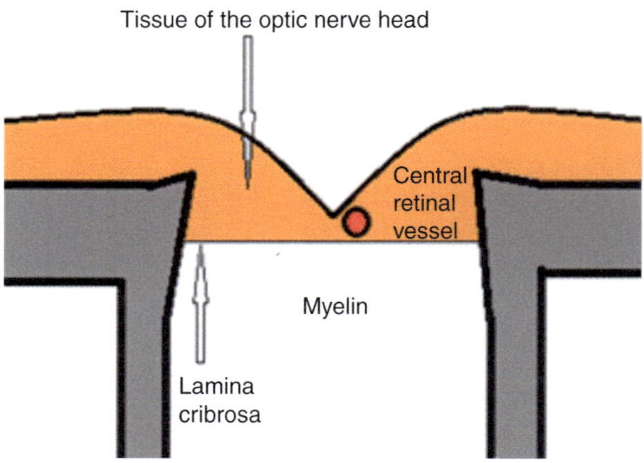

Fig. 10.1 The *pink color* of the optic nerve head depends on the hemoglobin contained in its capillaries. The observation light is reflected on the myelin, and that not absorbed by hemoglobin, mainly *red*, reaches the observer

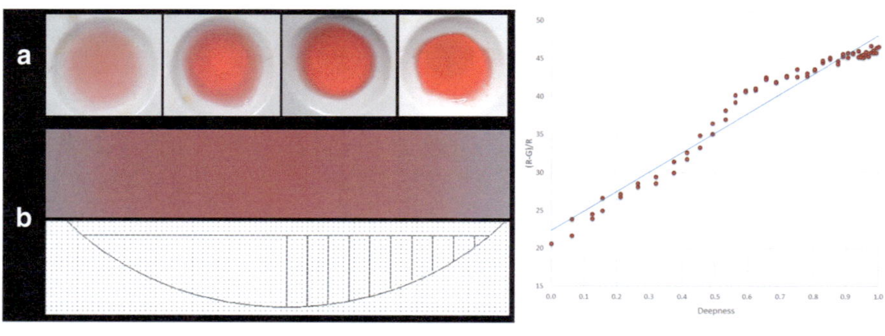

Fig. 10.2 If one photographs microplate wells containing dilutions of hemoglobin (**a**), the red and green components of the image will be proportional to the concentration and depth (**b**) of the layer through which the light passes, as shown in the graph on the right

10.2 Image Capture of the ONH and Delimitation of Boundaries, Vessels, and Cup

When a fundus image is captured with the intention of examining the retina, the ONH image often appears too white, without details. This is because it is a much paler structure than the rest of the fundus. For useful results and visualization of ONH details, it is necessary to underexpose the photograph, using a flash of lower intensity than usual. In a very bright image, the color levels of the camera detector reach their maximum value (255) and this saturation prevents seeing the chromatic characteristics of the tissue.

Initial versions of the Laguna ONhE program required manual definition of the ONH boundaries. Delimitation of the cup was not possible and, therefore, the ONH was divided into 24 regular sections by two circular lines at 1/3 and 2/3 of the radius, and four regularly spaced diameters. Analysis of all these sectors allowed us to calculate a glaucoma discriminant function (GDF) that has been shown to be useful for detecting the presence of perfusion defects characteristic of glaucoma, particularly affecting sectors 8 and 20. It even allows us to estimate the vertical cup/disc ratio without defining their precise form (Fig. 10.3).

A second version of the program allowed us to transpose the cup and disc boundaries obtained with OCT to a photographic image of the ONH, so that we could separately determine the amount of hemoglobin in the cup and in the various sectors of the neuroretinal rim (Fig. 10.4). Another version exploited the delimitation of these structures performed with a stereoscopic fundus camera to obtain similar information.

More recently these advances have allowed us to establish a relationship between the distribution of hemoglobin and the size and shape of the cup, so it has been possible to define its boundaries with great precision, without the need for OCT information or stereoscopic photography, simply using a conventional photograph.

Applying methods of image segmentation based on color patterns and identification of the components compatible with the shape of the ONH, it has been possible to automatically establish the boundaries of the ONH in 90 % of cases, without operator intervention. With the image of the ONH on the screen, a click of the mouse on the center of the ONH cues the program to automatically suggest the boundaries of the cup and disc, which must be accepted by the user (Fig. 10.5).

Incorrect delimitation of the boundaries with this automatic method is rare, but can occur especially in cases with areas of atrophy close to the ONH or other unusual morphology. In these cases the user can rectify the disc boundaries at their discretion. To do so an ellipse is projected on the ONH. The center of the ellipse and its shape can be changed using the mouse, until it fits the boundaries. When this configuration is confirmed, multiple points appear on radial axes, which can be adjusted one by one to fit the exact shape of the ONH (Fig. 10.6).

Once the ONH boundaries have been established, estimation of the cup is performed automatically in all cases, since automatic delimitation is generally more accurate than anything the user can achieve on a two-dimensional image. Similarly, internally, the program performs an automatic delimitation of the central retinal artery and vein and its main branches, excluding tissue information, and for use as a reference value of hemoglobin.

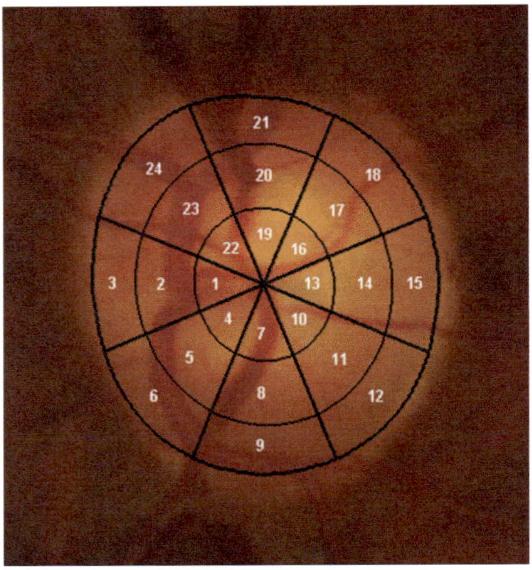

Fig. 10.3 Example of segmentation of the ONH in 24 sectors

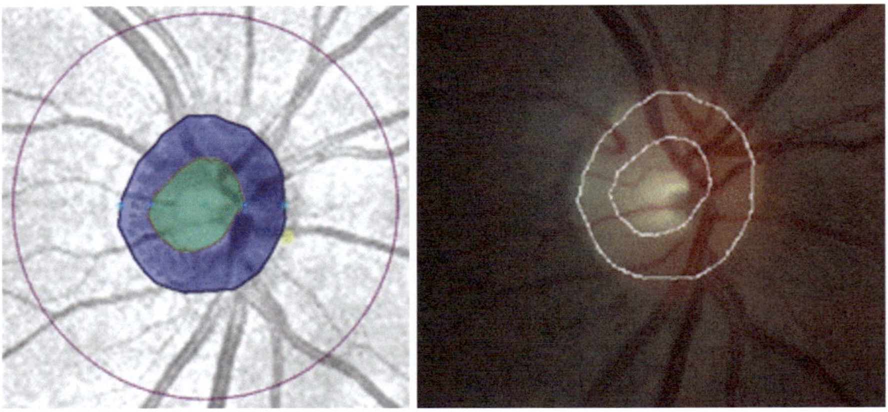

Fig. 10.4 Fusion of an OCT image (*left*) and a photograph of the ONH (*right*) to delimit the boundaries of the cup and disc

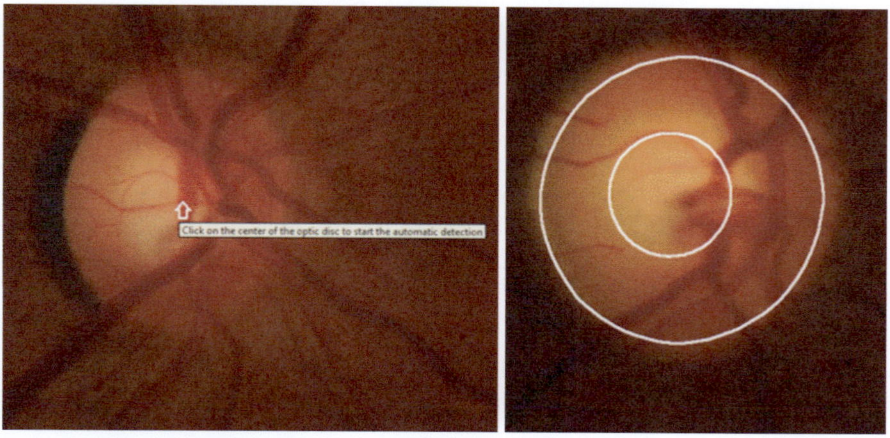

Fig. 10.5 By clicking on the center of the image (*left*), one obtains the cup and disc boundaries (*right*) which must be accepted

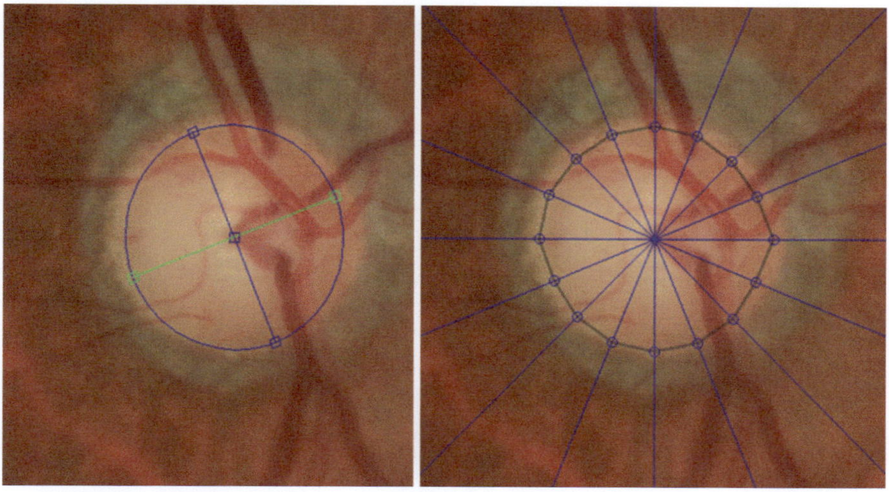

Fig. 10.6 Approximate delimitation using an ellipse (*left*) and fine-tuning using multiple radial points (*right*)

10.3 Hemoglobin Map

After boundary delimitation, the program automatically interprets whether the image is of a right or left eye, asking for user confirmation. It then shows the representative map of the presence of hemoglobin in each region of the ONH. A chromatic scale identifies these amounts of hemoglobin in percentages; 100 % corresponds to the central vessels of the retina. Warmer colors represent high densities of hemoglobin and cooler colors represent areas of lower perfusion or thin tissue, as in the case of cup (Figs. 10.7 and 10.8).

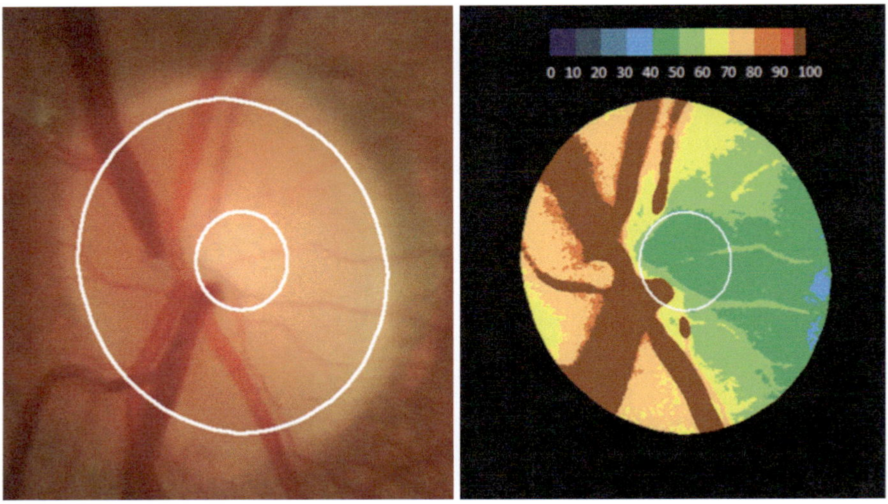

Fig. 10.7 Example of a hemoglobin map in a normal subject, with disc and cup delimitation

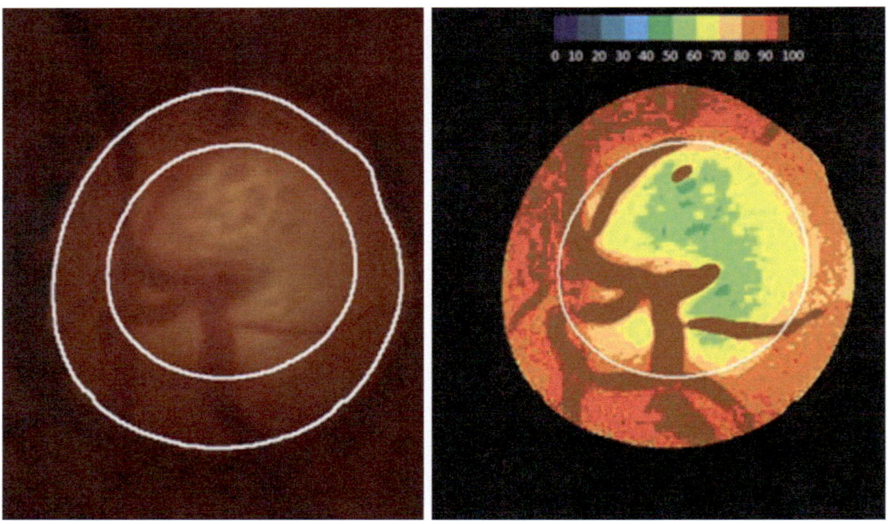

Fig. 10.8 Example of a hemoglobin map in glaucoma

10.4 Glaucoma Discriminant Function (GDF)

In glaucoma, it is well known that there is often greater deterioration of the ONH in areas close to the superior and inferior pole regions. Indeed, using the Laguna ONhE program, lower perfusion is usually found in the vicinity of its central vertical diameter, especially in the extreme and intermediate zones (e.g., sectors 8 and 20), as the subject loses tissue in the neuroretinal rim. Other regions, such as the temporal rim region (Sector 15), are more resistant to glaucomatous damage, which in effect show less impairment of perfusion.

The topographic distributions of hemoglobin allow us to estimate the vertical ratio cup/disc ratio as well as an index called "glaucoma discriminant function" (GDF) which has been shown to have high diagnostic capacity. This index tends to be positive in normal subjects and negative in glaucomatous subjects, which is useful for monitoring the disease. It has been adjusted for a specificity close to 95 %, so that negative values are infrequent in normal subjects, and highly negative values very infrequent (Figs. 10.9, 10.10 and 10.11).

Although the program attempts to compensate for the presence of cataracts, this circumstance may occasionally cause slight overestimation of hemoglobin. Moderate opacification of the lens has a negligible effect. Only with cataracts that require surgical intervention does this overestimation reach approximately 3–4 %. However, estimated cup/disc ratio and GDF index are not affected by the presence of this type of cataract (Fig. 10.12).

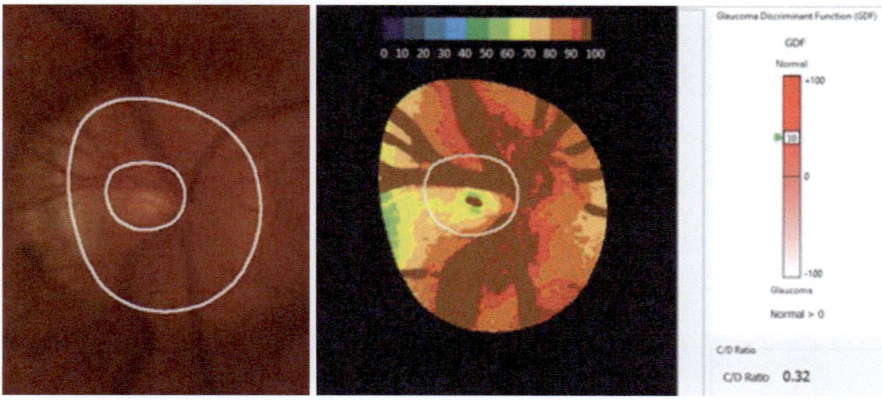

Fig. 10.9 Hemoglobin map and GDF in a normal case

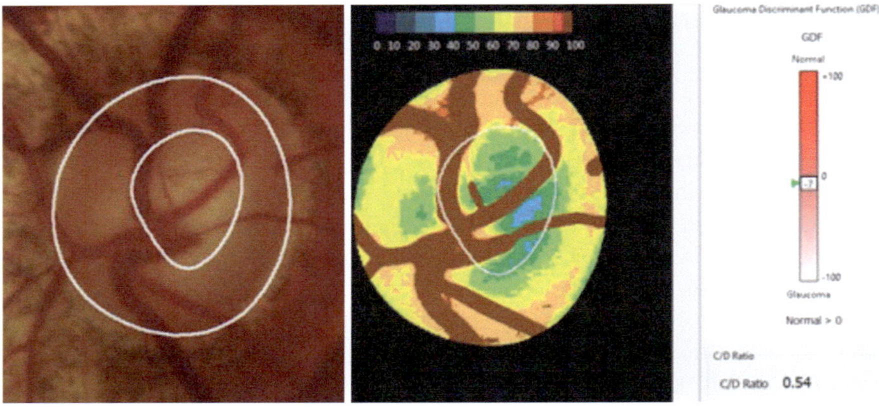

Fig. 10.10 Hemoglobin map and GDF in early glaucoma

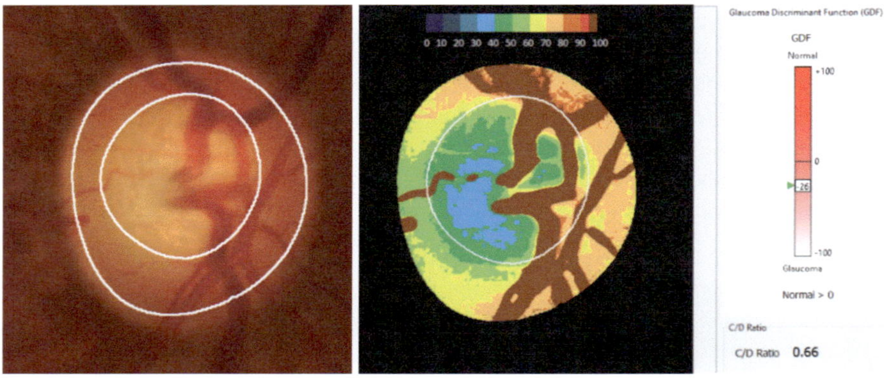

Fig. 10.11 Hemoglobin map and GDF in advanced glaucoma

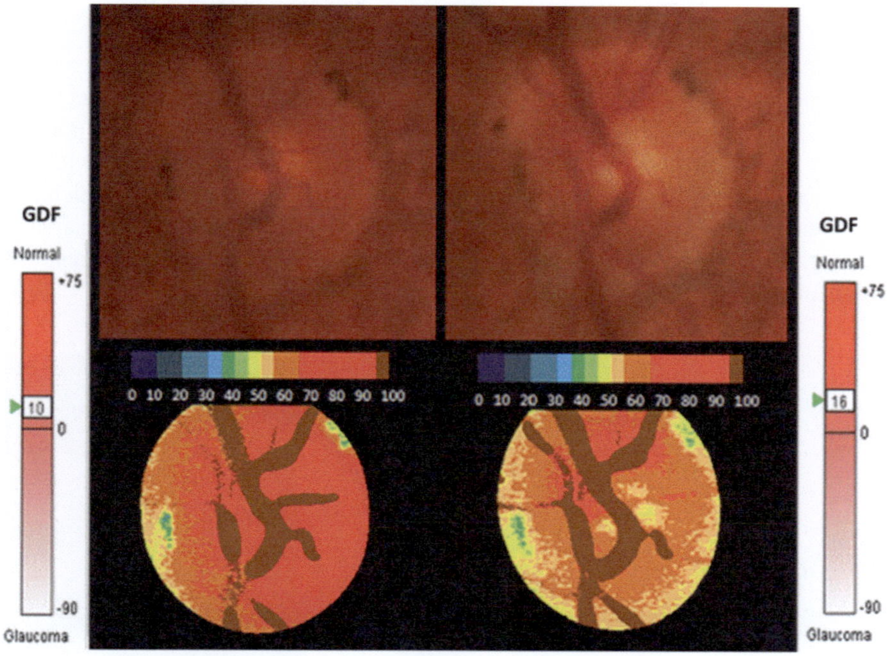

Fig. 10.12 Hemoglobin map and GDF before and after cataract operation in a patient with a normal optic nerve

10.5 Rim Hemoglobin

The program also provides information on the amount of hemoglobin present in the eight sectors into which the rim is usually divided, compared to the normal population. It has been shown that these perfusion data are better correlated with the patient's visual field sensitivity than mere measurement of the rim area, which can be obtained using OCT, for example. It has also been shown that rim surface area in many glaucoma patients is not only lost, but that hemoglobin content in the residual rim is often lower than normal (Fig. 10.13).

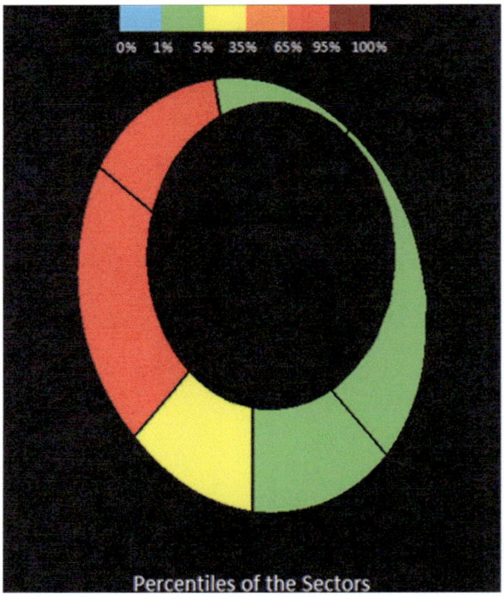

Fig. 10.13 Figure showing the percentile of rim hemoglobin data in the patient mentioned in Fig. 10.11, with respect to the normal population

10.6 TSNI Diagram

Another way to view the results is a diagram similar to that usually used to represent the thickness of the nerve fiber layer around the ONH. In this case the amount of hemoglobin present in the neuroretinal rim is represented starting with the temporal region and followed by the superior, nasal, and inferior regions (TSNI). The diagram simultaneously shows color-coded percentiles of these densities in the normal population, so they can be compared with those of the subject (Fig. 10.14).

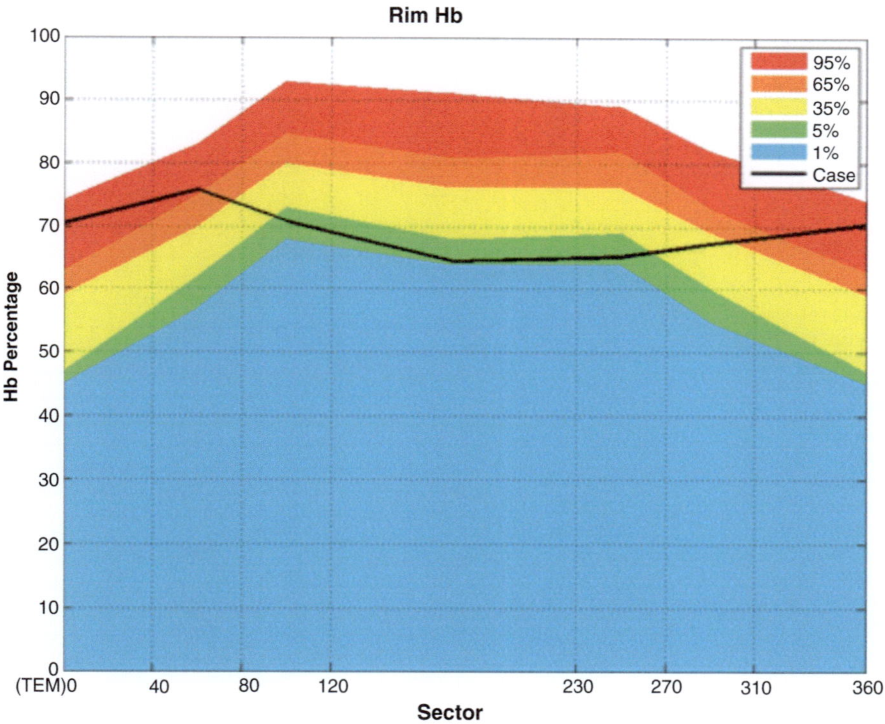

Fig. 10.14 TSNI diagram showing the amounts of hemoglobin in the rim of the same glaucomatous subject mentioned in Figs. 10.11 and 10.13

10.7 Sector Hemoglobin: Numerical Data

To calculate the GDF index and the vertical cup/disc ratio, the program divides the ONH into 24 sectors as previously described. The amounts of hemoglobin in each of these sectors, as well as those in the 8 sectors of the rim, are displayed in the form of a table, which also shows their percentile relative to that of the normal population (Fig. 10.15).

This information may be useful in other diseases such as optic neuritis where reduced perfusion may be found in different regions from those affected in glaucoma. In multiple sclerosis, for example, reduced perfusion is most frequently observed in area 15 or the temporal rim, which is not usually the case in glaucoma (Fig. 10.16).

Mean Hb		Percentiles of the Hb					
		0 - 1%	1 - 5%	5 - 35%	35 - 65%	65 - 95%	95 - 100%
Total	60.9			60.9			
Cup Hb	54.0			54.0			
Sector 311-40º (T)	70.4					70.4	
Sector 41-80º	75.8					75.8	
Sector 81-120º	70.9		70.9				
Sector 121-230º	64.4		64.4				
Sector 231-270º	65.2		65.2				
Sector 271-310º	67.3			67.3			
Sector 1	65.8			65.8			
Sector 2	55.6	55.6					
Sector 3 (N)	65.6			65.6			
Sector 4	68.1			68.1			
Sector 5	50.1	50.1					
Sector 6 (NI)	69.0			69.0			
Sector 7	68.0				68.0		
Sector 8	61.1			61.1			
Sector 9 (I)	75.0			75.0			
Sector 10	55.7				55.7		
Sector 11	64.4					64.4	
Sector 12 (TI)	71.4					71.4	
Sector 13	54.6				54.6		
Sector 14	64.0					64.0	
Sector 15 (T)	73.5						73.5
Sector 16	53.1			53.1			
Sector 17	62.0				62.0		
Sector 18 (TS)	78.7					78.7	
Sector 19	43.8			43.8			
Sector 20	49.5	49.5					
Sector 21 (S)	66.3	66.3					
Sector 22	48.9			48.9			
Sector 23	44.0	44.0					
Sector 24 (NS)	56.6	56.6					

Fig. 10.15 Table showing numerical results of the previous case

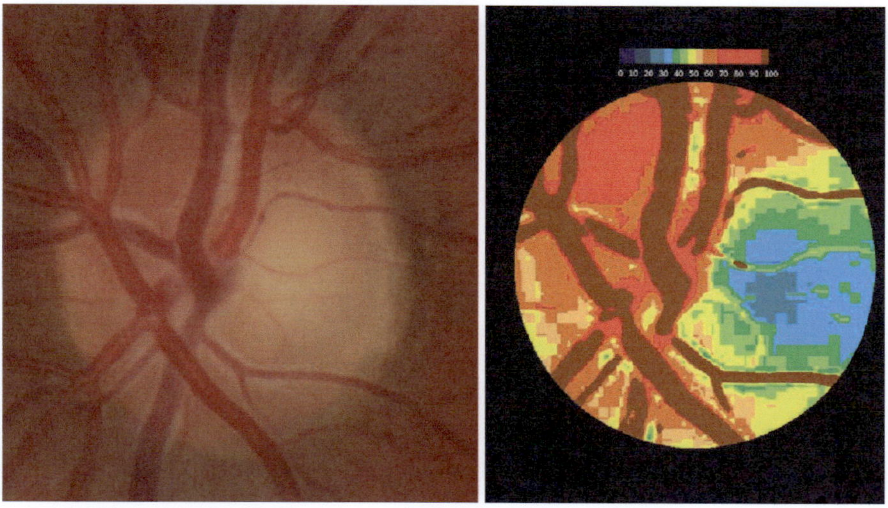

Fig. 10.16 Temporal perfusion defect in a case of optic neuritis due to multiple sclerosis

10.8 Data Export and Analysis

The total and sectorial index results and the diagnostic results of each test can be exported to an Excel file and printed out. This also facilitates statistical analysis of the results. The Excel spreadsheet includes graphic representations of patient data, which can be used in workshops and presentations (Fig. 10.17).

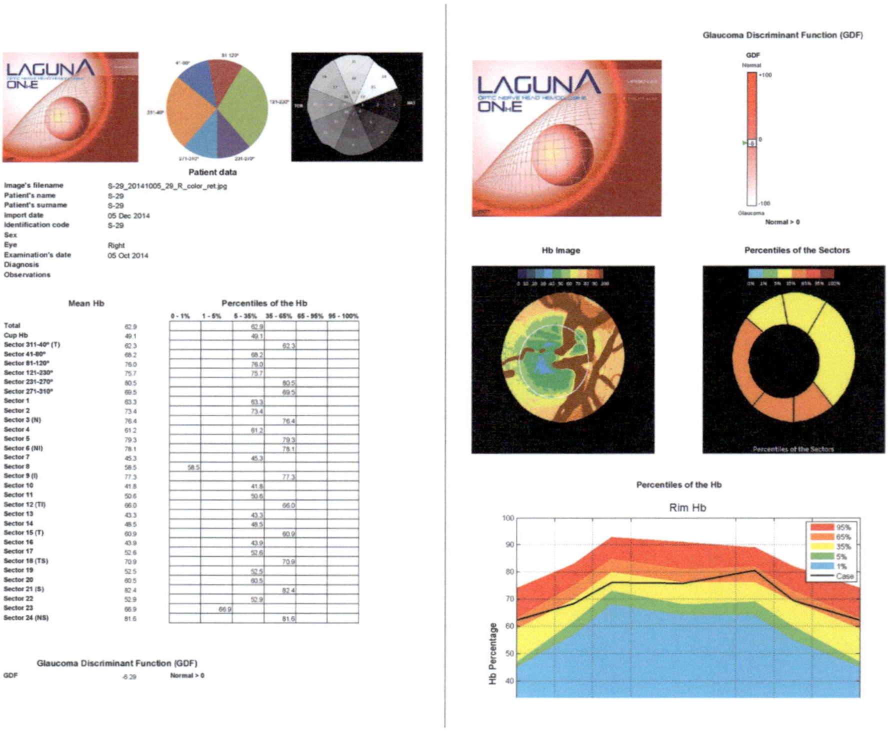

Fig. 10.17 Excel sheets showing results

10.9 Follow-Up

From the database of images for each patient, the tests can be recovered for overall analysis, and progression of the GDF index can be estimated by linear regression analysis (Fig. 10.18).

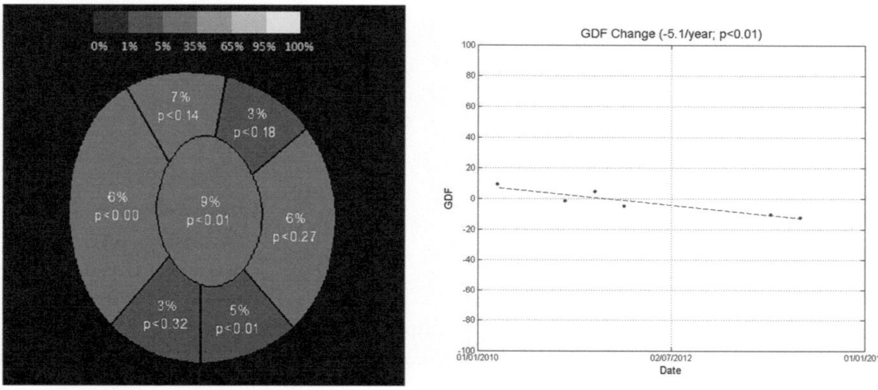

Fig. 10.18 Graphic representation of change in the amount of hemoglobin (*left*) and progression of GDF values (*right*)

Further Reading

1. Gonzalez de la Rosa M, Gonzalez-Hernandez M, Sigut J et al (2013) Measuring hemoglobin levels in the optic nerve head: comparisons with other structural and functional parameters of glaucoma. Invest Ophthalmol Vis Sci 54(1):482–489
2. Denniss J (2013) Estimation of hemoglobin levels in the optic nerve head for glaucoma management. Invest Ophthalmol Vis Sci 54(2):1515
3. Gonzalez de la Rosa M, Gonzalez-Hernandez M, Sigut J et al (2013) Author response: estimation of hemoglobin levels in the optic nerve head for glaucoma management. Invest Ophthalmol Vis Sci 54(3):2011–2012
4. Bambo MP, Garcia-Martin E, Perez-Olivan S et al (2013) Diagnostic ability of a new method for measuring haemoglobin levels in the optic nerve head in multiple sclerosis patients. Br J Ophthalmol 97(12):1543–1548
5. Bambo M, Garcia-Martin E, Perez-Olivan S et al (2014) Detecting optic atrophy in multiple sclerosis patients using new colorimetric analysis software: from idea to application. Semin Ophthalmol:1–4. doi:10.3109/08820538.2014.962171
6. Mendez-Hernandez C, Garcia-Feijoo J, Arribas-Pardo P et al (2014) Reproducibility of optic nerve head hemoglobin measures. J Glaucoma. 27 Oct 2014 [Epub ahead of print]. PMID: 25350818
7. Bambo MP, Garcia-Martin E, Satue M et al (2014) Measuring hemoglobin levels in the optic disc of Parkinson's disease patients using new colorimetric analysis software. Parkinsons Dis 2014:946540
8. Pena-Betancor C, Gonzalez-Hernandez M, Fumero-Batista F et al (2015) Estimation of the relative amount of hemoglobin in the cup and neuroretinal rim using stereoscopic color fundus images. Invest Ophthalmol Vis Sci 56(3):1562–1568
9. Bambo MP, Garcia-Martin E, Gutierrez-Ruiz F et al (2015) Analysis of optic disk color changes in Alzheimer's disease: a potential new biomarker. Clin Neurol Neurosurg 132:68–73

Chapter 11
Structure and Function Relationship in Glaucoma

Rizwan Malik and David F. Garway-Heath

11.1 Introduction

A clinician's assessment of a patient with glaucoma is based on risk assessment for disease (or disease progression), assimilation and integration of the results of visual field and imaging investigations with clinical findings. In some patients, this can be challenging. The decision-making process can be facilitated by an understanding of how visual field and structural measures are related and an understanding of reasons for discrepancy between the results of visual field and structural assessment. The aim of this chapter is to provide such an understanding. This chapter is formatted as a series of questions so that the reader can target areas most relevant to their interest or need.

R. Malik
Department of Glaucoma Theme, NIHR Biomedical Research Centre for Ophthalmology at Moorfields Eye Hospital and UCL Institute of Ophthalmology, London, UK
e-mail: rizimalik@googlemail.com

D.F. Garway-Heath (✉)
Department of Glaucoma Theme, NIHR Biomedical Research Centre for Ophthalmology at Moorfields Eye Hospital NHS Foundation Trust and UCL Institute of Ophthalmology, London, UK
e-mail: david.garway-heath@moorfields.nhs.uk

A. Ferreras (ed.), *Glaucoma Imaging*, DOI 10.1007/978-3-319-18959-8_11

11.2 How Is the Anatomy of the Retina and Optic Nerve Related?

A basic knowledge of optic nerve anatomy is helpful in predicting the location of visual field defects which arise from glaucomatous damage to the optic nerve head (also referred to as 'optic disc').

Retinal ganglion cells receive their input from amacrine and bipolar cells in the retina, which in turn receive their inputs from the photoreceptor cells (Fig. 11.1). The retinal ganglion cells are located in the ganglion cell layer, the innermost layer of the retina.

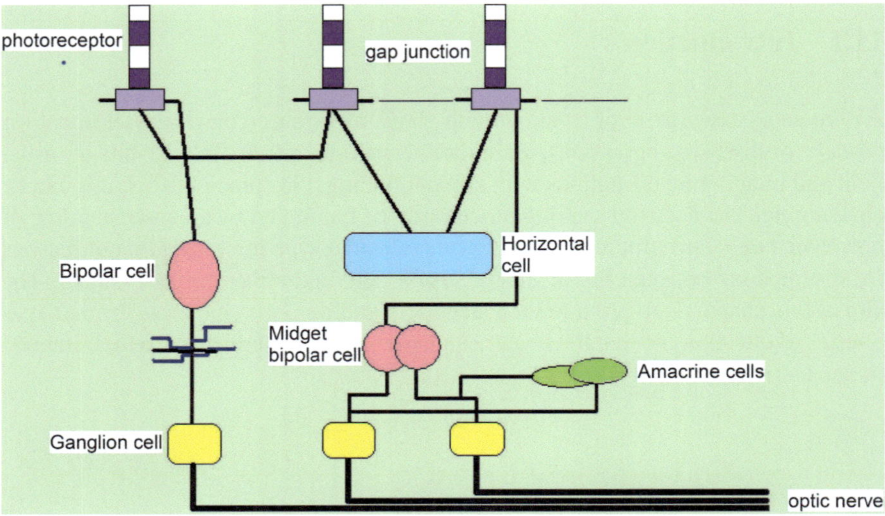

Fig. 11.1 Simplified diagram of the retina. The retinal ganglion cells receive their input from photoreceptor cells in their retina via a number of intermediate cells in the retina

The retinal ganglion cell axons travel forward towards the vitreous, turn direction to lie in the nerve fibre layer on the retinal surface, before entering the optic nerve head. Throughout the retina, there is a regular topographic arrangement, so that the fibres from the temporal retina enter the temporal optic nerve and fibres from the nasal retina enter the nasal optic nerve. The course of the nerve fibres in the retina varies depending on the location in the retina: the fibres in the temporal part of the retina tend to be arcuate and take a path around the fovea, above and below the temporal raphe; those in the nasal retina tend to radiate radially. The fibres travelling between the perifoveal region and the optic nerve form the papillomacular bundle (Fig. 11.2).

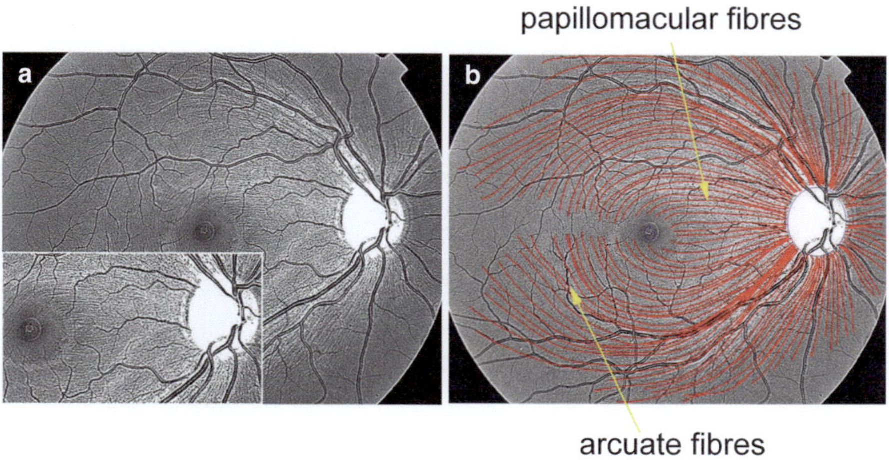

Fig. 11.2 (**a**) Retinal photograph taken with a blue filter with digital enhancement; (**b**) retinal nerve fibre bundles which have been traced back from the retina to their entry into the optic nerve [1]

11.3 What Is the 'Optic Nerve Head'?

The *optic nerve head* is composed of the surface nerve fibre layer, as well as the prelaminar, laminar and retrolaminar portions of the optic nerve [2] (Fig. 11.3). The optic disc and surface of the nerve fibre layer is visible clinically when examining the retina. The prelaminar and laminar portions of the nerve contain significant amount of glial tissue and connective tissue which contribute to residual rim tissue in advanced glaucoma. The lamina cribrosa is an important site of injury in glaucoma.

Spectral domain ocular coherence tomography of the optic nerve head has given new insights into the structures which correspond to the clinically viewed nerve head margin [3] (also see Fig. 11.14).

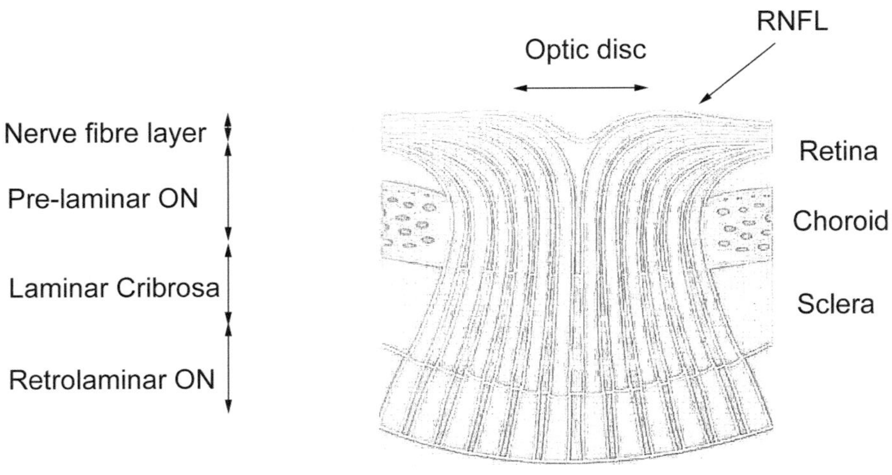

Fig. 11.3 Diagram of the optic nerve head. *ON* optic nerve, *RNFL* retinal nerve fibre layer

11.4 What Are the Pathophysiological Processes at a Cellular Level Responsible for Glaucoma?

Death of retinal ganglion cells and related axons from glaucomatous injury is multifactorial. Mechanical and ischaemic injury, in part from raised intraocular pressure, are key mechanisms. Abnormal immunity, inflammatory mediators and excessive glutamate production may also contribute [4] (Fig. 11.4).

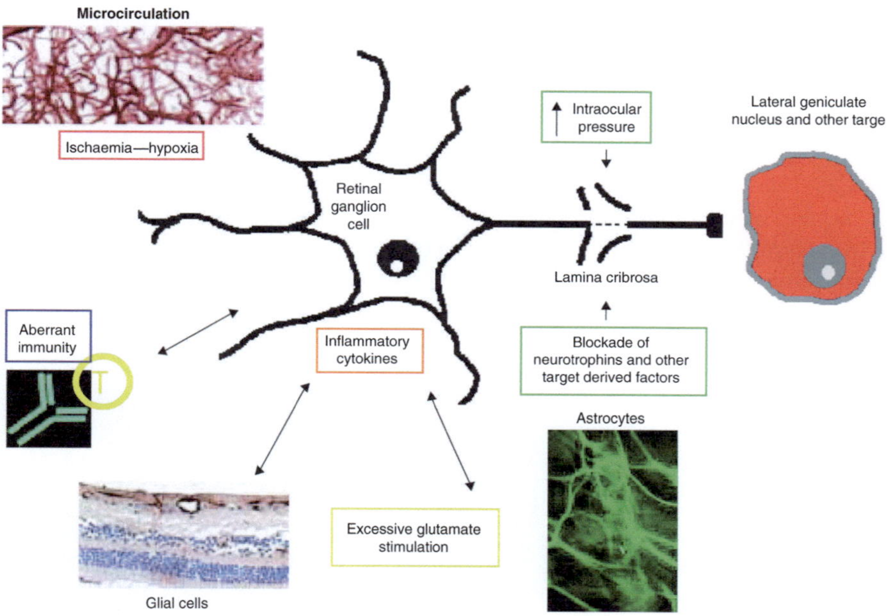

Fig. 11.4 Mechanisms of retinal ganglion cell death in glaucoma [4]. Reproduced from the *Lancet*, with permission from Elsevier

11.5 What Are Structural Measures for Glaucoma Assessment?

A structural measure for glaucoma assessment refers to measurements of the neuroretinal rim, retinal nerve fibre layer (RNFL) and the ganglion cell layer in the macula. The diagnosis of glaucoma is based on structural changes to the optic disc, specifically an enlargement of the optic disc cup and narrowing of the neuroretinal rim, with thinning of the RNFL which may be visible ophthalmoscopically. With advancing glaucoma, the neuroretinal rim exhibits progressive narrowing.

Whilst clinical examination of the optic disc and RNFL is essential, agreement between clinicians is often poor [5]. In other words, whilst one clinician may recognise an optic disc as glaucomatous, another may classify the same optic disc as healthy. Imaging of the optic disc and nerve fibre layer provides a more objective method of structural assessment. There are various imaging methods available, from optic disc photography to high resolution ocular coherence tomography (OCT), Fig. 11.6. Imaging modalities have been discussed in Chapters 7, 8, and 9. A number of measurements are provided by these devices. *Neuroretinal rim area* (*RA*) and *RNFL thickness*, and more recently *ganglion cell layer thickness*, are the most common structural measures used for comparison with functional measures.

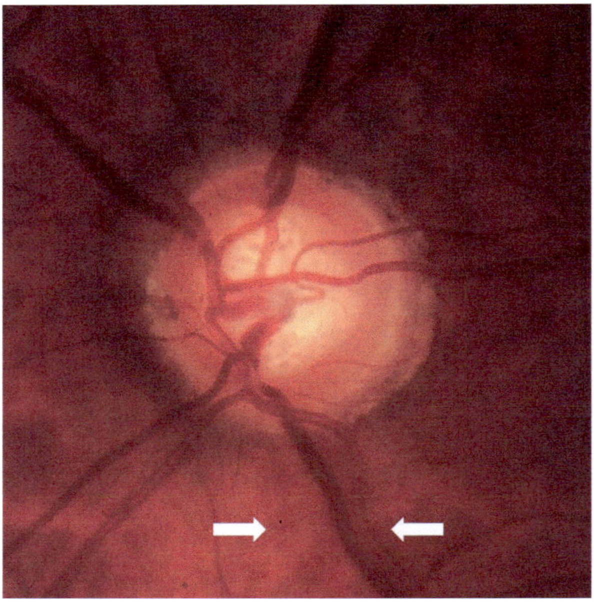

Fig. 11.5 Photograph of an optic disc with early inferior rim narrowing and a subtle retinal nerve fibre layer defect (*arrows*)

11.6 What Are Functional Measures for Glaucoma Assessment?

A variety of psychophysical and electrophysiological tests can be used to test the functional integrity of the visual system (Fig. 11.6). In clinical practice, visual field examination is the most widely used test and, for many, functional assessment in glaucoma is synonymous with visual field examination.

Although there are different forms of visual field test, standard automated perimetry is most common in clinical practice. This utilises a 'white' light on a less bright 'white background' to measure retinal sensitivity (in decibels, dB) at multiple locations. Glaucoma is characterised by defects (loss of sensitivity) in the visual field (Fig. 11.7); examination of the visual field is mandatory in patients who have, or are suspected to have, glaucoma. The location, shape, extent and depth of visual field defects depend on the location of optic disc damage and the stage of disease [6].

Tests to evaluate structure of the ONH		Tests to evaluate function of the ONH	
Test	**Example(s)**	**Test**	**Example(s)**
Stereoscopic Optic Nerve Head Photography	Donaldson camera Nidek 3Dx camera	**Visual acuity**	Snellen, LogMAR
Optic Nerve Head Morphometry-Planmietry	Discam	**Contrast sensitivity**	Pelli-Robson contrast sensitivity
Confocal scanning laser tomography	Heidelberg retinal tomograph, HRT	**Perimetry**	Standard automated (achromatic) perimetry Frequency doubling perimetry High-resolution perimetry Motion perimetry
		Colour vision	Ishihara colour plates
Scanning laser polarimetry	GDx	**Pupillometry**	RAPDx, ISCAN Pupillometry System
Ocular coherence tomography, OCT	Time-domain (Stratus OCT3) Fourier-domain / Spectral-domain OCT (Heidelberg Spectralis, RTVue, Cirrus)	**Electrophysiology**	Pattern electroretinogram Multifocal visual evoked potential Photopic negative response of flash ERG

Fig. 11.6 Structural and functional tests for glaucoma

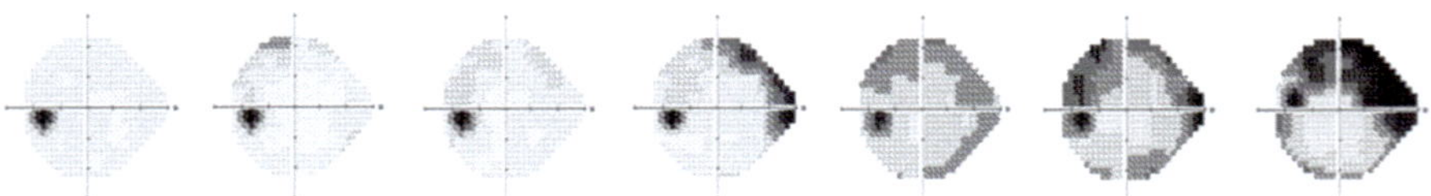

Fig. 11.7 Progressive visual field loss in glaucoma

11.7 Why Are Both Structure and Function Needed to Quantify Glaucoma?

Loss of retinal ganglion cells and related axons is associated with both structural damage and visual field loss in glaucoma and so it would be reasonable to expect a relationship between structure and function throughout the course of disease. In advanced glaucoma, structural and functional abnormalities are usually both apparent and there is high agreement between abnormal structure and abnormal function [7]. However, in earlier stages, identification of abnormality is often challenging. Structural abnormality may be detected before visual field abnormality in some patients whilst reproducible visual field loss may be detected first in other patients (Fig. 11.8) [8, 9]. This 'structure-function dissociation' has been demonstrated in a number of large studies in glaucoma (Fig. 11.9) [10–12].

There are a number of reasons for this seeming dissociation. Firstly, structural abnormality is often difficult to ascertain in optic discs which are abnormally large, small or tilted. In such patients, visual field abnormality may be the first detectable sign of glaucoma. Secondly, the agreement of abnormal structural and functional measures depends on the criteria used to define abnormality (Fig. 11.10).

Thirdly, both structural and [14], functional tests have significant test-retest variability [15, 16]. That is, a patient may have an abnormal result on one test, but a normal result on a subsequent test, and vice versa. For instance, in the Ocular Hypertension Treatment Study (OHTS), many patients who had developed reproducible glaucomatous visual field defects in two consecutive tests later performed a visual field test that was within normal limits [17]. The variability of visual field examination can be high (Fig. 11.11), especially in patients with established visual field loss [16]. In such patients, careful structural evaluation may provide the first reliable and consistent signs of glaucoma. More recently, it has become clear that the test-retest variability of structural measures can also be substantial [18]. When the results of structural and functional tests are consistent with the clinical impression, additional weight to the diagnosis is added. However, when the results of investigations are not consistent with clinical impression, tests should be repeated in the first instance. Interpretation of clinical investigations for glaucoma is further discussed below.

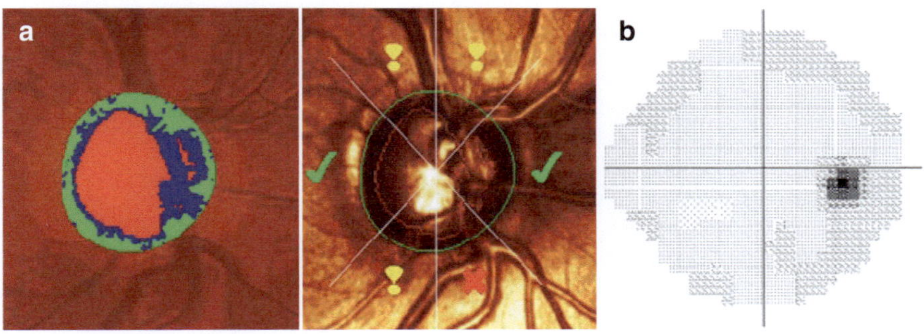

Fig. 11.8 'Structure-function dissociation': patient with (**a**) abnormal structure with confocal scanning laser tomography and (**b**) normal visual field

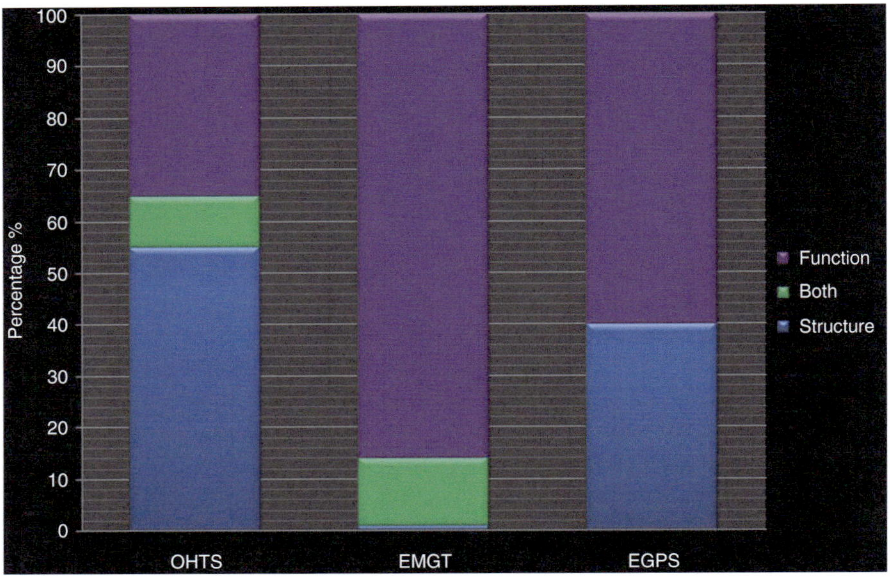

Fig. 11.9 Results of large studies showing the percentage of patients who first develop visual field or optic disc change (as defined by study criteria). *EGPS* European Glaucoma Prevention Study, *EMGT* Early Manifest Glaucoma Trial, *OHTS* Ocular Hypertension Treatment Study

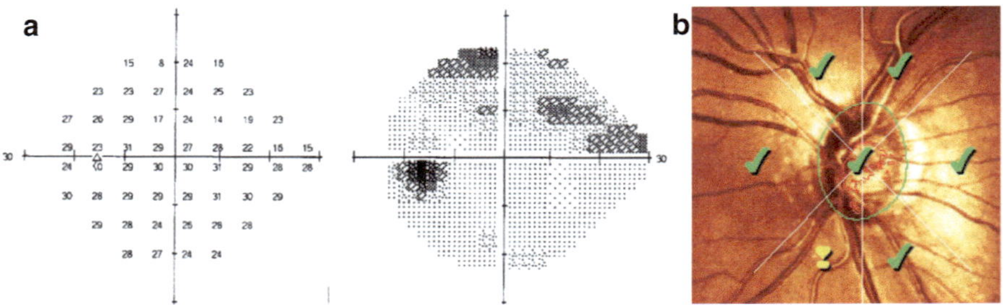

Fig. 11.10 'Agreement' between tests depends on the criteria used to define abnormality. In this patient with suspicious optic disc (**a**) and (**b**) reproducible visual field defect, the Moorfields Regression Analysis [13] from the Heidelberg Retina Tomograph, HRT3, gives a 'borderline' result. If this is regarded as 'abnormal', then the result is in agreement with the abnormal visual field. However, if the borderline result is treated as 'normal', then the two tests are seemingly discordant

11.8 Why Is Variability Important?

Variability is important because it is a significant factor contributing to discordance between structural and functional tests. *Intra-individual* (within-subject) variability can refer to test-retest variability or longitudinal variability, in which repeated measures are different despite no change in the underlying severity of glaucoma. These are sometimes referred to *short-* and *long-term fluctuation*, respectively. A third source of variability is variability across individuals, or *inter-individual variability*. So, for example, inter-individual structure/function variability occurs when two individuals with the same rim area can have different visual field sensitivity. This variability exists across both healthy individuals and patients with glaucoma. Variability is the main source of measurement 'noise' when attempting to identify the structure and function 'signal'. In fact, noise can account for the observed degree of discrepancy between structural and functional measures [19]. Trends in visual field measurements can be predicted with greater precision if the amount of variability at each level of sensitivity is accounted for [20].

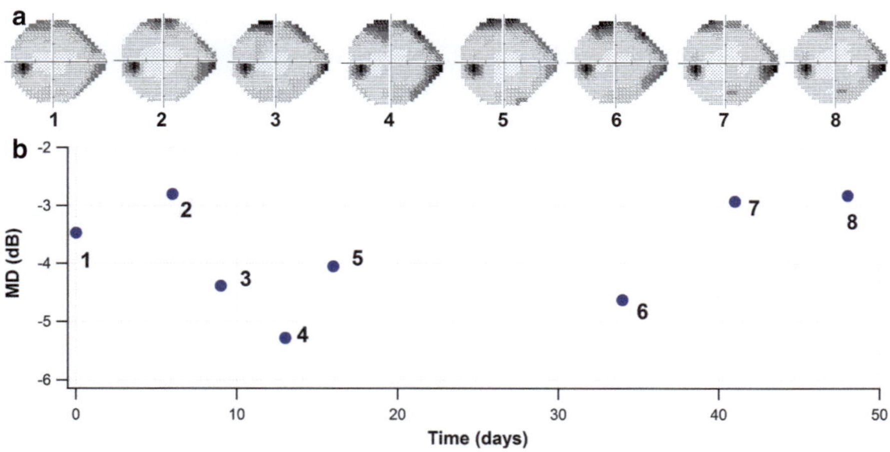

Fig. 11.11 Test-retest variability of visual fields. This patient had 6 repeat tests over a few weeks (**a**); The corresponding Mean Deviation, MD (dB) is shown in (**b**)

11.9 Are Structure and Function Quantitatively Related?

Despite measurement variability, visual field and structural measurements *are* related. A detailed description of the mathematical models that have been proposed to link structure and function has been published [21], but is beyond the scope of this chapter. However, a brief description aids the clinicians' understanding of how the two parameters may be related. This is useful for estimating the severity of glaucoma as well as identifying reasons for discordancy between structural and functional measurements.

Investigation of the longitudinal relationship between structure and function ('structure-function relationship') would need serial measurements over many years, which is difficult in practice. For this reason, cross-sectional measurements of structure and function for individuals with a range of glaucomatous disease are often studied. Inferences are then made about how these parameters may be related during the course of the disease process at an individual level.

A number of studies have concluded that a curvilinear relationship exists between visual field sensitivity (in dB) and rim area or RNFL thickness (in linear units) [22–24]. This implies that a given change in RA corresponds to a small change in visual field in early disease, whilst the same change in RA corresponds to a relatively larger change in visual field in more advanced disease, Fig. 11.12.

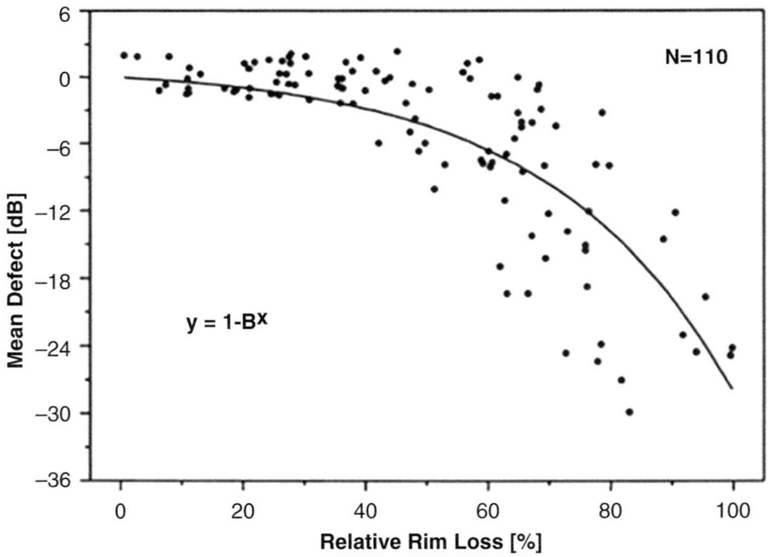

Fig. 11.12 Curvilinear relationship between visual field sensitivity (*dB*) and neuroretinal rim area loss (%) [22]

11.10 What Are the Simple Linear and Non-linear Models of Structure and Function?

The simple linear model predicts that visual field sensitivity (dB) and structural measures (or ganglion cell number) are linearly related when the visual field sensitivity is also plotted in linear units [23, 25–27]. It follows that if visual field sensitivity is plotted in dBs, the relationship is curvilinear [23, 25].

The non-linear model predicts that the relationship between dB visual field sensitivity and dB (logarithmic) ganglion cell number or structure is linear, but with a slope different from 1 [28]. This model has been derived from examining the relationship between visual field sensitivity and ganglion cell counts in monkey eyes at different retinal eccentricities [28, 29] (Fig. 11.13).

Both the simple linear and non-linear models are accepted models for relating structure and function.

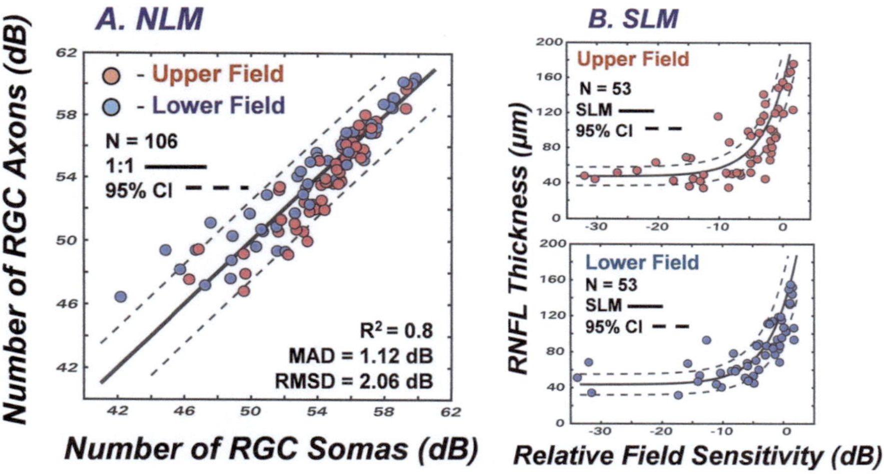

Fig. 11.13 Simple linear and non-linear structure-function models (Adapted from Harwerth et al. [29]). Reproduced from the *Progress in Retinal and Eye Research*, with permission from Elsevier

11.11 What Factors Influence the Quantitative Structure-Function Relationship?

Units of measurement, the stage (and range) of glaucoma severity studied and measurement variability all influence the nature of the structure-function relationship.

The non-linear relationship between structure and function may be an attribute of differing units of measurement: visual field sensitivity is conventionally measured in dB, which is logarithmic, whilst RA and RNFL thicknesses are measured in linear units. The relationship can be made more linear by plotting both structure and function in either linear or logarithmic units, as described above.

The range of disease severity studied can influence the inferred structure-function relationship. For a wide range of disease severity, the relationship is curvilinear. For a limited range of patients with early disease, the relationship appears more linear [30]. The relative range of measurements is different for structural and functional measurements. RA and RNFL thickness never drop to zero, even in eyes which are blind with glaucoma [31], because of non-neural tissue elements, whereas visual field sensitivity is extinguished in blind eyes.

Statistical methods used to assess whether a relationship exists between two measures, such as structure and function, involve fitting a line or curve to a scatterplot of data, such as visual field sensitivity versus RA or RNFL thickness. Conclusions regarding the structure-function relationship also depend on the statistical technique used to fit the data. Different conclusions can arise by using different techniques to fit the same data [32].

Visual field sensitivity, and therefore the structure-function relationship, is affected by stimulus parameters used to measure sensitivity [33]. So, the structure-function relationship also varies with stimulus size and retinal eccentricity.

11.12 Why Is the Structure-Function Relationship in the Macula Important?

The macula contains the highest density of retinal ganglion cells, and as such, has been the subject of much renewed interest in glaucoma [34–36]. Ganglion cell dysfunction may be evident, using electrophysiological techniques, in the macula when there is no visual field loss in the same region [37]. The macula may, therefore, provide a target for identifying early functional losses in some eyes. Standard stimuli used in perimetry may be too large, in relation to neural receptive field size [38], to tap into ganglion cell losses in the macula and optimisation of psychophysical stimuli for detection of field losses close to fixation, is the subject of current research [33].

11.13 Does the Structure-Function Relationship Provide an Insight into the Relationship Between Retinal Ganglion Cell Counts and Visual Field Sensitivity?

Structural measures are often assumed to represent retinal ganglion cell numbers and, as such, the structure-function relationship may give a valuable insight as to how visual field sensitivity changes with progressive ganglion cell loss. Relationships between RNFL thickness and visual field sensitivity [29] have been validated from ganglion cell counts in monkey eyes [28]. RA is related to retinal ganglion cell counts, but the relationship is only weak to moderate [39]. Therefore, conclusions from studies of the structure-function relationship, whilst often assumed to translate to the relationship between ganglion cell number and visual field sensitivity, should be interpreted with some caution.

Recently, novel spectral domain OCT-derived measures of rim tissue, such as minimum rim width (Fig. 11.14), have shown to be better for discriminating glaucomatous eyes from healthy eyes compared to conventional rim measures [40]. Minimum rim width is likely to provide a more accurate representation of neuronal loss in glaucoma than neuroretinal RA measured from photographic images. This is largely because the clinical disc margin has poor correspondence to the aperture in Bruch's membrane which transmits optic nerve [41].

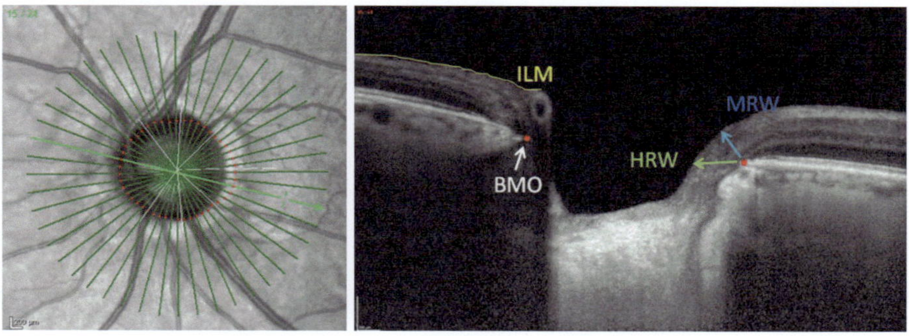

Fig. 11.14 Minimum rim width, MRW and Horizontal rim width, HRW are OCT-derived rim parameters and may better reflect neural loss in glaucoma than rim area (from confocal scanning laser tomography). *ILM* internal limiting membrane, *BMO* Bruch's membrane opening

11.14 Is There a Topographical Relationship Between Structure and Function?

A knowledge of the topographical relationship between the optic disc and corresponding region of the visual field is essential for discerning whether an abnormality (or change) in the visual field is due to glaucoma. The spatial relationship between visual field locations and the optic disc has been well studied [42–44]. The 'Garway-Heath map' (Fig. 11.15), provided the first complete description of this correspondence between conventional visual field locations and the optic disc by examining the path of discrete RNFL defects from red-free photographs [45]. Subsequently, a number of different correspondence maps have been published, with differing methodology, but similar overall findings [46–48]. The topographical map is useful clinically for relating optic disc changes to visual field loss and also have proved invaluable for research studies for quantifying the relationship between structure and function.

Whilst correspondence maps essentially provide an average description of the correspondence between optic disc sector and visual field, at an individual level the relationship is variable [1, 45, 47]. In other words, in one patient, a given location in the visual field may map to a specific sector of the optic disc, whilst in another patient, map to an adjacent sector. The precise correspondence depends on factors such as the position of the optic disc relative to the fovea, the degree of optic nerve tilt and axial length (Fig. 11.16) [1]. Consideration of these factors may reduce some of the structure/function variability across individuals and provide 'individualised' maps so that the location of visual field loss corresponding to optic nerve changes in a specific sector can be predicted more precisely.

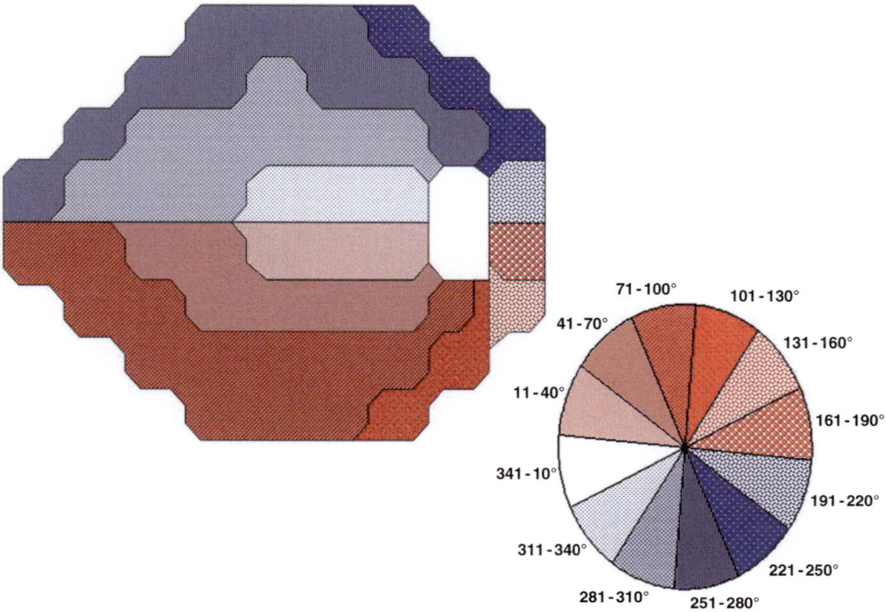

Fig. 11.15 Topographic correspondence between optic disc and visual field locations

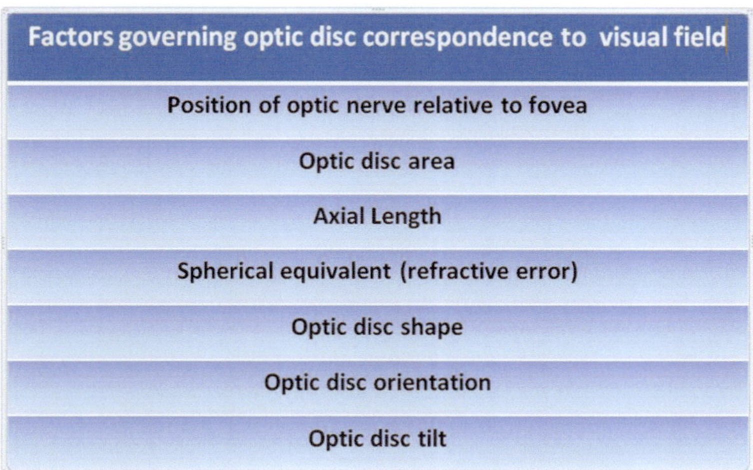

Fig. 11.16 Factors affecting the precise structure-function spatial correspondence

11.15 How Should the Results of Tests be Interpreted?

As a disease, the glaucoma in the early stages poses a unique diagnostic dilemma, in that there is a lack of a single definitive diagnostic test. Diagnosis is based on the clinician's impression. In essence, the likelihood a patient has glaucoma is gauged by assimilating findings from the history, examination and clinical investigations. The results of investigations which do not corroborate with a clinical impression should be questioned. Conversely, the results can add support to a diagnosis of glaucoma in suspect patients, when the diagnosis is in doubt.

In probabilistic terms, a history and clinical examination is used to estimate the *a priori* risk of glaucoma for a given patient [49]. The results of investigations then alter this *a priori* probability to derive a post-test probability (Fig. 11.17). For example, a patient with a suspicious optic disc and a positive family history for glaucoma, high intraocular pressure and a thinner cornea will have a higher pre-test probability of glaucoma than a patient with an absence of family history, normal IOP and thick cornea. An abnormal imaging result is unlikely to influence the post-test probability much for the latter scenario, in which the pre-test probability for glaucoma is low.

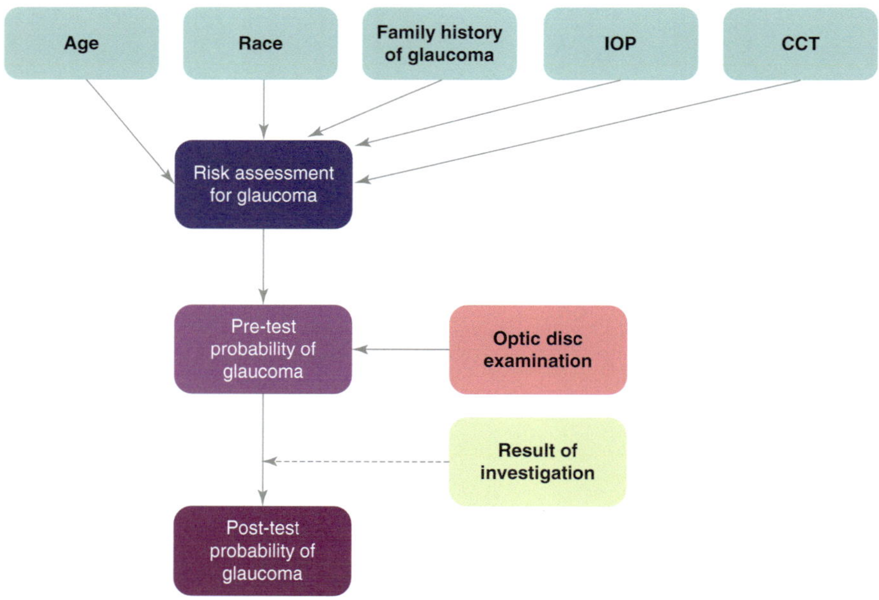

Fig. 11.17 Interpreting tests for glaucoma. The result of an investigation should only be considered in conjunction with a clinical impression. *IOP* intraocular pressure, *CCT* central corneal thickness

11.16 Can Structural and Functional Tests Be Integrated for Glaucoma Assessment?

In recent years, there has been a move to integrate structural and functional tests to facilitate clinical decision making in patients with glaucoma. Bayesian methodology has been applied, using the results of confocal laser scanning tomography to predict a trend in visual field change (Fig. 11.18) [50].

Although imaging and perimetric test results can be displayed simultaneously on a common platform (Fig. 11.19), there is no agreed method for integrating the results of these investigations. However, this is subject of contemporary research. Indices derived from both visual field and OCT have been reported to be sensitive for identifying progression [51].

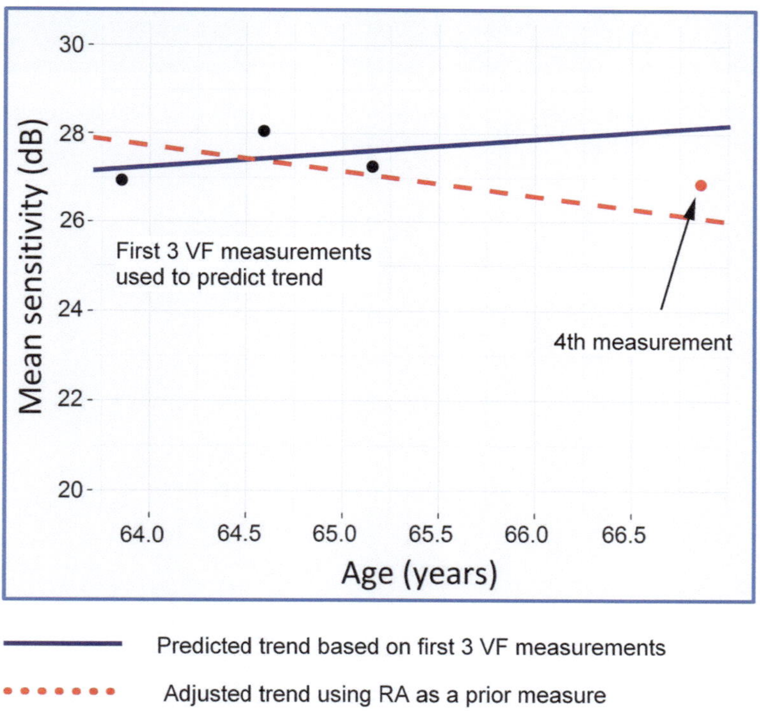

Fig. 11.18 Using rim area as a 'prior' for estimating the trend in visual field sensitivity

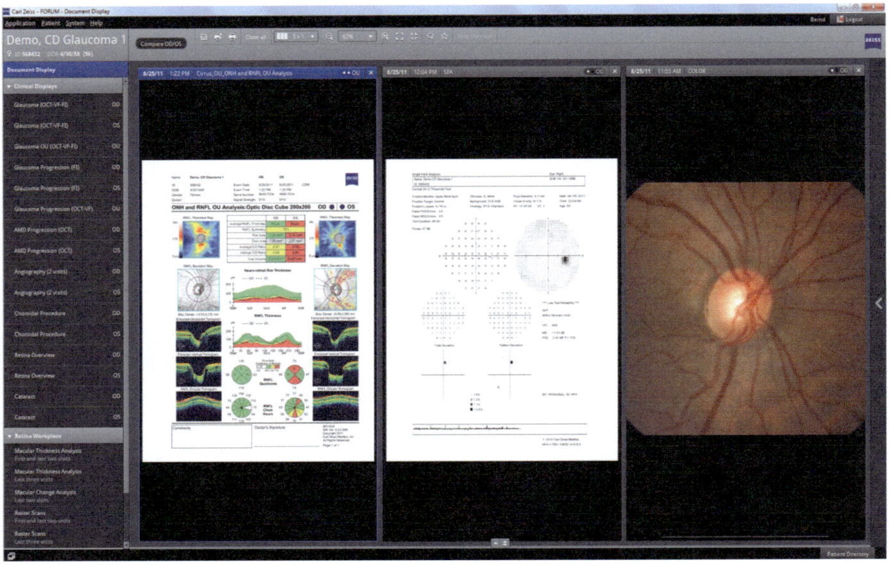

Fig. 11.19 FORUM is an example of results of imaging, and visual field investigations are displayed on a common platform (Courtesy of Zeiss)

References

1. Lamparter J, Russell RA, Zhu H et al (2013) The influence of intersubject variability in ocular anatomical variables on the mapping of retinal locations to the retinal nerve fiber layer and optic nerve head. Invest Ophthalmol Vis Sci 54(9):6074–6082
2. Hayreh SS (2011) Structure of the optic nerve. Ischaemic optic neuropathies. Springer, Heidelberg
3. Chauhan BC, Burgoyne CF (2013) From clinical examination of the optic disc to clinical assessment of the optic nerve head: a paradigm change. Am J Ophthalmol 156(2):218–27 e2
4. Weinreb RN, Khaw PT (2004) Primary open-angle glaucoma. Lancet 363(9422):1711–1720
5. Reus NJ, Lemij HG, Garway-Heath DF et al (2010) Clinical assessment of stereoscopic optic disc photographs for glaucoma: the European Optic Disc Assessment Trial. Ophthalmology 117(4):717–723
6. Araie M (1995) Pattern of visual field defects in normal-tension and high-tension glaucoma. Curr Opin Ophthalmol 6(2):36–45
7. Stroux A, Korth M, Junemann A et al (2003) A statistical model for the evaluation of sensory tests in glaucoma, depending on optic disc damage. Invest Ophthalmol Vis Sci 44(7): 2879–2884
8. Strouthidis NG, Scott A, Peter NM, Garway-Heath DF (2006) Optic disc and visual field progression in ocular hypertensive subjects: detection rates, specificity, and agreement. Invest Ophthalmol Vis Sci 47(7):2904–2910
9. Artes PH, Chauhan BC (2005) Longitudinal changes in the visual field and optic disc in glaucoma. Prog Retin Eye Res 24(3):333–354
10. Miglior S, Zeyen T, Pfeiffer N et al (2005) Results of the European glaucoma prevention study. Ophthalmology 112(3):366–375
11. Heijl A, Bengtsson B, Hyman L, Leske MC (2009) Natural history of open-angle glaucoma. Ophthalmology 116(12):2271–2276
12. Gordon MO, Beiser JA, Brandt JD et al (2002) The Ocular Hypertension Treatment Study: baseline factors that predict the onset of primary open-angle glaucoma. Arch Ophthalmol 120(6):714–720; discussion 829–830
13. Wollstein G, Garway-Heath DF, Hitchings RA (1998) Identification of early glaucoma cases with the scanning laser ophthalmoscope. Ophthalmology 105(8):1557–1563
14. Chauhan BC, LeBlanc RP, McCormick TA, Rogers JB (1994) Test-retest variability of topographic measurements with confocal scanning laser tomography in patients with glaucoma and control subjects. Am J Ophthalmol 118(1):9–15
15. Artes PH, Iwase A, Ohno Y, Kitazawa Y, Chauhan BC (2002) Properties of perimetric threshold estimates from Full Threshold, SITA Standard, and SITA Fast strategies. Invest Ophthalmol Vis Sci 43(8):2654–2659
16. Heijl A, Lindgren A, Lindgren G (1989) Test-retest variability in glaucomatous visual fields. Am J Ophthalmol 108(2):130–135
17. Keltner JL, Johnson CA, Quigg JM et al (2000) Confirmation of visual field abnormalities in the Ocular Hypertension Treatment Study. Ocular Hypertension Treatment Study Group. Arch Ophthalmol 118(9):1187–1194
18. Tan JC, Garway-Heath DF, Hitchings RA (2003) Variability across the optic nerve head in scanning laser tomography. Br J Ophthalmol 87(5):557–559
19. Crabb DP, Owen VMF, Garway-Heath DF (2007) Poor agreement between current tests of structural and functional progression in glaucoma can be explained by measurement noise. ARVO E-abstract 1615. Inves Ophthalmol Vis Sci 48:1615
20. Zhu H, Russell RA, Saunders LJ et al (2014) Detecting changes in retinal function: analysis with Non-stationary Weibull error regression and spatial enhancement (ANSWERS). PLoS One 9(1), e85654
21. Malik R, Swanson WH, Garway-Heath DF (2012) 'Structure-function relationship' in glaucoma: past thinking and current concepts. Clin Experiment Ophthalmol 40(4):369–380

22. Bartz-Schmidt KU, Thumann G, Jonescu-Cuypers CP, Krieglstein GK (1999) Quantitative morphologic and functional evaluation of the optic nerve head in chronic open-angle glaucoma. Surv Ophthalmol 44(Suppl 1):S41–S53
23. Garway-Heath DF, Holder GE, Fitzke FW, Hitchings RA (2002) Relationship between electrophysiological, psychophysical, and anatomical measurements in glaucoma. Invest Ophthalmol Vis Sci 43(7):2213–2220
24. Ajtony C, Balla Z, Somoskeoy S, Kovacs B (2007) Relationship between visual field sensitivity and retinal nerve fiber layer thickness as measured by optical coherence tomography. Invest Ophthalmol Vis Sci 48(1):258–263
25. Garway-Heath DF, Caprioli J, Fitzke FW, Hitchings RA (2000) Scaling the hill of vision: the physiological relationship between light sensitivity and ganglion cell numbers. Invest Ophthalmol Vis Sci 41(7):1774–1782
26. Swanson WH, Felius J, Pan F (2004) Perimetric defects and ganglion cell damage: interpreting linear relations using a two-stage neural model. Invest Ophthalmol Vis Sci 45(2):466–472
27. Hood DC, Greenstein VC, Odel JG et al (2002) Visual field defects and multifocal visual evoked potentials: evidence of a linear relationship. Arch Ophthalmol 120(12):1672–1681
28. Harwerth RS, Carter-Dawson L, Smith EL 3rd et al (2004) Neural losses correlated with visual losses in clinical perimetry. Invest Ophthalmol Vis Sci 45(9):3152–3160
29. Harwerth RS, Wheat JL, Fredette MJ, Anderson DR (2010) Linking structure and function in glaucoma. Prog Retin Eye Res 29(4):249–271
30. Malik R, Swanson WH, Nicolela MT (2014) Structure and function relationships in glaucoma. In: Shaarawy TM, Sherwood MB, Hitchings RA, Crowston JG (eds) Glaucoma, 2nd edn. Elsevier, Oxford
31. Sihota R, Sony P, Gupta V, Dada T, Singh R (2006) Diagnostic capability of optical coherence tomography in evaluating the degree of glaucomatous retinal nerve fiber damage. Invest Ophthalmol Vis Sci 47(5):2006–2010
32. Marin-Franch I, Malik R, Crabb DP, Swanson WH (2013) Choice of statistical method influences apparent association between structure and function in glaucoma. Invest Ophthalmol Vis Sci 54(6):4189–4196
33. Redmond T, Garway-Heath DF, Zlatkova MB, Anderson RS (2010) Sensitivity loss in early glaucoma can be mapped to an enlargement of the area of complete spatial summation. Invest Ophthalmol Vis Sci 51(12):6540–6548
34. Hood DC, Slobodnick A, Raza AS, de Moraes CG, Teng CC, Ritch R (2014) Early glaucoma involves both deep local, and shallow widespread, retinal nerve fiber damage of the macular region. Invest Ophthalmol Vis Sci 55(2):632–649
35. Hood DC, Raza AS, de Moraes CG, Liebmann JM, Ritch R (2013) Glaucomatous damage of the macula. Prog Retin Eye Res 32:1–21
36. Luo X, Patel NB, Rajagopalan LP, Harwerth RS, Frishman LJ (2014) Relation between macular retinal ganglion cell/inner plexiform layer thickness and multifocal electroretinogram measures in experimental glaucoma. Invest Ophthalmol Vis Sci 55(7):4512–4524
37. Bach M, Sulimma F, Gerling J (1997) Little correlation of the pattern electroretinogram (PERG) and visual field measures in early glaucoma. Doc Ophthalmol 94(3):253–263
38. Wilson ME (1970) Invariant features of spatial summation with changing locus in the visual field. J Physiol 207(3):611–622
39. Varma R, Quigley HA, Pease ME (1992) Changes in optic disk characteristics and number of nerve fibers in experimental glaucoma. Am J Ophthalmol 114(5):554–559
40. Chauhan BC, O'Leary N, Almobarak FA et al (2013) Enhanced detection of open-angle glaucoma with an anatomically accurate optical coherence tomography-derived neuroretinal rim parameter. Ophthalmology 120(3):535–543
41. Reis AS, Sharpe GP, Yang H et al (2012) Optic disc margin anatomy in patients with glaucoma and normal controls with spectral domain optical coherence tomography. Ophthalmology 119(4):738–747

42. Weber J, Dannheim F, Dannheim D (1990) The topographical relationship between optic disc and visual field in glaucoma. Acta Ophthalmol (Copenh) 68(5):568–574
43. Wirtschafter JD, Becker WL, Howe JB, Younge BR (1982) Glaucoma visual field analysis by computed profile of nerve fiber function in optic disc sectors. Ophthalmology 89(3):255–267
44. Read RM, Spaeth GL (1974) The practical clinical appraisal of the optic disc in glaucoma: the natural history of cup progression and some specific disc-field correlations. Trans Am Acad Ophthalmol Otolaryngol 78(2):OP255–OP274
45. Garway-Heath DF, Poinoosawmy D, Fitzke FW, Hitchings RA (2000) Mapping the visual field to the optic disc in normal tension glaucoma eyes. Ophthalmology 107(10):1809–1815
46. Gardiner SK, Johnson CA, Cioffi GA (2005) Evaluation of the structure-function relationship in glaucoma. Invest Ophthalmol Vis Sci 46(10):3712–3717
47. Jansonius NM, Nevalainen J, Selig B et al (2009) A mathematical description of nerve fiber bundle trajectories and their variability in the human retina. Vision Res 49(17):2157–2163
48. Denniss J, McKendrick AM, Turpin A (2012) An anatomically customizable computational model relating the visual field to the optic nerve head in individual eyes. Invest Ophthalmol Vis Sci 53(11):6981–6990
49. Garway-Heath DF, Friedman DS (2006) How should results from clinical tests be integrated into the diagnostic process? Ophthalmology 113(9):1479–1480
50. Russell RA, Malik R, Chauhan BC, Crabb DP, Garway-Heath DF (2012) Improved estimates of visual field progression using bayesian linear regression to integrate structural information in patients with ocular hypertension. Invest Ophthalmol Vis Sci 53(6):2760–2769
51. Medeiros FA, Zangwill LM, Anderson DR et al (2012) Estimating the rate of retinal ganglion cell loss in glaucoma. Am J Ophthalmol 154(5):814–24 e1

Chapter 12
Assessment of Structural Glaucoma Progression

Francesco Oddone

12.1 Introduction

Glaucoma is a group of chronic, progressive optic neuropathies with in common morphological changes that take place along the visual pathway from the retinal ganglion cell layer to the brain. Associated with these changes, there is a progressive decay of the visual function in the form of visual field loss that can eventually, in absence of treatment, lead to blindness.

The detection of morphological glaucomatous changes over time is a complex clinical task. The complexity arises from different factors: the rate of change may vary generously from patient to patient as well as within the same patient over time, the morphological changes commonly do not match, neither chronologically or in magnitude, the functional changes, and ultimately we lack an accurate reference test against which the accuracy of new testing strategies can be assessed. Moreover, we need to consider another factor contributing to the complexity, and this is represented by the rapidly evolving technology that impairs the possibility for the clinician to rely on consistent consecutive tests over time making the task of detecting changes even more arduous.

In this scenario, in order to maximize the likelihood to detect morphological glaucoma progression, the clinician should be knowledgeable about qualitative methods of detecting changes, to become knowledgeable about the statistical progression analysis strategies and algorithms, and to be always up to date with the technological advancements.

F. Oddone, MD, PhD
Glaucoma Research Unit, IRCCS Fondazione G.B.Bietti, Rome, Italy
e-mail: oddonef@gmail.com

A. Ferreras (ed.), *Glaucoma Imaging*, DOI 10.1007/978-3-319-18959-8_12

12.2 Morphological Changes During Glaucoma

Glaucoma determines, at the eye level, characteristic changes of the morphology of the optic nerve head (ONH) and a progressive thinning of the retinal nerve fiber layer (RNFL) and of the ganglion cell layer (GCL).

Morphological glaucomatous changes that can be assessed at the optic nerve head level are represented by a focal and/or generalized narrowing of the neuroretinal rim that determines a focal or generalized enlargement of the optic disc cup.

12.3 Detecting Structural Progression Qualitatively

Morphological glaucomatous changes that can be assessed qualitatively are represented by ONH and RNFL changes. Changes of the optic nerve head are represented by a focal and/or generalized narrowing of the neuroretinal rim (Fig. 12.1) that determines a focal or generalized enlargement of the optic disc cup, while changes of the RNFL are represented by the onset or the enlargement of wedge shaped RNFL defects.

These changes can be qualitatively appreciated either directly at the slit lamp, by high magnification ophthalmoscopy, or by means of consecutive monoscopic or stereoscopic photographs. Ophthalmoscopy for detecting glaucoma progression is limited by the high grade of subjectivity and by the lack of a reliable reference comparator to establish whether changes have occurred or not. Drawings in the patients' note can be helpful but again subjectivity and lack of reliability are issues of major concern. Nevertheless ophthalmoscopy has one advantage over fundus photographs that even the most advanced technologies are lacking, that is the capability of assessing the color of the fundus feature (e.g. pallor) despite assessing whether pallor is changed over time is a difficult task even for an expert clinician.

Monoscopic or stereoscopic high magnification fundus photography still represents the gold standard for detecting structural changes over time in glaucoma. Despite also the qualitative assessment of fundus photographs suffers from the problem of subjectivity, there are structural changes that can be best detected by this method. In fact, ONH changes are often accompanied by changes in the relative position and visibility of the main ONH and peripapillary vessels. Baring of a vessel previously sustained by neural tissue is a clear sign of neuroretinal rim thinning and glaucoma progression (Figs. 12.1 and 12.2) and the currently available imaging devices are not yet capable of analyzing vessels characteristics.

12.3.1 Baring Vessels

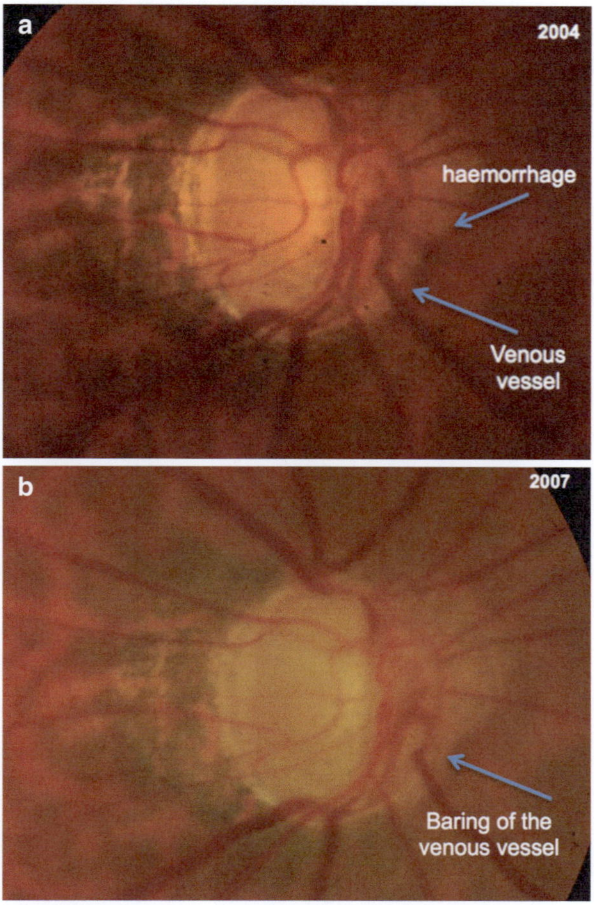

Fig. 12.1 (**a**) Right ONH photograph taken in 2004. A splinter hemorrhage of the disc is clearly visible in the infero-nasal quadrant. (**b**) in the same quadrant 3 years later is clearly visible a marker of structural progression represented by the baring of a major venous vessel

12.3.2 ONH Hemorrhages

ONH hemorrhages are not pathognomonic of glaucoma, but when they occur in a glaucomatous eye they are a good predictive sign of future progression of the visual field damage [1]. ONH hemorrhages can be only appreciated by qualitative methods such as ophthalmoscopy or fundus photography but not by the high-tech imaging devices (Figs. 12.1, 12.2, 12.3, 12.4).

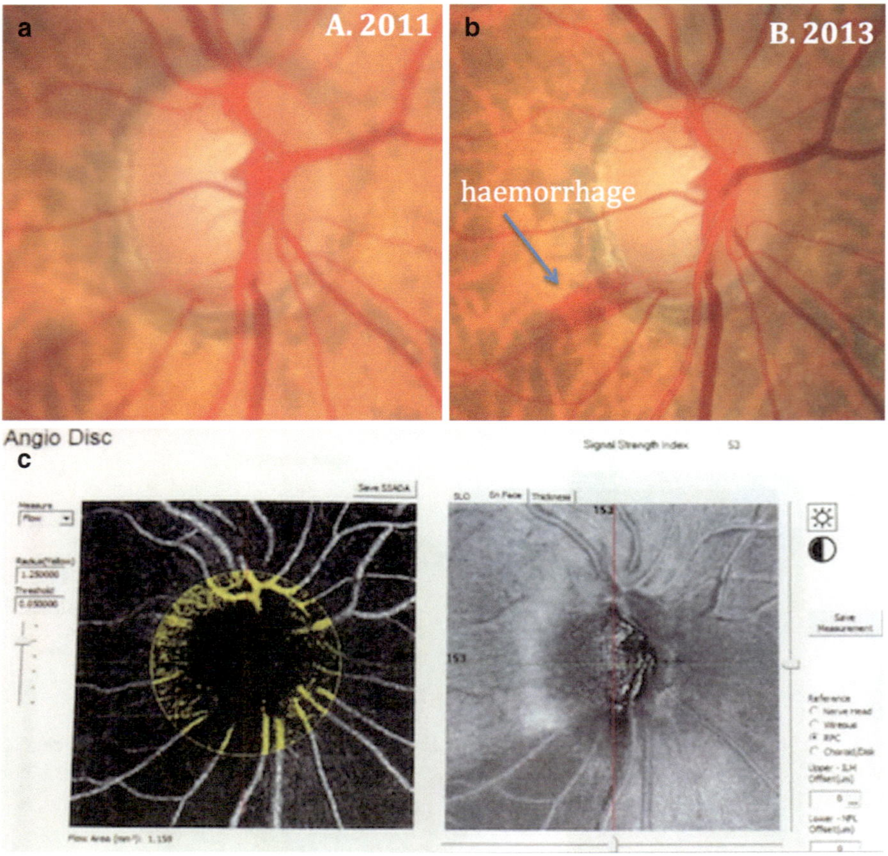

Fig. 12.2 (**a**) Right ONH photograph taken in 2011. An enlargement of the optic disc cup is evident associated with a focal narrowing of the rim in the infero-temporal quadrant (notching) with signs of probable past splinter hemorrhages. (**b**) In the same quadrant 2 years later is clearly visible a recurrent splinter hemorrhage. (**c**) Corresponding ONH OCT angiography acquired in 2014 showing an area of reduced flow in the same quadrant. (**d**) Corresponding progression of the visual field damage

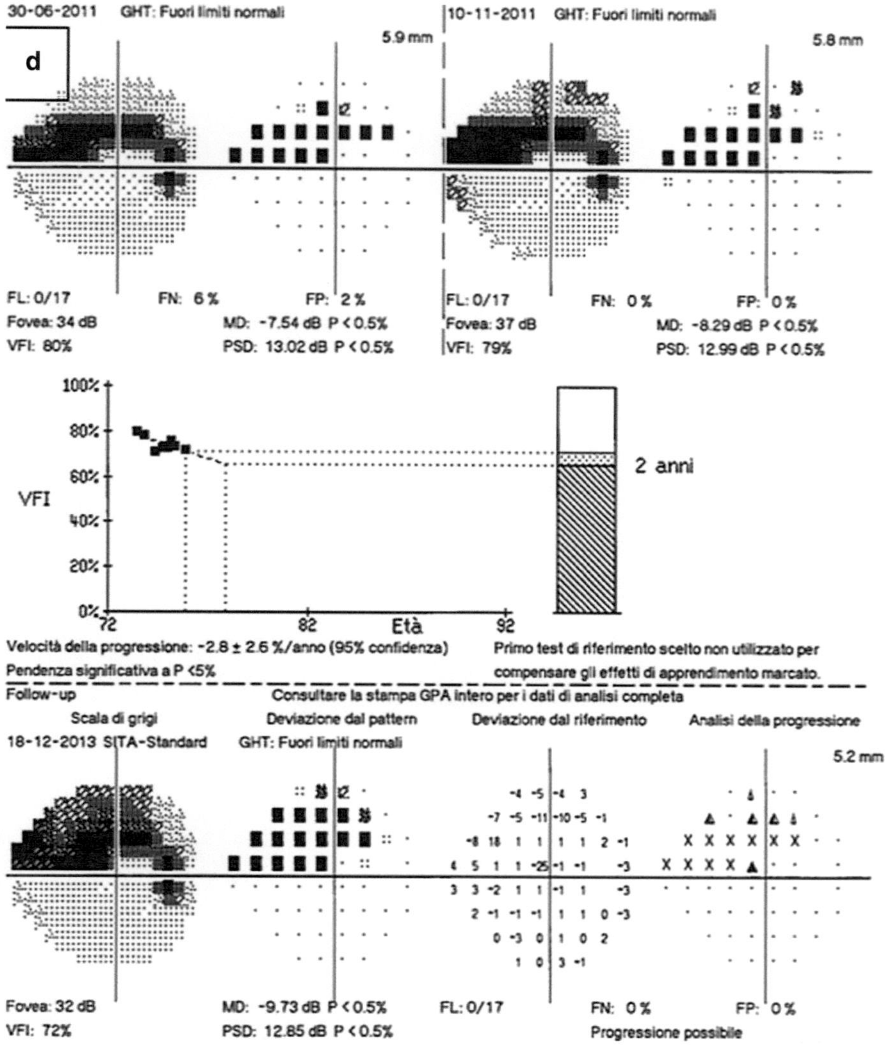

Fig. 12.2 (continued)

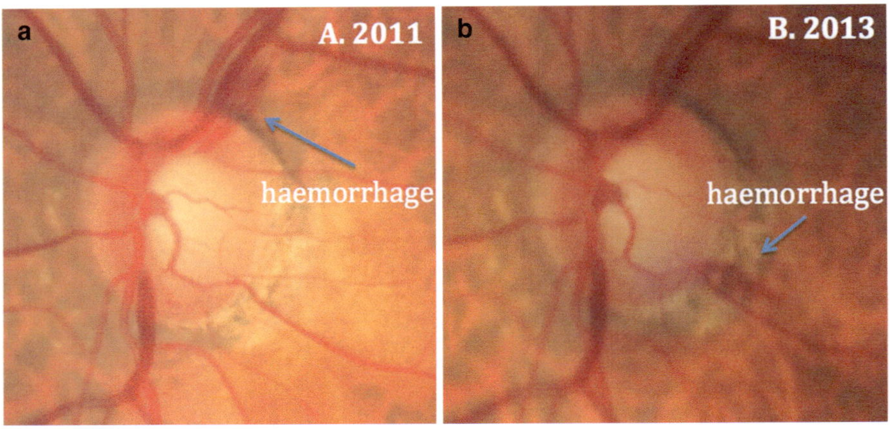

Fig. 12.3 Left eye, same patient of Fig. 12.2. (**a**) Left ONH photograph taken in 2014. A splinter hemorrhage is visible in the supero-temporal quadrant. (**b**) Few months later the supero-temporal hemorrhage is reabsorbed and a new one appeared in the infero-temporal quadrant. (**c**) Corresponding progression of the visual field damage

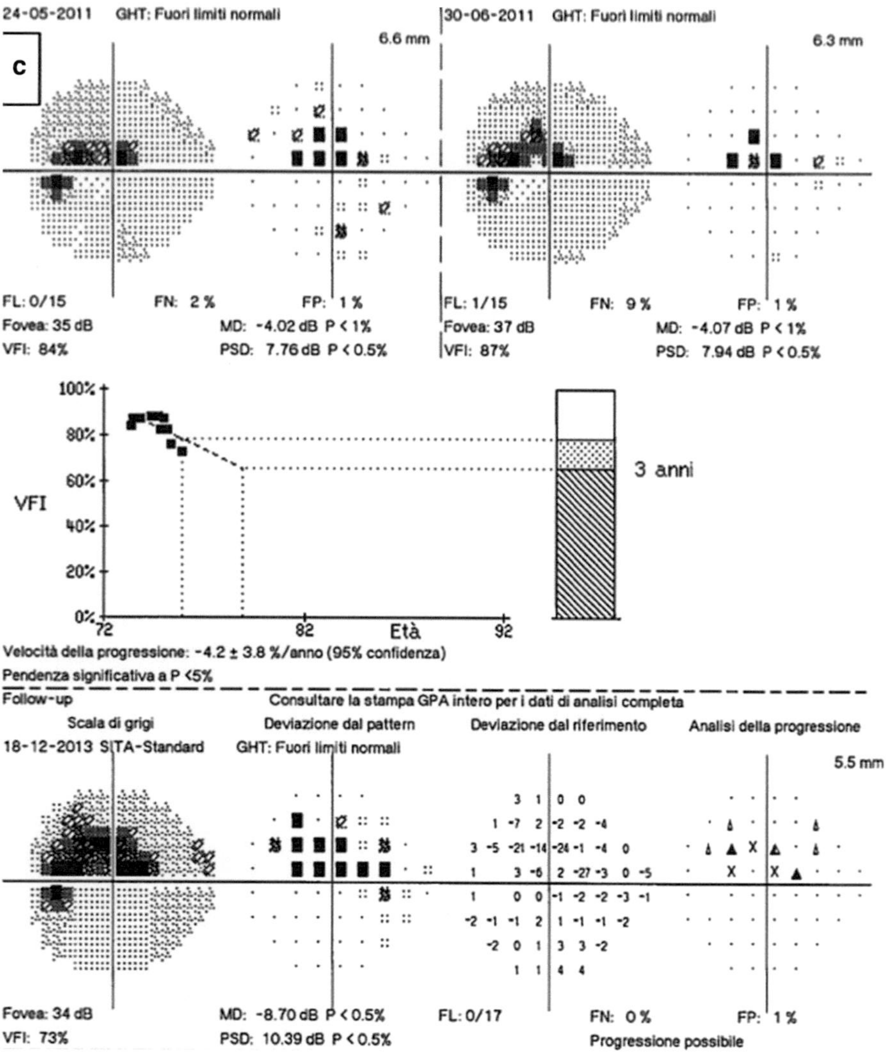

Fig. 12.3 (continued)

12.4 Detecting Structural Progression Quantitatively

12.4.1 Statistical Approaches

Progressive changes over time of a biological parameter can be studied either with an event analysis approach or with a trend analysis approach. Both approaches are valid, but they are not interchangeable since they provide different information.

Event analysis is based on the statistical comparison of a follow-up test with a baseline reference test, and if the difference between the two exceeds the threshold of the test-retest variability the follow-up test is flagged as progressed. The strength of this approach is that a relatively small number of consecutive examinations is required to perform the analysis (usually 4, including a confirmation test), while the major limitation is represented by the lack of information about the rate of change over time (Figs. 12.4, 12.5, 12.6, 12.7, 12.8, 12.9, 12.10).

The trend analysis approach does not need a baseline reference test but take into account the whole series of examinations performed over time that is fitted into a regression model which enable the calculation of the rate of change and its statistical significance. The major limitation of the trend analysis approach is represented by the higher number of examinations required for the analysis to be reliable (minimum 6). Nevertheless, newly proposed frequency of testing algorithms may reduce this number and improve accuracy [2, 3].

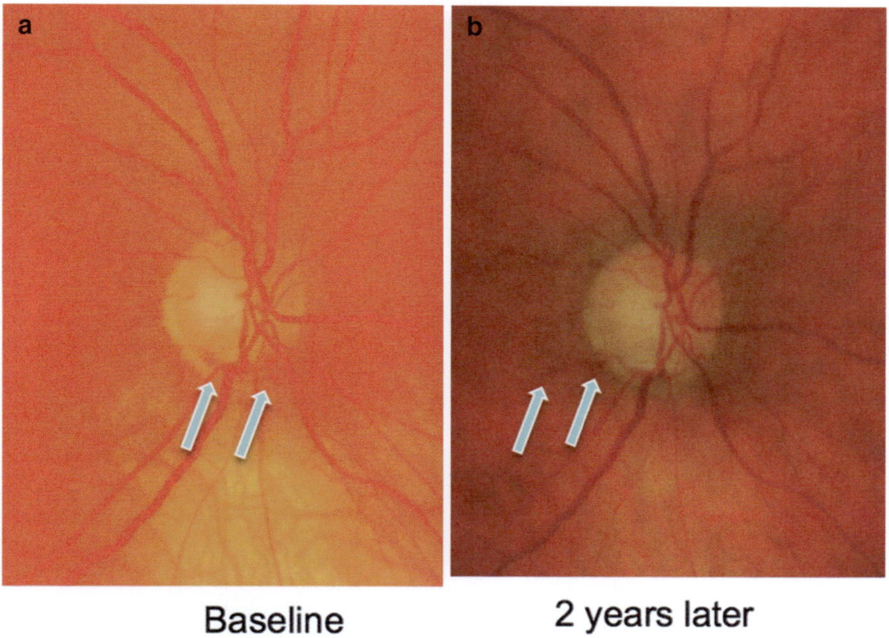

Fig. 12.4 (**a**) Baseline right ONH photograph showing splinter hemorrhages at the inferior pole. (**b**) Right ONH photograph showing structural damage occurring at the inferior pole in 2 years of follow-up. (**c**) Cirrus-HD OCT Guided Progression Analysis printout (Carl Zeiss Meditec, Dublin, USA). The trend analysis of the superior RNFL thickness shows statistically significant progression (*red dot*). The inferior RNFL thickness trend analysis shows no significant changes. This is related to a common artifact called "floor effect" that occurs in advanced damaged ONH/RNFL when OCT cannot detect further thinning of an already very thin residual tissue. In advanced cases, imaging might not represent the method of choice for monitoring further progression. (**d**) Cirrus-HD OCT Guided Progression Analysis printout (Carl Zeiss Meditec, Dublin, USA). The event analysis shows a statistically possible loss in the superior quadrant at the 5th follow-up test confirmed and flagged as likely loss at the 6th test. Event analysis approach to detect progression compares each single follow-up test with the baseline. If the difference between the two exceeds the threshold of the test-retest variability, the follow-up test is flagged as possible progression. If this is confirmed, the following test is flagged as likely progression. The event analysis does not provide estimates of rate of change. (**e**) Corresponding visual field progression

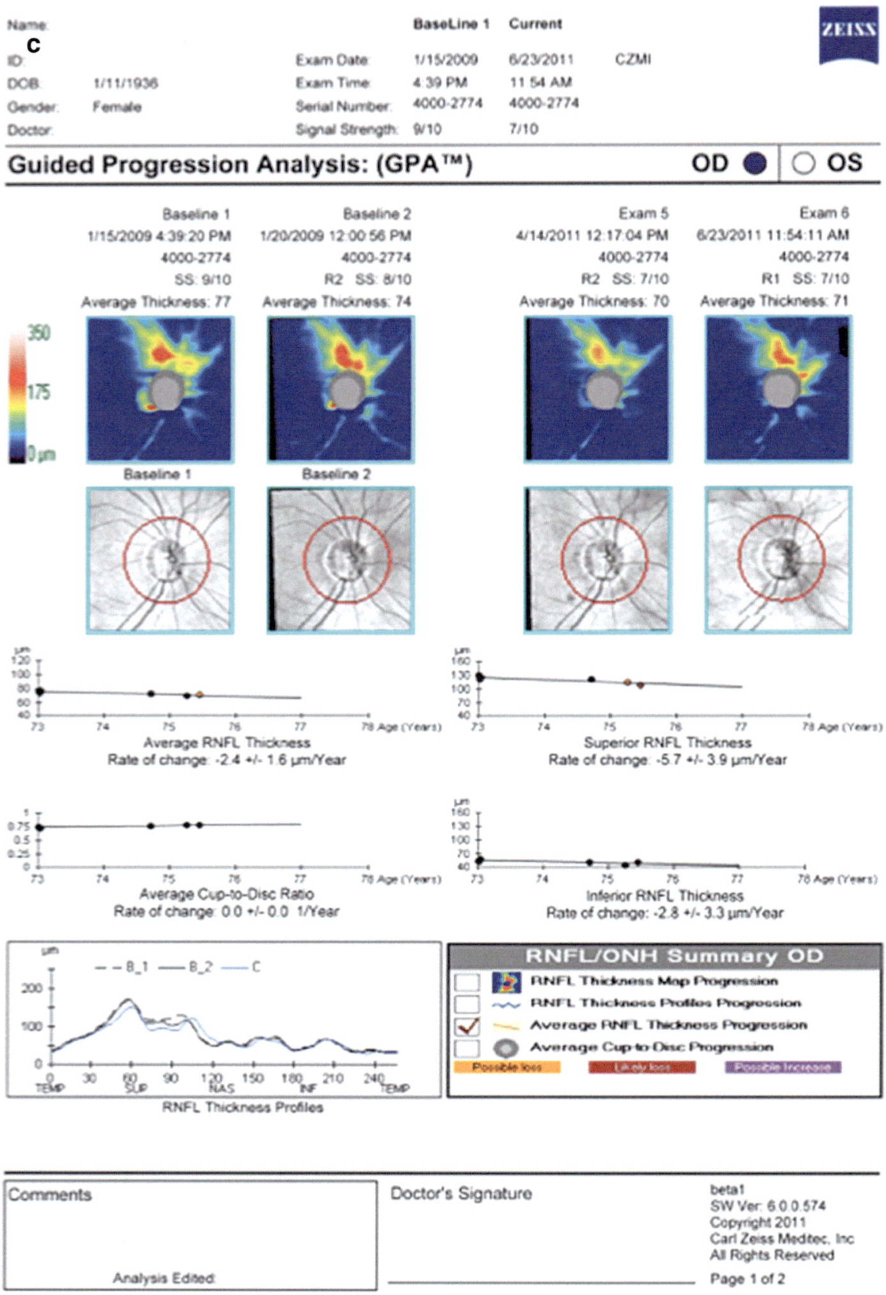

Fig. 12.4 (continued)

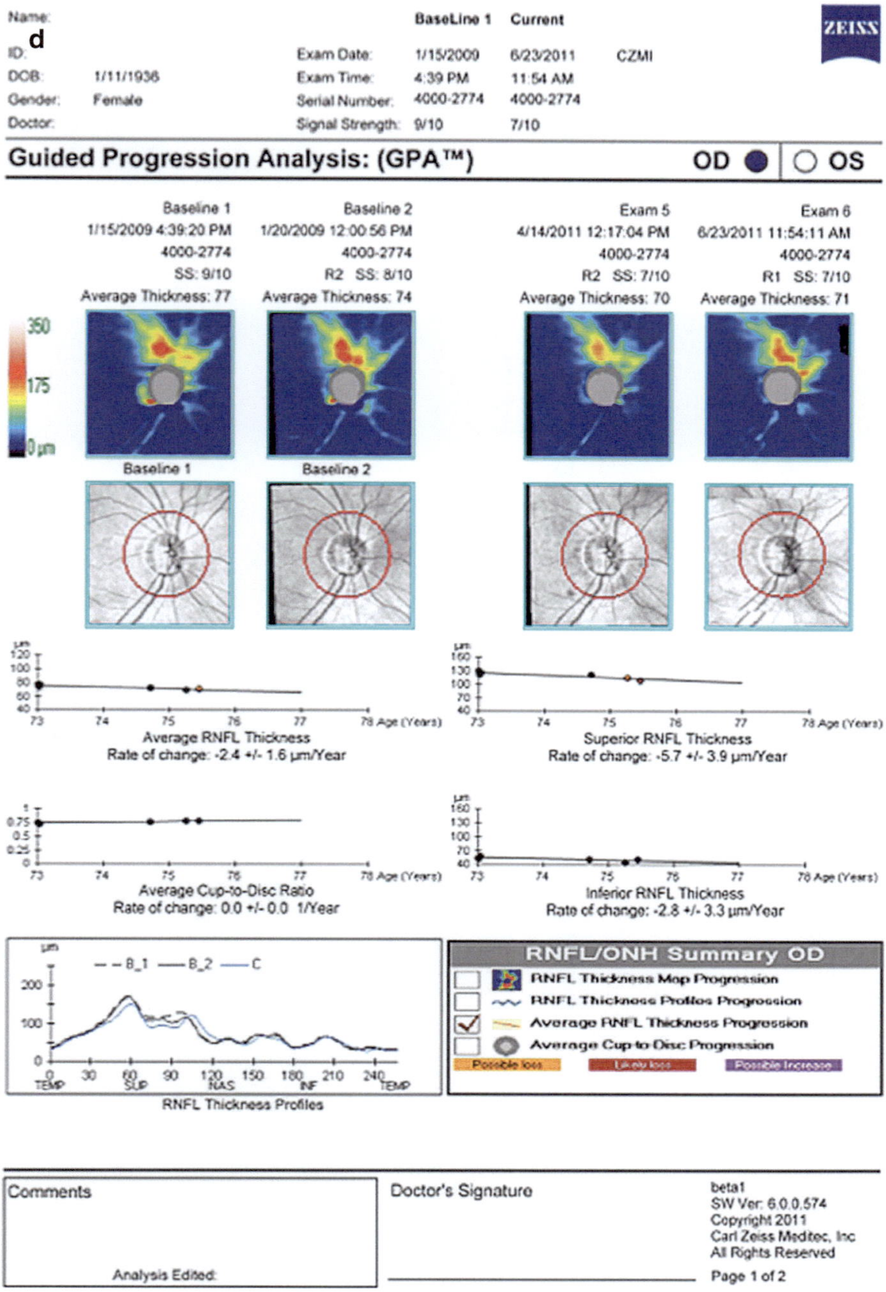

Fig. 12.4 (continued)

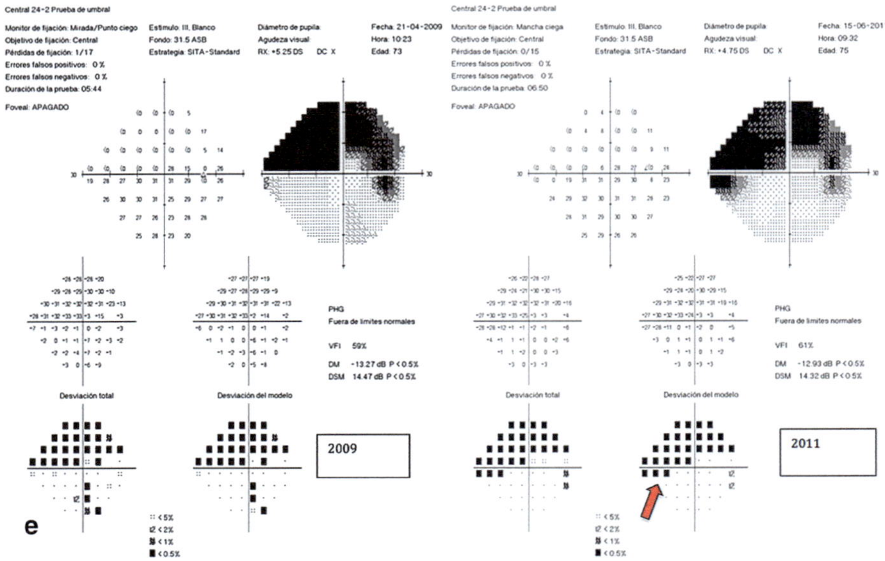

Fig. 12.4 (continued)

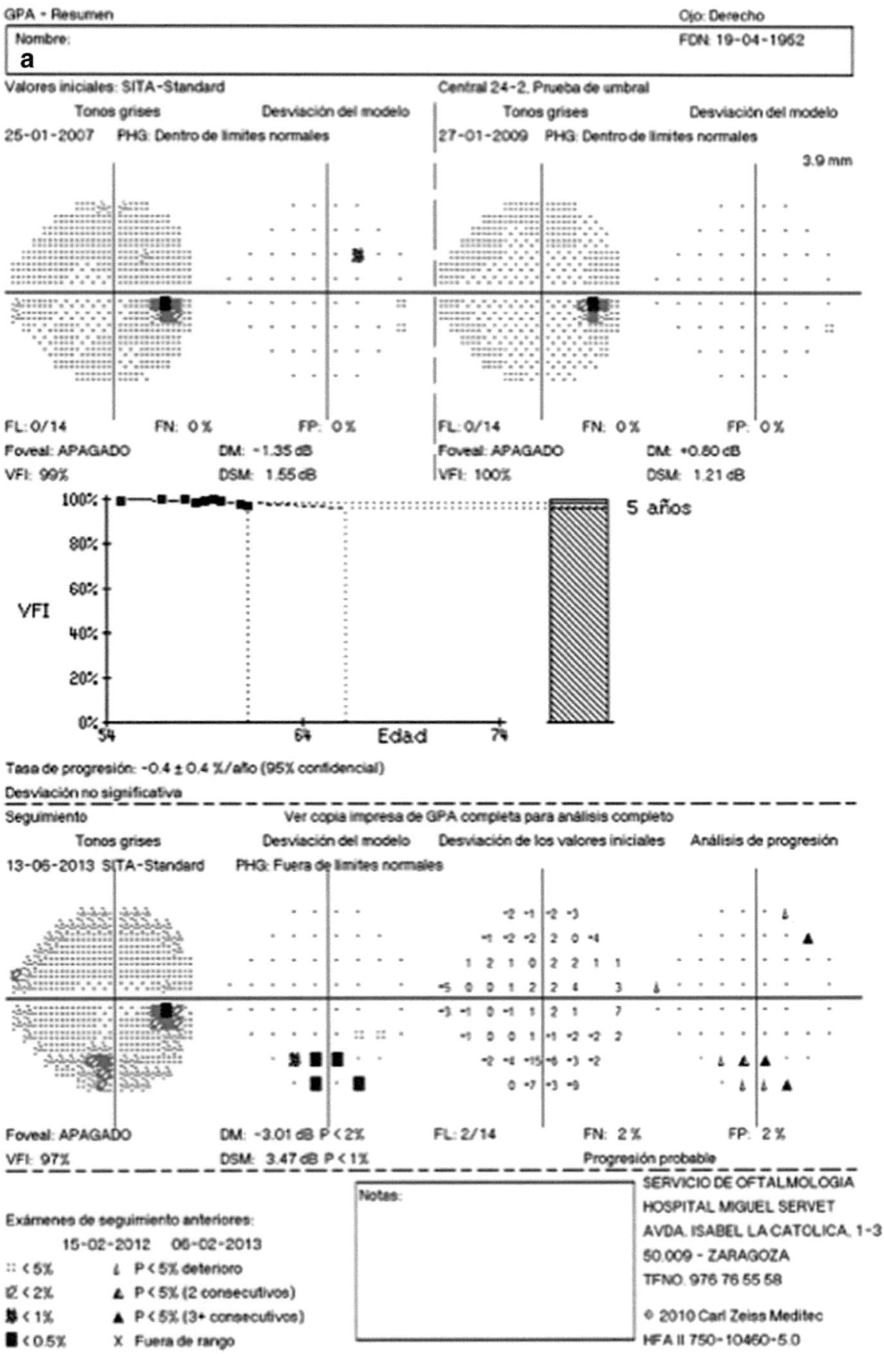

Fig. 12.5 (**a**) Visual field index (VFI) progression analysis is showing a stable trend between 2007 and 2013. The event analysis (bottom right of the printout) shows test locations flagged as likely progressing. (**b**) The Cirrus-HD OCT GPA trend analysis (Carl Zeiss Meditec, Dublin, USA) shows a likely progression of the average, superior, and inferior RNFL thickness. The TSNIT graph at the bottom left of the page shows the areas of change. (**c**) The Cirrus-HD OCT GPA event analysis shows a likely progression in the two last follow-up tests

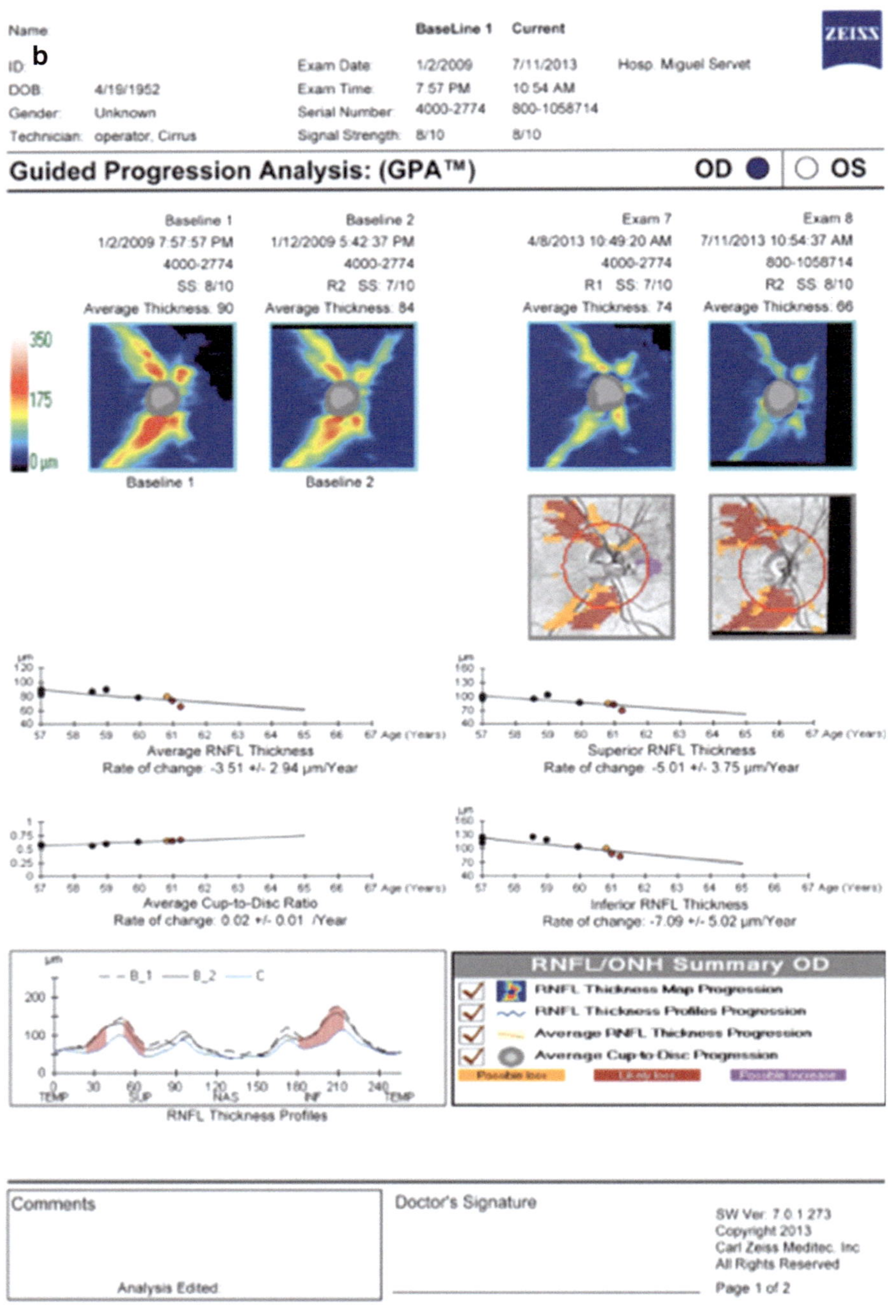

Fig. 12.5 (continued)

Name: **C**
ID:
DOB: 4/19/1952
Gender: Unknown
Technician: operator, Cirrus

	BaseLine 1	Current
Exam Date:	1/2/2009	7/11/2013
Exam Time:	7:57 PM	10:54 AM
Serial Number:	4000-2774	800-1058714
Signal Strength:	8/10	8/10

Hosp. Miguel Servet

ZEISS

Guided Progression Analysis: (GPA™)

OD ● | ○ OS

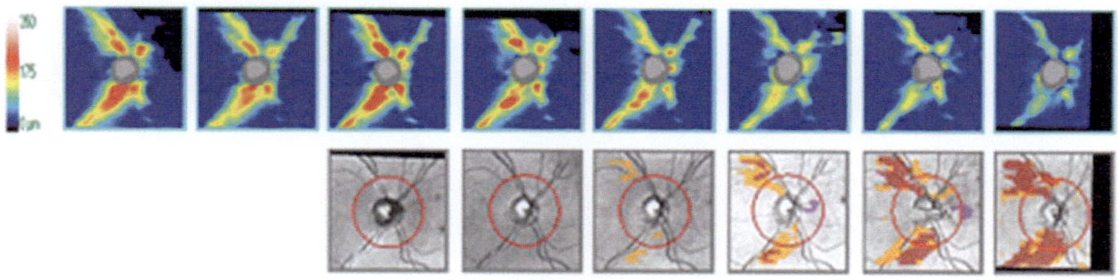

RNFL and ONH Summary Parameters

		Exam Date/Time	Serial Number	Registration Method	SS	Avg RNFL Thickness (µm)	Inf Quadrant RNFL (µm)	Sup Quadrant RNFL (µm)	Rim Area (mm²)	Average Cup-to-Disc Ratio	Vertical Cup-to-Disc Ratio	Cup Volume (mm³)
Baseline1:	1	1/2/2009 7:57:57 PM	4000-2774		8/10	90	124	103	1.18	0.59	0.55	0.277
Baseline2:	2	1/12/2009 5:42:37 PM	4000-2774	R2	7/10	84	113	96	1.20	0.58	0.54	0.275
	3	11/9/2010 10:41:59 AM	4000-2774	R2	6/10	87	125	95	1.21	0.58	0.56	0.257
	4	4/8/2011 12:16:42 PM	4000-2774	R1	7/10	90	119	104	1.12	0.61	0.58	0.299
	5	3/29/2012 1:15:30 PM	4000-2774	R1	7/10	78	104	87	1.07	0.64	0.65	0.307
	6	2/7/2013 1:03:45 PM	4000-2774	R1	8/10	80	100	85	1.08	0.67	0.67	0.381
	7	4/8/2013 10:49:20 AM	4000-2774	R1	7/10	74	89	84	1.12	0.66	0.63	0.282
Current:	8	7/11/2013 10:54:37 AM	800-1058714	R2	8/10	66	83	70	1.02	0.68	0.67	0.370

Registration Methods
R2 - Registration based on translation and rotation of OCT fundus
R1 - Registration based only on translation of disc center

Likely Loss
Possible Loss

Compared to baseline, statistically significant loss of tissue detected. For Average RNFL, Superior RNFL, Inferior RNFL, Rim Area the values have decreased. For Cup-to-Disc Ratios and Cup Volume values have increased.

Possible Increase

Compared to baseline, statistically significant increase detected. For Average RNFL, Superior RNFL, Inferior RNFL, Rim Area values have increased. For Cup-to-Disc Ratios and Cup Volume values have decreased.

Comments

Analysis Edited:

Doctor's Signature

SW Ver: 7.0.1.273

Page 2 of 2

Fig. 12.5 (continued)

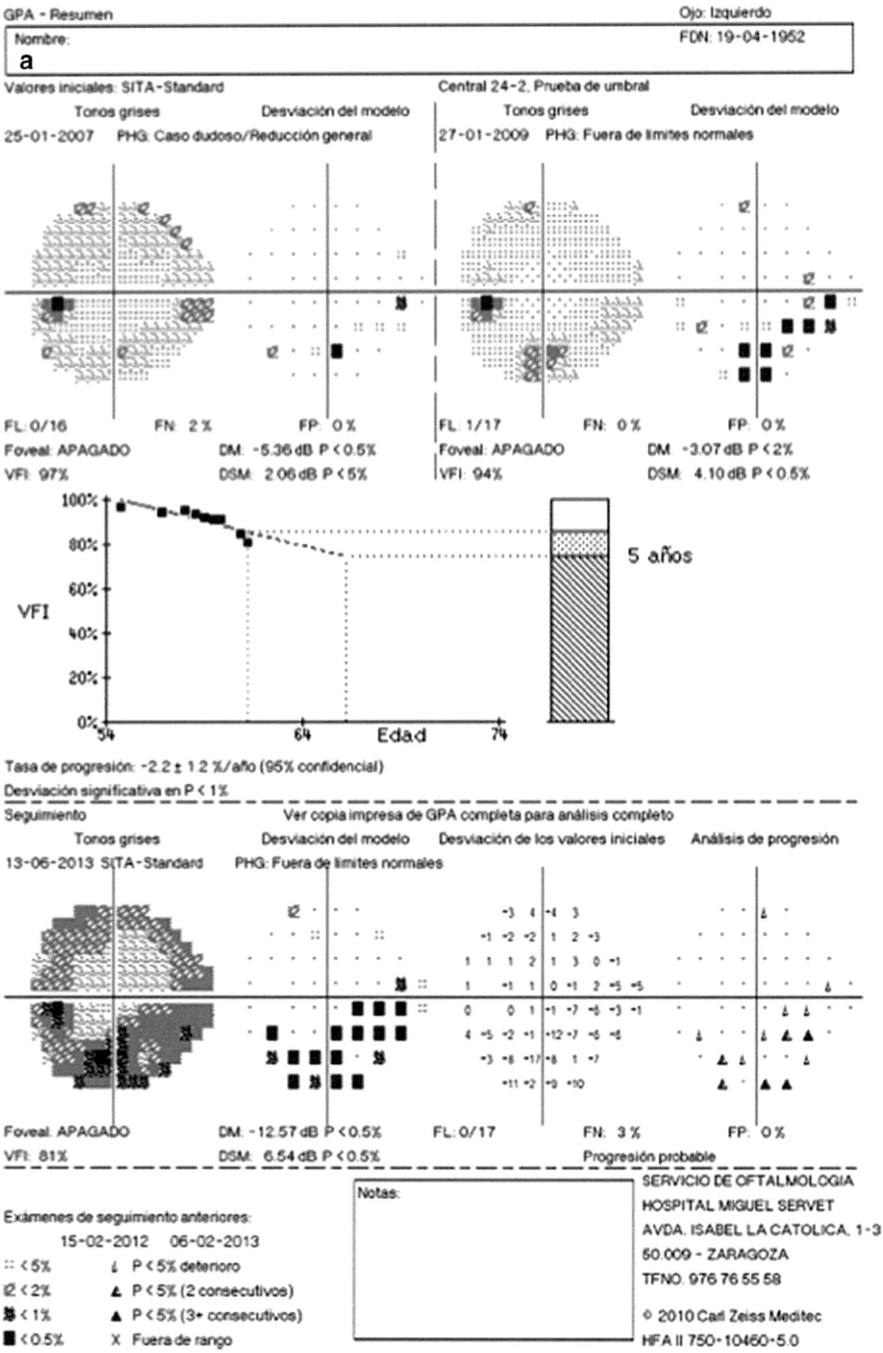

Fig. 12.6 (**a**) Visual field progression analysis is showing significant progression between 2007 and 2013 with both approaches (trend and event analysis). (**b**) The Cirrus-HD OCT GPA trend analysis (Carl Zeiss Meditec, Dublin, USA) shows a likely progression of the average, superior, and inferior RNFL thickness. The TSNIT graph at the bottom left of the page shows the areas of change. (**c**) The Cirrus-HD OCT GPA event analysis shows a likely progression in the two last follow-up tests

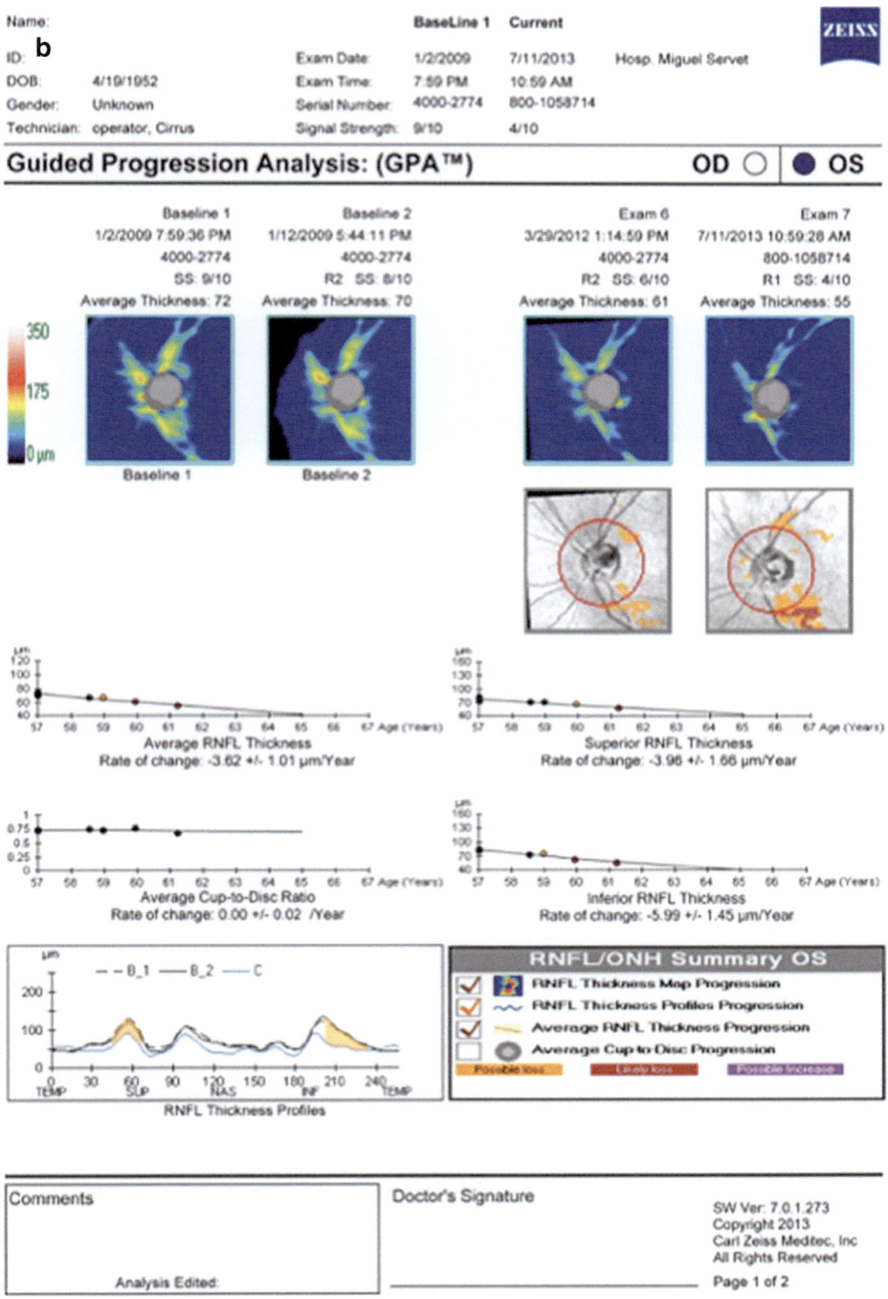

Fig. 12.6 (continued)

			BaseLine 1	Current		
Name:						ZEISS
ID:	C	Exam Date:	1/2/2009	7/11/2013	Hosp. Miguel Servet	
DOB:	4/19/1952	Exam Time:	7:59 PM	10:59 AM		
Gender:	Unknown	Serial Number:	4000-2774	800-1058714		
Technician:	operator, Cirrus	Signal Strength:	9/10	4/10		

Guided Progression Analysis: (GPA™)

OD ○ ● OS

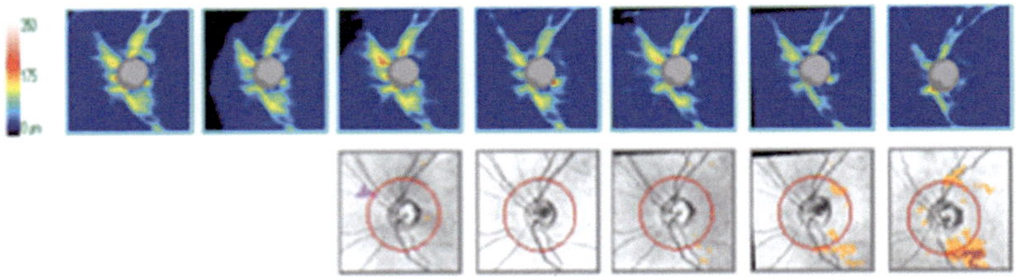

RNFL and ONH Summary Parameters

		Exam Date/Time	Serial Number	Registration Method	SS	Avg RNFL Thickness (µm)	Inf Quadrant RNFL (µm)	Sup Quadrant RNFL (µm)	Rim Area (mm²)	Average Cup-to-Disc Ratio	Vertical Cup-to-Disc Ratio	Cup Volume (mm³)
Baseline1:	1	1/2/2009 7:59:36 PM	4000-2774		9/10	72	83	82	0.94	0.74	0.70	0.596
Baseline2:	2	1/12/2009 5:44:11 PM	4000-2774	R2	8/10	70	86	75	0.97	0.73	0.70	0.580
	3	1/19/2009 10:54:06 AM	4000-2774	R2	8/10	73	84	75	0.98	0.73	0.68	0.551
	4	11/9/2010 10:42:46 AM	4000-2774	R1	8/10	67	74	71	0.89	0.75	0.75	0.586
	5	4/8/2011 12:16:11 PM	4000-2774	R2	6/10	67	76	71	0.93	0.74	0.73	0.563
	6	3/29/2012 1:14:59 PM	4000-2774	R2	6/10	61	63	67	0.88	0.76	0.75	0.609
Current:	7	7/11/2013 10:59:28 AM	800-1058714	R1	4/10	55	57	58	1.18	0.68	0.68	0.408

Registration Methods
R2 - Registration based on translation and rotation of OCT fundus
R1 - Registration based only on translation of disc center

Likely Loss
Possible Loss

Compared to baseline, statistically significant loss of tissue detected. For Average RNFL, Superior RNFL, Inferior RNFL, Rim Area the values have decreased. For Cup-to-Disc Ratios and Cup Volume values have increased.

Possible Increase

Compared to baseline, statistically significant increase detected. For Average RNFL, Superior RNFL, Inferior RNFL, Rim Area values have increased. For Cup-to-Disc Ratios and Cup Volume values have decreased.

Comments

Analysis Edited:

Doctor's Signature

SW Ver: 7.0.1.273

Page 2 of 2

Fig. 12.6 (continued)

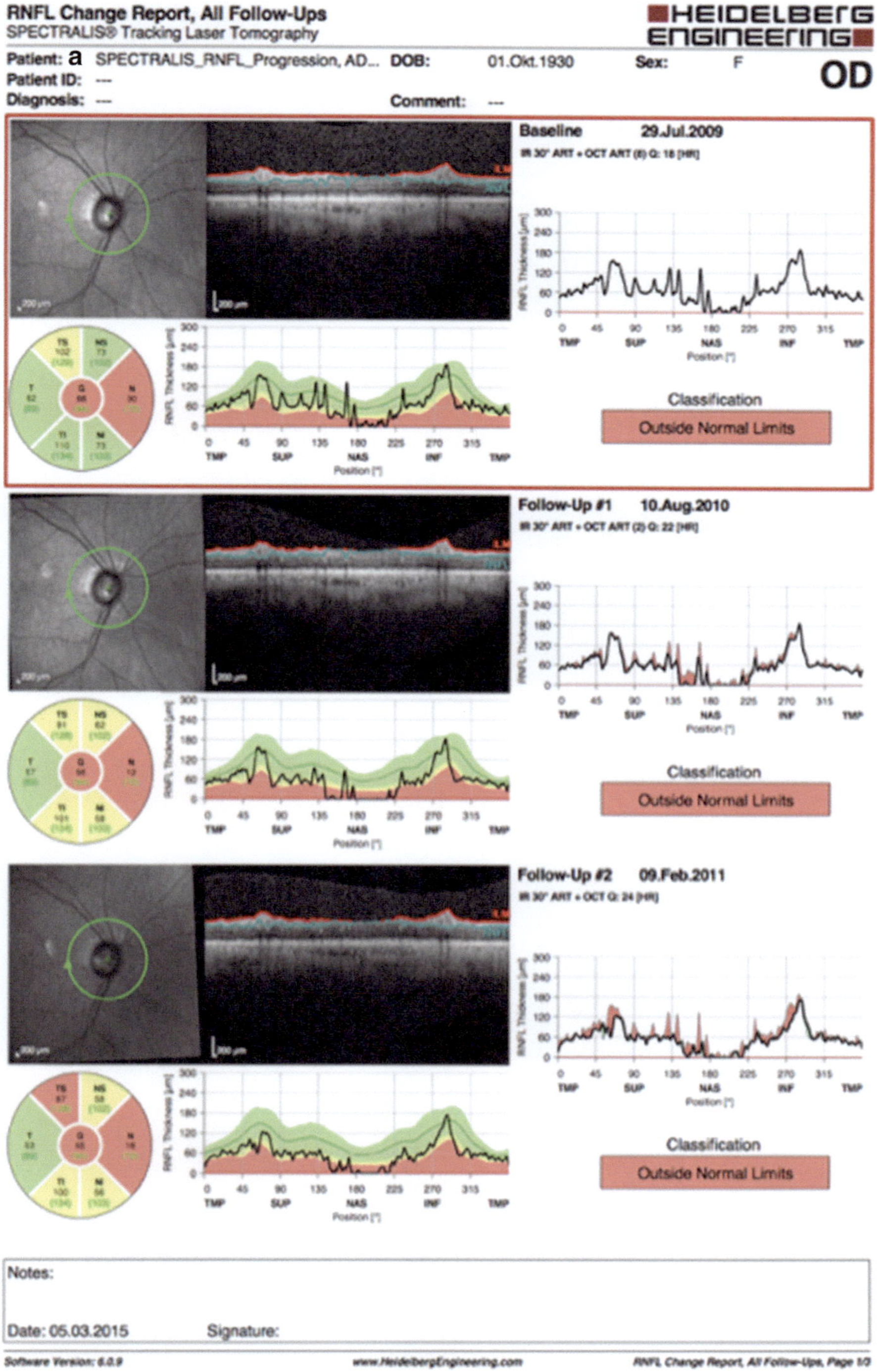

Fig. 12.7 (**a–c**) show the progression printouts from baseline to follow-up #9 for a RNFL circle scan performed by the Heidelberg Spectralis OCT. Apart from the usual classifications, on the right-hand side a difference graph is shown highlighting differences between individual exams (*red indicating* a decrease, *green* an increase) in the thickness values

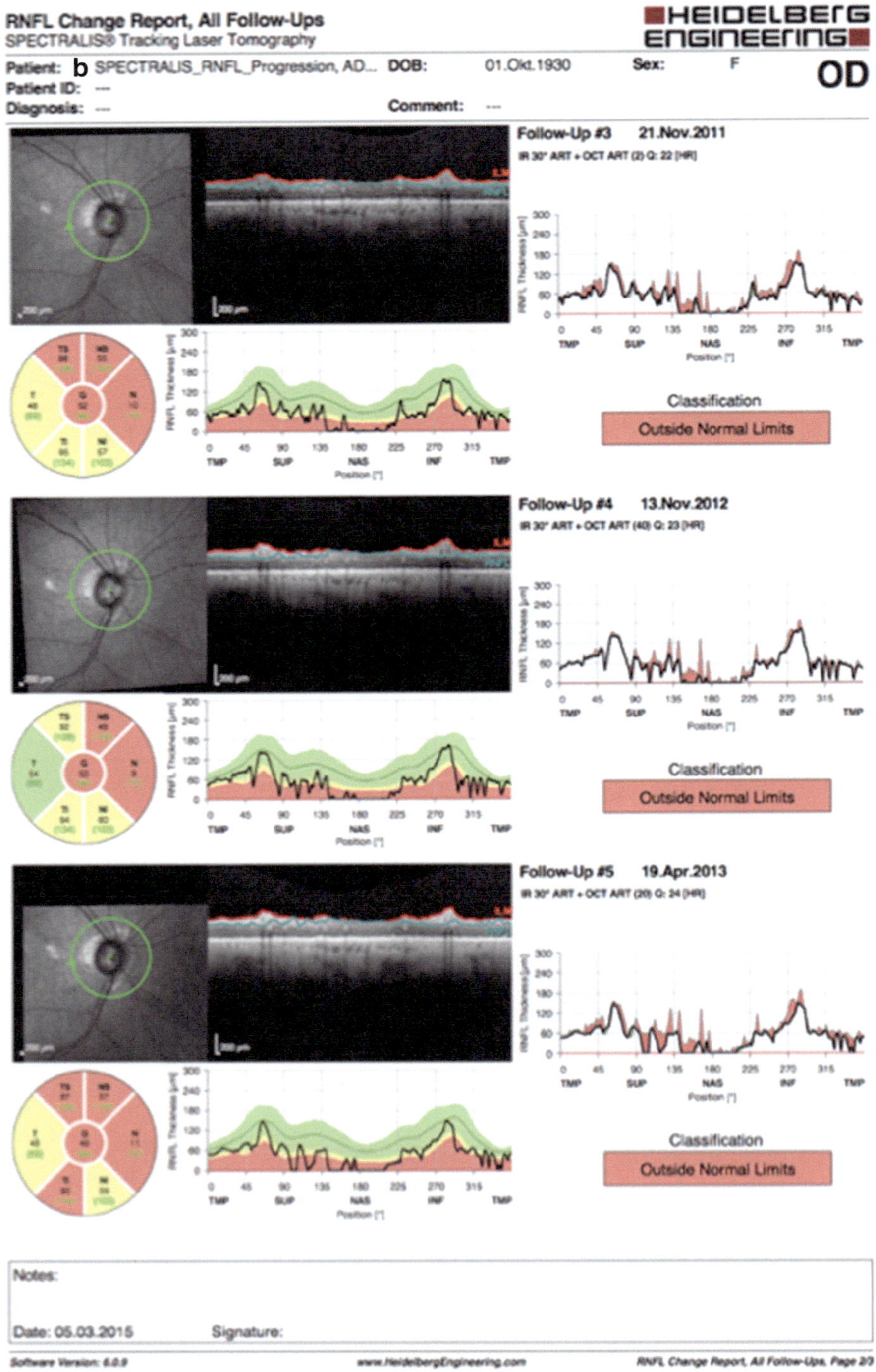

Fig. 12.7 (continued)

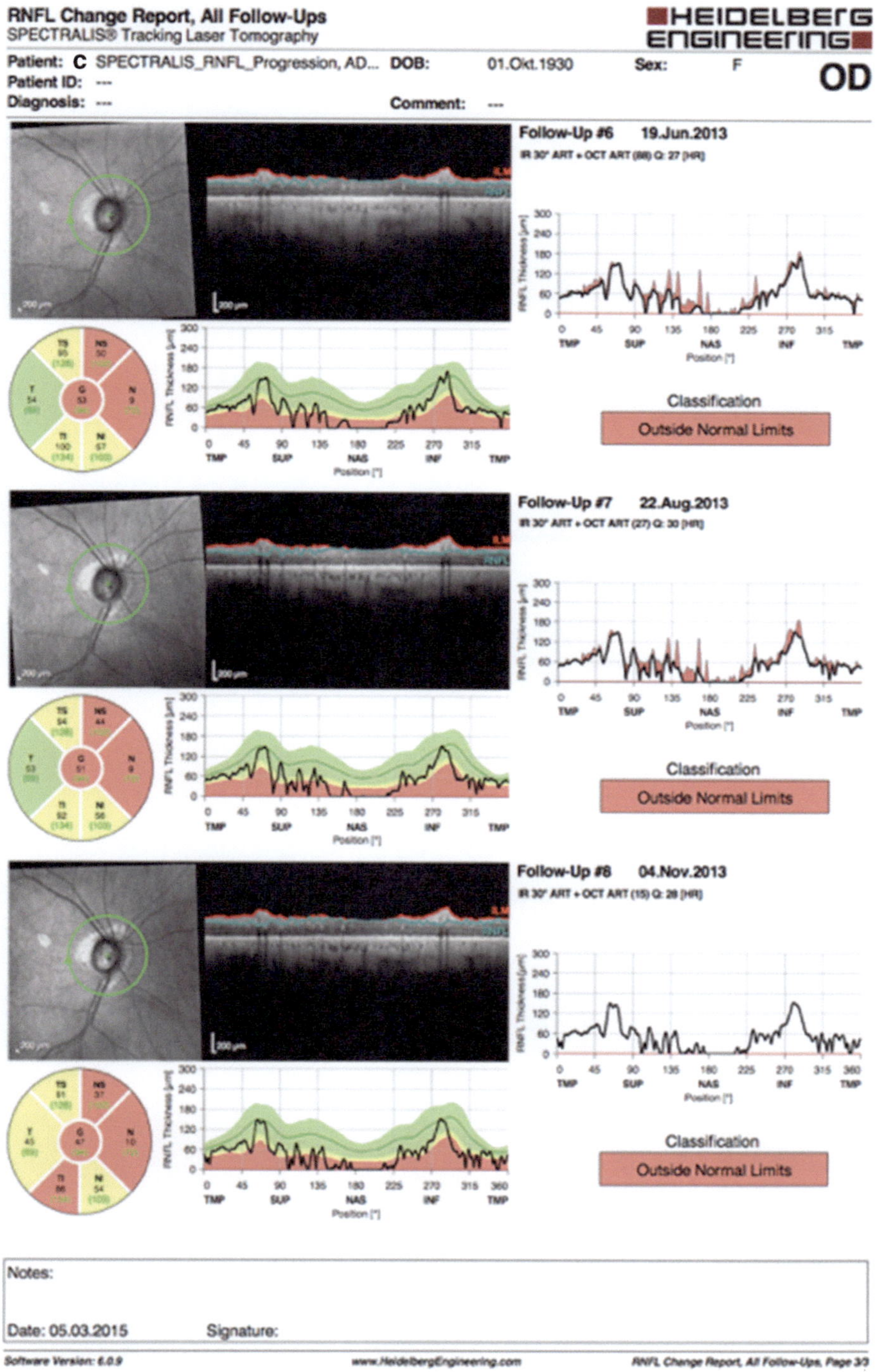

Fig. 12.7 (continued)

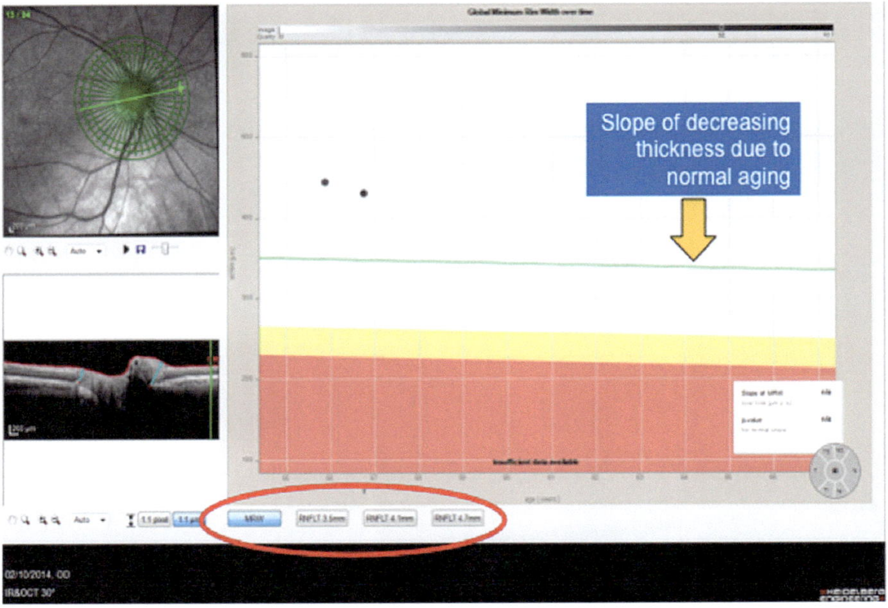

Fig. 12.8 The new Glaucoma Module Premium Edition of the Spectralis OCT2 (Heidelberg Engineering, Heidelberg, Germany) provides new paradigms for ONH analysis and for diagnosing progression. The glaucoma progression analysis provides comparison to the normal aging slope (*green line*), and the rim or any of the RNFL parameters can be selected looking at its changes globally or by sector

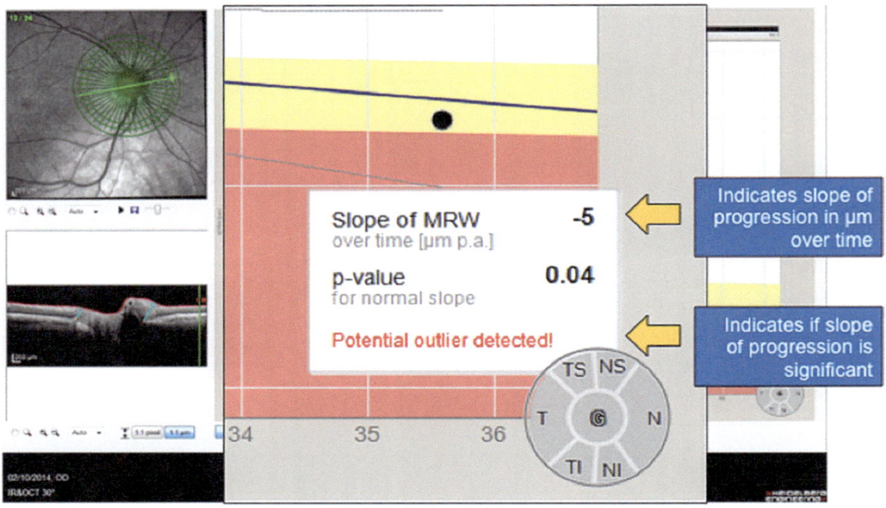

Fig. 12.9 The new Spectralis OCT2 Glaucoma progression analysis shows the slope of change in microns per annum and also gives a probability value

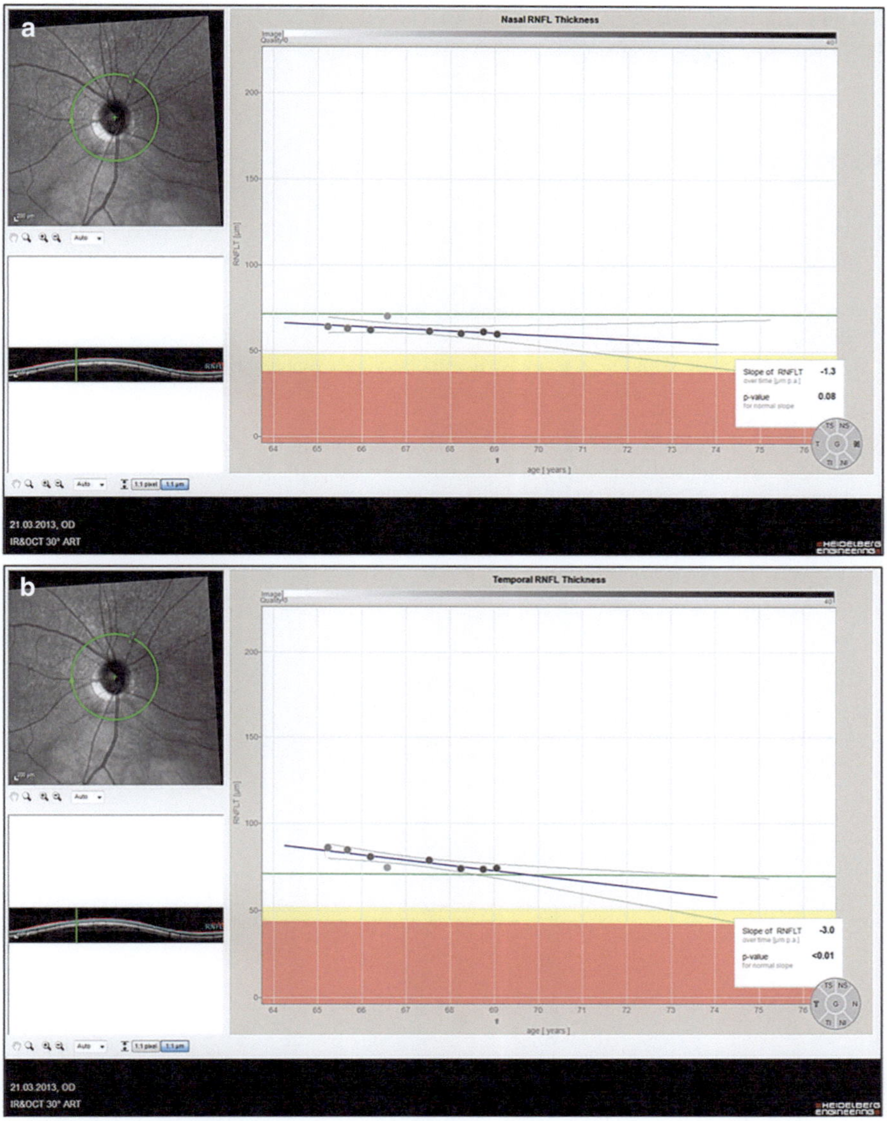

Fig. 12.10 (**a**, **b**) show the new possibility to analyze individual sectors over time and compare them to a normative age corrected database. This is especially interesting, since here also the slope of nerve fiber loss and its comparison to the loss due to normal aging (*p* value) are compared and thus give a good guideline to the clinician on whether this change differs significantly from the normal aging, thus indicating a possible pathological decrease

Acknowledgement The work for this author was supported by the Italian Ministry of Health and by Fondazione Roma

References

1. Medeiros FA, Alencar LM, Sample PA, Zangwill LM, Susanna R Jr, Weinreb RN (2010) The relationship between intraocular pressure reduction and rates of progressive visual field loss in eyes with optic disc hemorrhage. Ophthalmology 117(11):2061–6
2. Crabb DP, Russell RA, Malik R, Anand N, Baker H, Boodhna T, Bronze C, Fung SSM, Garway-Heath DF, Glen FC, Hernández R, Kirwan JF, Lemer C, McNaught AI, Viswanathan AC. Frequency of visual field testing when monitoring patients newly diagnosed with glaucoma: mixed methods and modelling. Southampton (UK): NIHR Journals Library; 2014 Aug. PubMed PMID: 25642569.
3. Zhu H, Russell RA, Saunders LJ, Ceccon S, Garway-Heath DF, Crabb DP (2014) Detecting changes in retinal function: analysis with non-stationary Weibull error regression and spatial enhancement (ANSWERS). PLoS One 9(1), e85654

MIX
Papier aus verantwortungsvollen Quellen
Paper from responsible sources
FSC® C105338

If you have any concerns about our products,
you can contact us on
ProductSafety@springernature.com

In case Publisher is established outside the EU,
the EU authorized representative is:
Springer Nature Customer Service Center GmbH
Europaplatz 3, 69115 Heidelberg, Germany

Printed by Libri Plureos GmbH
in Hamburg, Germany